Epidemiology

Beyond the Basics

Moyses Szklo, MD, DrPH
Professor of Epidemiology
School of Hygiene and Public Health
Johns Hopkins University
Baltimore, Maryland

F. Javier Nieto, MD, PhD
Professor and Chair
Department of Population Health Sciences
University of Wisconsin Medical School
Madison, Wisconsin

JONES AND BARTLETT PUBLISHERS
Sudbury, Massachusetts
BOSTON   TORONTO   LONDON   SINGAPORE

World Headquarters
Jones and Bartlett
Publishers
40 Tall Pine Drive
Sudbury, MA 01776
978-443-5000
info@jbpub.com
www.jbpub.com

Jones and Bartlett
Publishers Canada
2406 Nikanna Road
Mississauga, ON L5C
2W6
CANADA

Jones and Bartlett
Publishers International
Barb House, Barb Mews
London W6 7PA
UK

Copyright © 2004 by Jones and Bartlett Publishers, Inc.
Originally published by Aspen Publishers, © 2000.

Library of Congress Cataloging-in-Publication Data
Szklo, M. (Moyses)
Epidemiology: beyond the basics/
Moyses Szklo, F. Javier Nieto.
p. cm.
Includes bibliographical references and index.
ISBN 0-7637-4722-X
1. Epidemiology. I. Nieto, F. Javier. II. Title.
RA651.S97 1999
614.4—dc21
99-29768
CIP

Production Credits
Publisher: Michael Brown
Associate Editor: Chambers Moore
Production Manager: Amy Rose
Associate Production Editor: Karen C. Ferreira
Associate Marketing Manager: Joy Stark-Vancs
Manufacturing Buyer: Amy Bacus
Printing and Binding: Malloy, Inc.
Cover Printing: Malloy, Inc.

Printed in the United States of America
07 06 05   10 9 8 7 6 5 4 3

To Hilda and Marion

Table of Contents

Foreword ix
Preface xi
Acknowledgments xv

PART I—INTRODUCTION 1

**Chapter 1—Basic Study Designs in Analytical
　　　　　Epidemiology** 3
　1.1　Introduction: Descriptive and Analytical Epidemiology 3
　1.2　Analysis of Age, Birth Cohort, and Period Effects 4
　1.3　Ecologic Studies 17
　1.4　Studies Based on Individuals as Observation Units 23

**PART II—MEASURES OF DISEASE OCCURRENCE AND
　　　　　ASSOCIATION** 53

Chapter 2—Measuring Disease Occurrence 55
　2.1　Introduction: Basic Elements of Epidemiologic Inference—
　　　　Defining and Counting Disease Outcomes 55
　2.2　Measures of Incidence 58
　2.3　Measures of Prevalence 85
　2.4　Odds 87

Chapter 3—Measuring Associations Between Exposures and Outcomes 91
3.1 Introduction 91
3.2 Measuring Associations in a Cohort Study 91
3.3 Cross-Sectional Studies: Point Prevalence Rate Ratio 105
3.4 Measuring Associations in Case-Control Studies 106
3.5 Assessing the Strength of Associations 118

PART III—THREATS TO VALIDITY AND ISSUES OF INTERPRETATION 123

Chapter 4—Understanding Lack of Validity: Bias 125
4.1 Overview 125
4.2 Selection Bias 128
4.3 Information Bias 135
4.4 Combined Selection/Information Biases 153
4.5 Biases in Reporting Study Results: Publication Bias 169

Chapter 5—Identifying Noncausal Associations: Confounding 177
5.1 Introduction 177
5.2 The Nature of the Association Between the Confounder, the Exposure, and the Outcome 180
5.3 Assessing the Presence of Confounding 190
5.4 Additional Issues Related to Confounding 197
5.5 Conclusion 209

Chapter 6—Defining and Assessing Heterogeneity of Effects: Interaction 211
6.1 Introduction 211
6.2 How Is Effect Measured? 212
6.3 Strategies To Evaluate Interaction 213
6.4 Assessment of Interaction in Case-Control Studies 223
6.5 More on the Interchangeability of the Definitions of Interaction 233
6.6 Which Is the Relevant Model: Additive Versus Multiplicative Interaction? 235
6.7 The Nature and Reciprocity of Interaction 237
6.8 Interaction, Confounding Effect, and Adjustment 241
6.9 Statistical Modeling and Statistical Tests for Interaction 243

6.10 Interpreting Interaction 243
6.11 Interaction and Search for New Risk Factors in
      Low-Risk Groups 249
6.12 Interaction and "Representativeness" of Associations 251

PART IV—DEALING WITH THREATS TO VALIDITY 255

Chapter 7—Stratification and Adjustment:
      Multivariate Analysis in Epidemiology 257
7.1 Introduction 257
7.2 Stratification and Adjustment Techniques To
     Disentangle Confounding. 258
7.3 Adjustment Methods Based on Stratification 265
7.4 Multiple Regression Techniques for Adjustment 280
7.5 Incomplete Adjustment: Residual Confounding 328
7.6 Overadjustment. 331
7.7 Conclusion 333

Chapter 8—Quality Assurance and Control. 343
8.1 Introduction 343
8.2 Quality Assurance 344
8.3 Quality Control. 350
8.4 Indices of Validity and Reliability. 362
8.5 Regression to the Mean. 401

PART V—ISSUES OF REPORTING 405

Chapter 9—Communicating Results of Epidemiologic
      Studies. 407
9.1 Introduction 407
9.2 What To Report 407
9.3 How To Report. 413
9.4 Conclusion 429

Appendix A—Standard Errors, Confidence Intervals,
      and Hypothesis Testing for Selected
      Measures of Risk and Measures of
      Association 431
Appendix B—Test for Trend (Dose Response) 459
Appendix C—Test of Homogeneity of Stratified
      Estimates (Test for Interaction) 463

**Appendix D—Quality Assurance and Quality
     Control Procedures Manual for
     Blood Pressure Measurement and
     Blood/Urine Collection in the
     ARIC Study** 467
**Appendix E—Calculation of the Intraclass
     Correlation Coefficient** 479

Index 483
About the Authors 495

Foreword

The role of epidemiology, its concepts, and its methods have been receiving increased attention and recognition by people in academic medicine, governmental agencies, and industry and by policy makers. This has resulted in the publication of numerous books and the offering of many graduate programs, including half a dozen summer sessions. These efforts are aimed at preparing students and practitioners of public health and medicine to respond to this increased demand by giving them the necessary skills and knowledge to do so.

There are a number of books on epidemiology written at the introductory level and still other books devoted to specific areas of application, but there are few books done at the advanced level. This volume, *Epidemiology: Beyond the Basics,* is significant because it truly fills a gap that has long existed for an intermediate-level book.

In this book you will learn something about cohort and nested case-control studies, birth cohort analysis, ecological studies, cumulative incidence, measures of association, confounding, interaction, reliability and validity measures, and more. You will find a clear explanation of the various forms of bias so frequently encountered in epidemiology and the different ways of avoiding them or at least addressing them effectively.

Complex concepts such as confounding, interactions, and statistical modeling are presented in a way that makes them not only easily understood but also not quickly forgotten. This is accomplished by the authors' liberal use of graphics and diagrams, examples, and clear writing. The reader will gain a good understanding of epidemiologic methods and their useful role in the medical and public health sciences.

The health professional of the future will need to have a broad understanding of methodological issues as well as critical insights into their proper application in order to investigate the cause of disease and develop and test intervention strategies. Whether the goal is to find the cause of disease, to evaluate the impact of a program on the health status of a population, or to develop an appropriate policy, epidemiology is the science to call into action.

Michel A. Ibrahim, MD, PhD
Professor of Epidemiology and Social Medicine
University of North Carolina at Chapel Hill
Chapel Hill, North Carolina

Preface

This book was conceived as an intermediate epidemiology text-book. As such, it explores and discusses key epidemiologic concepts and basic methods in more depth than that found in basic textbooks on epidemiology.

As an intermediate methods text, this book is expected to have a heterogeneous readership. Some potential readers are epidemiology students who may use it as a bridge between basic and more advanced epidemiologic methods. Other readers may include those who would like to advance their knowledge beyond the basic epidemiologic principles and methods but who are not statistically minded and are thus reluctant to tackle the many excellent textbooks that strongly focus on epidemiology's quantitative aspects. Although the demonstration of many epidemiologic concepts and methods needs to rely on statistical formulations, these formulations are extensively supported in this book by real-life examples throughout, hopefully making their logic intuitively easier to follow. The practicing epidemiologist, too, may find selected portions of this book useful for an understanding of concepts beyond basics. Thus, the common denominators for the intended readers are familiarity with the basic strategies of analytic epidemiology and a desire to increase the level of understanding of several notions that are more or less (and naturally so) insufficiently covered in many basic textbooks. The way in which this textbook is organized should make this readily apparent.

In Chapter 1, the basic observational epidemiologic research strategies are reviewed, including those based on studies of both groups and individuals. Although descriptive epidemiology is not the focus of this book, birth cohort analysis is discussed in some depth in this chapter, as this approach is rarely covered in detail in basic textbooks. Another topic in the interface between descriptive and analytical epidemiology, namely ecological studies, is also discussed, with a view toward extending its discussion beyond the possibility of inferential (ecological) bias. Next, the chapter reviews observational studies based on individuals as units of observation—that is, cohort and case-control studies. Different types of case-control design are reviewed (case-based, case-control studies within a defined cohort). The strategy of matching as an approach to achieve pre–data collection comparability is also briefly discussed.

Chapters 2 and 3 cover issues of measurement of outcome frequency and measures of association. In Chapter 2, absolute measures of outcome frequency and their calculation methods are reviewed, including the person-time approach for the calculation of incidence density and both the classical life table and the Kaplan-Meier method for the calculation of cumulative incidence. Chapter 3 deals with measures of association, including those based on relative (eg, relative risk, odds ratio) and absolute (attributable risk) differences. The connections between measures of association obtained in cohort and case-control studies are emphasized. In particular, a description is given of the different measures of association (ie, odds ratio, relative risk, rate ratio) that can be obtained in case-control studies as a function of the control selection strategies that were introduced in Chapter 1.

Chapters 4 and 5 are devoted to threats to the validity of epidemiologic studies, namely bias and confounding. In Chapter 4, the most common types of bias are discussed, including both selection and information bias. In the discussion of information bias, simple examples are given to improve the understanding of the phenomenon of misclassification resulting from less than perfect sensitivity and specificity of the approaches used for ascertaining exposure, outcome, and/or confounding variables. This chapter also provides a discussion of cross-sectional biases and biases associated with evaluation of screening procedures; for the latter, a simple approach to estimate lead time bias is given that may be useful for those involved in evaluative studies of this sort. In Chapter 5, the concept of confounding is introduced, and approaches to evaluate confounding are reviewed. Special issues related to confounding are discussed, including residual confounding and the role of statistical significance in the evaluation of confounding effects.

Interaction (effect modification) is discussed in Chapter 6. The chapter discusses the concept of interaction, emphasizing its pragmatic application as well as the strategies to evaluate the presence of additive and multiplicative interactions. Practical issues discussed in this chapter include whether to adjust when interaction is suspected and the importance of the additive model in public health.

The last three chapters are devoted to approaches to handle threats to the validity of epidemiologic results. In Chapter 7, strategies for the adjustment of confounding factors are presented, including both the more parsimonious approaches (eg, direct adjustment, Mantel-Haenszel) and the more complex (eg, multiple regression). Emphasis is placed on the selection of the method that is most appropriate for the study design used (eg, Cox proportional hazards for the analysis of survival data or Poisson regression for the analysis of rates per person-time). Chapter 8 reviews the basic quality control strategies for the prevention and control of measurement error and bias. Both qualitative and quantitative approaches used in quality control are discussed. The most often used analytic strategies for estimating validity and reliability of data obtained in epidemiologic studies are reviewed (eg, unweighted and weighted kappa, correlation coefficients) in this chapter. Finally, in Chapter 9, the key issue of communication of results of epidemiologic studies is discussed. Examples of common mistakes made when reporting epidemiologic data are given as a way to stress the importance of clarity in such reports.

Some appendixes are also provided. Appendixes A, B, C, and E describe selected statistical procedures (eg, standard errors and confidence levels, trend test, test of heterogeneity of effects, intraclass correlation) to help the reader more thoroughly evaluate the measures of risk and association discussed in the text and to expose him or her to procedures that, while relatively simple, are not available in many statistical packages used by epidemiology students and practitioners. Finally, Appendix D includes two sections on quality assurance and control procedures taken from the corresponding manual of the Atherosclerosis Risk and Communities (ARIC) Study as examples of real-life applications of some of the procedures discussed in Chapter 8.

Readers are encouraged to use the Web page for this book: http:// publichealth.jbpub.com/epidemiology/szklo to e-mail us to point out errors or unclear passages or to suggest other improvements. All significant contributions will be acknowledged in the next edition. Any corrections to errors in the text will be posted on the Web page.

Acknowledgments

This book is an outgrowth of an intermediate epidemiology course (informally known as "Epi-2") taught by the authors at the Johns Hopkins School of Public Health. Over the years this course has benefited from significant intellectual input of many faculty, including, among others, George W. Comstock, Helen Abbey, James Tonascia, and Mary Meyer. The authors especially acknowledge George W. Comstock, a mentor to both of us, who has been involved with the course for several decades and is still co-teaching it with us. His in-depth knowledge of epidemiologic methods and wisdom over the years have been instrumental to our professional growth. Dr. Comstock also kindly provided many of the materials and examples used in the last chapter of this book.

Our department's present and past chairmen, Jon Samet and Leon Gordis, consistently have supported this endeavor, for which we are deeply appreciative. Our gratitude also is extended to our good friends Alfonso Mele, Paolo Pasquini, Rosa Maria Corona, and to other colleagues from the Italian Superior Health Institute's Division of Epidemiology who kindly provided key logistical support during a sabbatical leave taken by one of us (MS) when the first drafts of many of the chapters were written.

We are indebted to several colleagues, including Eliseo Guallar, Joseph Coresh, and Woody Chambless, who read partial sections of the text or provided guidance in solving conceptual or statistical riddles, and to Michael Silverberg for his careful reading of the manuscript and useful editorial and substantive suggestions. We also thank the reviewers, especially Ana Diez-Roux and Eyal Shahar, to whom an early version of the text was sent by Aspen Publishers, for their painstaking review and pointed criticisms and suggestions for changes, many of which were incorporated in the text. We also are grateful to Jingzhong Ding for his help with the development of graphics and tables and to Rodney Palmer for his administrative assistance.

To have had the privilege of teaching "Epi-2" for so many years made us realize how much we have learned from our students, to whom we are deeply grateful. Finally, without the support and extraordinary patience of all members of our families, we could not have devoted so much time and effort into writing this book.

PART I

Introduction

CHAPTER 1

Basic Study Designs in Analytical Epidemiology

descriptive- available data ; rates vs. demographics

1.1 INTRODUCTION: DESCRIPTIVE AND ANALYTICAL EPIDEMIOLOGY

Epidemiology is traditionally defined as the study of the distribution and determinants of health-related states or events in specified populations and the application of this study to control health problems.[1] Epidemiology has been classified as either "descriptive" or "analytic." In general terms, *descriptive epidemiology* makes use of available data to examine how rates (eg, mortality) vary according to demographic variables (eg, those obtained from censuses). When the distribution of rates is not uniform according to person, time, and place, the epidemiologist is able not only to define high-risk groups for prevention purposes (eg, hypertension is more prevalent in US blacks than in whites, thus defining blacks as a high-risk group) but also to generate causal hypotheses based on the classical agent-host-environment paradigm (eg, the hypothesis that an environmental factor to which blacks are exposed, such as excessive salt intake, is responsible for their higher risk of hypertension).

A thorough review of descriptive epidemiologic approaches can be readily found in numerous sources.[2,3] For this reason, and given the overall scope of this book, this chapter focuses on study designs that are relevant to *analytical epidemiology*. The single exception is found in Section 1.2 of this chapter, in which a special type of descriptive strategy, the *analysis of birth cohorts,* is briefly discussed. The reasons for this exception are as follows: (1) although the assessment of birth cohort data often shares with other descriptive approaches a reliance on information that is usually available, it requires the application of an analytical approach with a level of complexity usually not found in

3

descriptive epidemiology; and (2) this type of analysis is often key for the understanding of the observed association between age (often strongly associated with the occurrence of many diseases as well as their determinants) and disease in cross-sectional analyses. (An additional, more pragmatical reason is that birth cohort analysis is usually not discussed in detail in basic textbooks.)

Hypotheses of associations of suspected risk factor exposures with health outcomes are assessed in analytic epidemiologic studies. Although some of the concepts discussed in subsequent chapters, such as measures of association and interaction, are also relevant to experimental studies (randomized clinical trials), the main focus of this textbook is *observational* epidemiology.

Two general strategies are used for the assessment of associations in observational studies: (1) studies using populations or groups of individuals as units of observation—the so-called ecologic studies—and (2) studies using individuals as observation units, which include the prospective (or cohort), the case-control, and the cross-sectional study designs.

1.2   ANALYSIS OF AGE, BIRTH COHORT, AND PERIOD EFFECTS

Health surveys conducted in population samples usually include participants over a wide age range. Age is a strong risk factor for many health outcomes and is also frequently associated with numerous exposures. Thus, even if the effect of age is not among the primary objectives of the study, it is often important to assess its relation with exposures and outcomes, given its potentially important confounding effects.

Table 1–1 shows the results of a hypothetical cross-sectional study conducted in 1995 to assess the prevalence rates of a disease Y according to age. (A more strict use of the term "rate" as a measure of the occurrence of incident events is defined in Section 2.2.2. This term is also widely used in a more general sense to refer to proportions such as prevalence.[1] It is in this more general sense that the term is used here and in other parts of the book.) In Figure 1–1, these results are plotted at the midpoints of 10-year age groups (eg, for ages 30–39, at 35 years; for ages 40–49, at 45 years; and so on). These data show that the prevalence of Y in this population decreases with age. Does this mean that the prevalence rates of Y decrease *as individuals age*? Not necessarily. For many disease processes, exposures have cumulative effects that are expressed over long periods of time. Long latency peri-

Table 1–1 Hypothetical Data from a Cross-Sectional Study of Prevalence of Disease Y in a Population, by Age, 1995

Age Group (Years)	Midpoint (Years)	1995 Prevalence (per 1000)
30–39	35	45
40–49	45	40
50–59	55	36
60–69	65	31
70–79	75	27

ods and cumulative effects characterize, for example, numerous exposure/disease associations, including smoking/lung cancer, radiation/ thyroid cancer, and saturated fat intake/atherosclerotic disease. Thus, the health status of a person who is 50 years old at the time of the survey may be partially dependent on this person's past exposures (eg, smoking during early adulthood). This variability of past exposures in successive generations (birth cohorts*) can distort the appar-

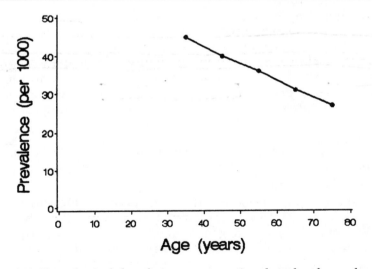

Figure 1–1 Hypothetical data from a cross-sectional study of prevalence of disease Y in a population, by age, 1995 (based on data from Table 1–1).

Birth cohort: "(from Latin *cohors,* warriors, the tenth part of a legion) the component of the population born during a particular period and identified by period of birth so that its characteristics (eg, causes of death and numbers still living) can be ascertained as it enters successive time and age periods."[1]

ent associations between age and health outcomes that are observed at any given point in time. This concept can be illustrated as follows.

Assume that the same investigator who collected the data shown in Table 1-1 is able to recover data from previous surveys conducted in the same population in 1965, 1975, and 1985. The resulting data are presented in Table 1-2 and Figure 1-2 and show consistent trends of decreasing prevalence of Y with age in each of these surveys. Consider now plotting these data using a different approach, as shown in Figure 1-3. The dots in Figure 1-3 are at the same places as in Figure 1-2, except that the lines are connected by *birth cohort* (the 1995 survey is also plotted in Figure 1-3). Each of the broken lines represents a birth cohort converging to the 1995 survey. For example, the "youngest" age point in the 1995 cross-sectional curve represents the rate of disease Y for individuals aged 30 to 39 years (average 35 years) who were born between 1955 and 1964: that is, in 1960 on average. Individuals in this 1960 birth cohort were on average 10 years younger, that is, 25 years of age at the time of the 1985 survey and 15 years of age at the time of the 1975 survey. The line for the 1960 birth cohort thus represents how the prevalence of Y changes with increasing age for individuals born, on average, in 1960. Evidently, the cohort pattern shown in Figure 1-3 is very different from that suggested by the cross-sectional data and is consistent for all birth cohorts shown in the figure in that it suggests that the prevalence of Y actually *increases* as people age. The fact that the inverse trend is observed in the cross-sectional data is due to a strong "cohort effect" in this example: that is, the prevalence of Y is strongly determined by the year of birth

Table 1–2 Hypothetical Data from a Series of Cross-Sectional Studies of Prevalence of Disease Y in a Population, by Age and Survey Date (Calendar Time), 1965 to 1995

Age Group (Years)	Midpoint (Years)	Survey Date			
		1965	1975	1985	1995
		Prevalence (per 1000)			
10–19	15	17	28		
20–29	25	14	23	35	
30–39	35	12	19	30	45
40–49	45	10	18	26	40
50–59	55		15	22	36
60–69	65			20	31
70–79	75				27

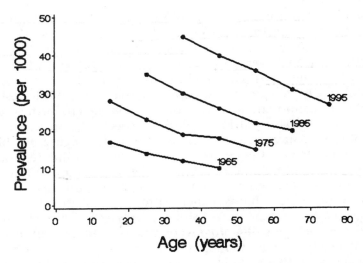

Figure 1–2 Hypothetical data from a series of cross-sectional studies of prevalence of disease Y (per 1000) in a population, by age, and survey date (calendar time), 1965, 1975, 1985, and 1995 (based on data from Table 1–2).

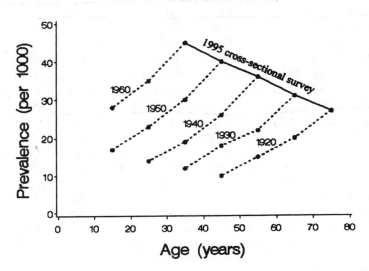

Figure 1–3 Plotting of the data in Figure 1–2 by birth cohort (see also Table 1–3). The dotted lines represent the different birth cohorts (from 1920 to 1960) as they converge to the 1995 cross-sectional survey (solid line, as in Figure 1–1).

of the person. For any given age, the prevalence rate is higher in younger (more recent) than in older cohorts. Thus, in the 1995 cross-sectional survey (Figure 1–1), the older subjects come from birth cohorts with relatively lower rates, whereas the youngest come from the cohorts with higher rates. This can be clearly seen in Figure 1–3 by selecting one age (eg, 45 years) and observing that the rate is lowest for the 1920 birth cohort and increases for each subsequent birth cohort: that is, the 1930, 1940, and 1950 cohorts, respectively. An alternative display of these data is shown in Figure 1–4. In this figure, the birth cohorts are plotted on the abscissa (*x* axis), and each line represents the change across birth cohorts for a given age group. Often, the choice among these alternative graphical representations is a matter of personal preference: that is, which pattern the investigator wishes to emphasize. Whereas Figure 1–4 shows trends according to birth cohorts more explicitly (eg, for any given age group, there is an increasing prevalence from older to more recent cohorts), Figure 1–3 has an intuitive appeal in that each line represents a birth cohort as it ages. As long as one pays careful attention to the labeling of the graph, any of these displays is appropriate to identify cohort patterns. Note that the same patterns displayed in Figures 1–3 and 1–4 can be seen in Table 1–2, moving downward to examine cross-sectional trends and diagonally from left to right to examine birth cohort trends. An alternative and probably more easily readable tabular display of the same data for the purpose of detecting trends according to birth cohort is shown in Table 1–3, which allows the examination of trends according to age ("age effect") within each birth cohort (horizontal lines in Table 1–3). Additionally, and in agreement with Figure 1–4, prevalence rates increase for each age group in Table 1–3 from older to more recent cohorts (cohort effect) (detected by moving one's eyes from the top to the bottom of each age group column in Table 1–3).

Thus, the data in the above example are simultaneously affected by two strong effects: cohort effect and age effect (for definitions, see Exhibit 1–1). These two trends are jointly responsible for the seemingly paradoxical trend observed in the cross-sectional analyses in this hypothetical example (Figures 1–1 and 1–2), in which the rates seem to *decrease* with age. The fact that more recent cohorts have substantially higher rates (cohort effect) overwhelms the increase due to age and explains the cross-sectional pattern.

In addition to cohort and age effects, patterns of rates can be influenced by the so-called "period effect." The term *period effect* is frequently used to refer to a global shift or change in trends that affects the rates across birth cohorts and age groups (Exhibit 1–1). Any phe-

Cross sectional trends
& Birth cohort trends

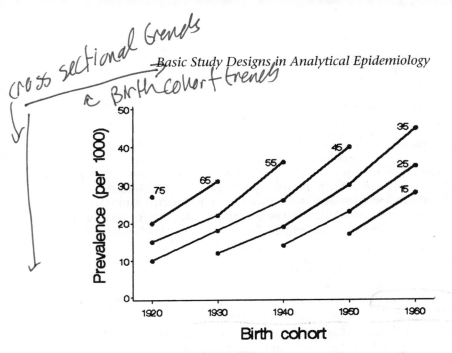

Figure 1–4 Alternative display of the data in Figures 1–2 and 1–3. Birth cohorts are represented in the *x* axis. The lines represent age groups (labeled using the midpoints, in years).

nomenon occurring at a specific point in time (or during a specific period) that affects an entire population (or a significant segment of it), such as a war, a new treatment, or a massive migration, can produce this change independently of age and birth cohort. A hypothetical example is shown in Figure 1–5. This figure shows data similar to those used in the previous example (eg, Figure 1–3), except that in this case the rates level off in 1985 for all cohorts: that is, when the

Table 1–3 Rearrangement of the Data Shown in Table 1–2 by Birth Cohort

Birth Cohort Range	Midpoint	Age Group (Midpoint, in Years)						
		15	25	35	45	55	65	75
		Prevalence (per 1000)						
1915–24	1920				10	15	20	27
1925–34	1930			12	18	22	31	
1935–44	1940		14	19	26	36		
1945–54	1950	17	23	30	40			
1955–64	1960	28	35	45				

Exhibit 1–1 Definitions of Age, Cohort, and Period Effects

Age effect:	Change in the rate of a condition according to age, irrespective of birth cohort and calendar time
Cohort effect:	Change in the rate of a condition according to year of birth, irrespective of age and calendar time
Period effect:	Change in the rate of a condition affecting an entire population at some point in time, irrespective of age and Birth Cohort

1960 cohort is 25 years old on the average, when the 1950 cohort is 35 years old, and so on.

Period effects on prevalence rates can occur, for example, when new medications or preventive interventions are introduced for diseases that previously had poor prognoses, as in the case of the introduction of insulin, antibiotics, and polio vaccines.

It is important to understand that the so-called birth cohort effects may have little to do with the circumstances surrounding the time of birth of a given cohort of individuals. Rather, cohort effects may result from the lifetime experience (including, but not limited to, those

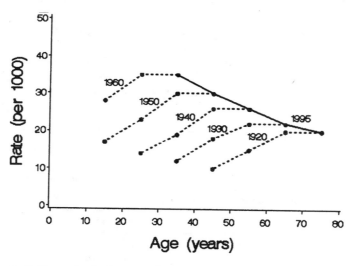

Figure 1–5 Hypothetical example of period effect: an event happened in 1985 that affected all birth cohorts (1920 through 1960) in a similar way and slowed down the rate of increase with age. The solid line represents the observed cross-sectional age pattern in 1995.

surrounding birth) of the individuals born at a given point in time that influence the disease or outcome of interest. For example, currently observed patterns of association between age and coronary heart disease may result from cohort effects related to changes in diet (eg, fat intake) or smoking habits of adolescent and young adults over time. It is well known that early coronary atherosclerotic lesions ("fatty streaks") frequently develop in the first decade of life[4]; in middle and older ages, some of these lesions may evolve into raised atherosclerotic lesions, eventually leading to thrombosis, lumen occlusion, and the resulting clinically manifest acute ischemic events. Thus, a young adult's dietary and/or smoking habits may influence early atherosclerosis development and subsequent coronary risk. If changes in these habits occur in the population over time, successive birth cohorts necessarily go through changing degrees of exposure to early atherogenic factors, which will determine in part future cross-sectional patterns of association of age with coronary heart disease.

Another way to understand the concept of cohort effects is as the result of an *interaction* between age and calendar time. The concept of interaction is discussed in detail in Chapter 6 of this book. In simple terms, it means that a given variable (eg, calendar time in the case of a cohort effect) *modifies the strength or the nature of an association* between another variable (eg, age) and an outcome (eg, coronary atherosclerosis). In the above example, it means that the age-related atherosclerosis development changes over time as a result of changing risk factors (eg, dietary/smoking habits of young adults). In other words, calendar time–related changes in risk factors modify the association between age and atherosclerosis.

Cohort-age-period analyses can be applied not only to prevalence data but also to incidence and mortality data. A classical example is Wade Hampton Frost's study of age patterns of tuberculosis mortality.[5] Figure 1–6 presents two graphs from Frost's landmark paper. With regard to Figure 1–6A, Frost[5(p94)] noted that

> looking at the 1930 curve, the impression given is that nowadays an individual encounters his greatest risk of death from tuberculosis between the ages of 50 and 60. But this is not really so; the people making up the 1930 age group 30 to 60 have, in earlier life, passed through *greater* mortality risk. (emphasis in original)

To demonstrate this, Frost displayed the birth cohort data shown in Figure 1–6B, which show that for cohorts born in 1870 through 1890, the risk of tuberculosis death after the first few years of life is actually highest at age 20 to 30 years.

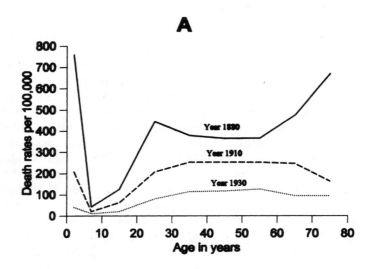

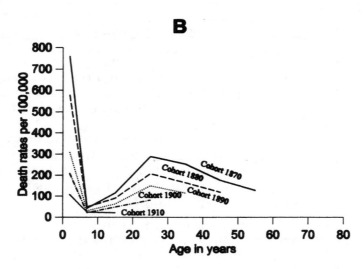

Figure 1–6 Frost's analysis of age in relation to tuberculosis mortality (males only). **A**: Massachusetts death rates from tuberculosis, by age, 1880, 1910, 1930. **B**: Massachusetts death rates from tuberculosis, by age, in successive 10-year cohorts. *Source:* Reprinted with permission from WH Frost, The Age-Selection of Tuberculosis Mortality in Successive Decades, *American Journal of Hygiene,* Vol 30, pp 91–96, © 1939.

Another, more recent, example is shown in Figure 1–7, based on an analysis of age, cohort, and period effects on the incidence of colorectal cancer in a region of Spain.[6] Note that in these figures, birth cohorts are placed on the *x* axis (as in Figure 1–4). These figures show strong cohort effects: for each age group, the incidence rates of colorectal cancer tend to increase from older to more recent birth cohorts. An age effect is also evident, since for each birth cohort (for any given year-of-birth value in the horizontal axis), the rates are higher for older than for younger individuals. Note also that, probably because of the wide range of rates that needed to be plotted, a logarithmic scale was used in the ordinate. (For further discussion of the use of logarithmic versus arithmetic scales, see Chapter 9, Section 9.3.5.)

An additional example of age-cohort-period analysis of incidence data is shown in Figure 1–8. This figure shows incidence of dementia

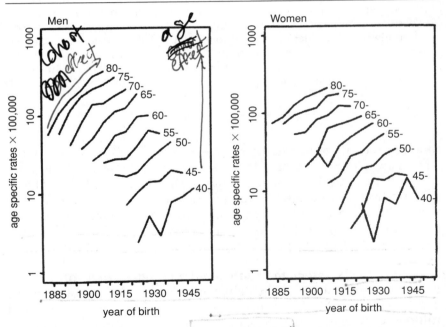

Figure 1–7 Trends in age-specific incidence rates of colorectal cancer in Navarra and Zaragoza (Spain). *Source:* Reprinted with permission from G. López-Abente et al, Age-Period-Cohort Modeling of Colorectal Cancer Incidence and Mortality in Spain, *Cancer Epidemiology, Biomarkers, and Prevention,* Vol 6, pp 999–1005, © 1997, American Association for Cancer Research, Inc.

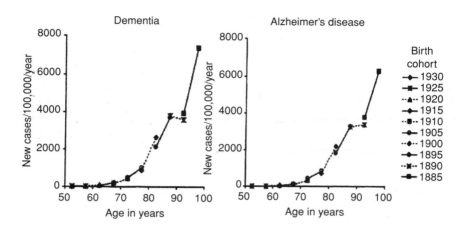

Figure 1–8 Five-year average incidence rates of dementia (new cases per 100,000 person-years) by age and birth cohort, both sexes combined, Rochester, Minnesota. For each birth cohort, two points are represented corresponding to the incidence in 1975 to 1979 and 1980 to 1984, respectively. *Source:* Reprinted with permission from WA Rocca et al, Incidence of Dementia and Alzheimer's Disease: A Reanalysis of the Rochester, Minnesota 1975–1984 Data, *American Journal of Epidemiology,* Vol 148, No 1, pp 51–62, © 1998.

among residents of Rochester, Minnesota, from 1975 through 1984.[7] This is an example in which there is a strong age effect—that is, rates increase dramatically with age for all birth cohorts—but virtually no cohort effect, as indicated by the practically overlapping data for the successive birth cohort pairs for any given age group. It should be manifest from Figure 1–8 that, in the absence of cohort effects, the same age patterns of rates are found in cross-sectional and cohort curves.

Period effects associated with incidence rates tend to be more prominent for diseases for which the cumulative effects of previous exposures are relatively unimportant, such as infectious diseases and injuries. Conversely, in chronic diseases such as cancer and cardiovascular diseases, cumulative effects are usually important, and thus cohort effects tend to affect incidence rates to a greater extent than period effects.

Finally, these methods can also be used to study variables other than disease rates. An example is the analysis of age-related changes in serum cholesterol levels shown in Figure 1–9, based on data from the Florida Geriatric Research Program, an ongoing program designed to provide free medical screening for the elderly.[8] This figure reveals slight cohort effects, in that serum cholesterol levels tend to be higher in older than in more recent birth cohorts for most age groups. A J- or U-shape age pattern is also seen: that is, for each birth cohort, serum cholesterol tends to first decrease or remain stable with increasing age and to achieve its maximum value in the oldest members of the cohort. Although at a first glance this pattern might be considered an "age effect," note that, for each cohort, the maximum cholesterol values in the oldest age group coincide with a single point in calendar time: 1985 through 1987 (ie, for the 1909–1911 birth cohort at 76 years of age, for the 1906–1908 cohort at 79 years of age, and so on), leading Newschaffer et al to observe that

> a period effect is suggested by a consistent change in curve height at a given time point over all cohorts. . . . Therefore, based on simple visual inspection of the curves, it is not possible to attribute the consistent U-shaped increase in cholesterol to aging, since some of this shape may be accounted for by period effects.[8(p26)]

In complex situations such as that illustrated in the preceding discussion, multiple regression techniques can be used to disentangle the age, cohort, and period effects. Describing these techniques in detail is beyond the scope of this book. (A general discussion of multiple regression methods is presented in Chapter 7, Section 7.4.2). The interested reader can find examples and further references in the original papers from the above-cited examples (eg, López-Abente et al[6] and Newschaffer et al[8]).

Finally, it should be emphasized that birth cohort effects may affect associations between disease outcomes and variables other than age. Consider, for example, a case-control study (see Section 1.4.2) in which cases and controls are closely matched by age (see Section 1.4.5). Assume that, in this study, cases are.identified over a 10-year span (eg, from 1960 through 1969) and controls at the end of the accrual of cases. In this study, age per se does not act as a confounder, as cases and controls are matched on age (see Section 5.2.2); however, the fact that cases and controls are identified from different birth cohorts may affect the assessment of variables, such as educational level, that may have changed rapidly across birth cohorts. In this case, birth cohort, but not age, would confound the association between education and the disease of interest.

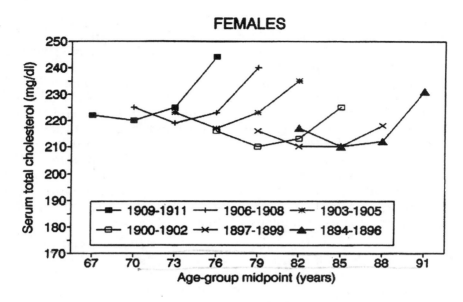

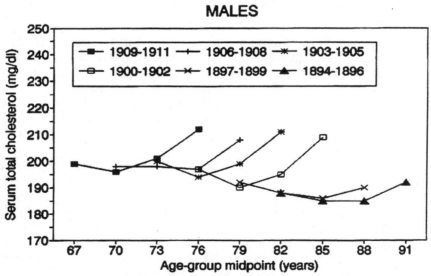

Figure 1–9 Sex-specific mean serum cholesterol levels by age and birth cohort: longitudinal data from the Florida Research Program, Dunedin County, Florida, 1976 to 1987. *Source:* Reprinted with permission from CJ Newschaffer, TL Bush, and WE Hale, Aging and Total Cholesterol Levels: Cohort, Period, and Survivorship Effects, *American Journal of Epidemiology,* Vol 136, pp 23–34, © 1992.

1.3 ECOLOGIC STUDIES

The units of observation in an ecologic study are usually geographically defined populations (such as countries or regions within a country) or the same geographically defined population at different points in time. Mean values* for both a given postulated risk factor and the outcome of interest are obtained for each observation unit for comparison purposes. Typically, the analysis of ecological data involves plotting the risk factor and outcome values for all observation units to assess whether a relationship is evident. For example, Figure 1–10 displays the death rates for coronary heart disease in men from 16 cohorts included in the Seven Countries Study plotted against the corresponding estimates of mean fat intake (percent calories from fat).[9] A positive relation between these two variables is suggested by these data, as there is a tendency for the death rates to be higher in countries having higher average saturated fat intakes.

Different types of variables can be used in ecological studies,[10] which are briefly summarized as follows:

- *Aggregate measures* that summarize the characteristics of individuals within a group as the mean value of a certain parameter, or the proportion of the population or group of interest with a certain characteristic. Examples include the rate of a given disease, average amount of fat intake (Figure 1–10), proportion of smokers, and median income.
- *Environmental measures* that represent physical characteristics of the geographic location for the group of interest. Individuals within the group may have different degrees of exposure to a given characteristic, which could theoretically be measured. Examples include air pollution intensity and hours of sunlight.
- *Global measures* that represent characteristics of the group that are not reducible to characteristics of individuals (ie, that do not have analogues at the individual level). Examples include the type of political or health care system, a certain regulation or law, and the presence and magnitude of health inequalities.

In a traditional ecologic study, two ecologic variables are contrasted to examine their possible association. Typically, an ecologic measure of exposure and an aggregate measure of disease or mortality are compared (eg, Figure 1–10). These ecological measures can also be used in

---

*A mean value can be calculated for both continuous and discrete (eg, dichotomous) variables. A rate or a proportion is a mean value when individual values are dichotomous.

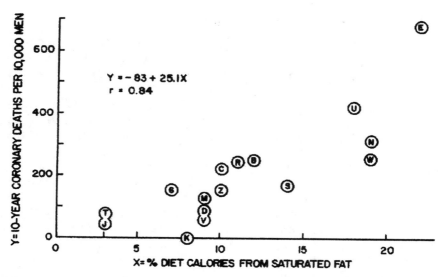

Figure 1–10 Example of an ecological study. Ten-year coronary death rates of the cohorts from the Seven Countries Study plotted against the percentage of dietary calories supplied by saturated fatty acids. Cohorts: B, Belgrade; C, Crevalcore; D, Dalmatia; E, East Finland; G, Corfu; J, Ushibuka; K, Crete; M, Montegiorgio; N, Zuphen; R, Rome railroad; S, Slavonia; T, Tanushimaru; U, American railroad; V, Velika Krsna; W, West Finland; Z, Zrenjanin. Shown in the figure are the correlation coefficient r and the linear regression coefficients (see Chapter 7, Section 7.4.1) corresponding to this plot. *Source:* Reprinted with permission from *Seven Countries: A Multivariate Analysis of Death and Coronary Heart Disease,* by A Keys, Cambridge, Mass: Harvard University Press, copyright © 1980 by the President and Fellows of Harvard College.

studies of individuals (ie, cross-sectional, case-control, or cohort studies; see Section 1.4) in which the investigator chooses to define exposure using an ecologic criterion on the basis of its expected superior construct validity.* For example, to examine the relationship between socioeconomic status and prevalent cardiovascular disease in individuals, the investigator may choose an aggregate indicator of socioeconomic status (eg, median family income in the neighborhood) to de-

---

*Construct validity is the extent to which an operational variable (eg, weight) accurately represents the phenomenon it purports to represent (eg, nutritional status).

fine the socioeconomic status of each individual, rather than, for example, his or her (individual) educational level or income. Furthermore, both individual and aggregate measures can be combined in *multilevel analyses* as when examining the joint effect of individuals' and aggregate levels of income and education in relation to prevalent cardiovascular disease.[11]

Although an ecologic association may accurately reflect a causal connection between a suspected risk factor and a disease (eg, the positive association between fat intake and coronary heart disease [CHD] depicted in Figure 1–10), the phenomenon of *ecologic fallacy* is often invoked as limiting the use of ecologic correlations as bona fide tests of etiologic hypotheses. The ecological fallacy (or *aggregation bias*) has been defined as "the bias that may occur because an association observed between variables on an aggregate level does not necessarily represent the association that exists at an individual level."[1] The phenomenon of ecologic fallacy is schematically illustrated in Figure 1–11, based on an example proposed by Diez-Roux.[12] In a hypothetical ecologic study examining the relationship between per capita income and the risk of motor vehicle injuries in three hypothetical populations composed of seven individuals each, a positive correlation between mean income and risk of injuries is observed. However, a close inspection of *individual* values reveals that cases occur exclusively in persons with low income (<US $20,000). In this extreme example of ecologic fallacy, the association detected when using populations as observation units—namely, that higher mean income relates to a higher risk of motor vehicle injuries—has a direction diametrically opposed to that expressing the relationship between income and motor vehicle injuries in individuals—namely, that higher individual income relates to a lower injury risk. Thus, the conclusion from the ecological analysis that a higher income is a risk factor for motor vehicle injuries may well be fallacious (see below).

Another example of a situation in which this type of fallacy may have occurred is given by an ecological study that showed a direct (positive) correlation between the percentage of the population that was Protestant and suicide rates in a number of Prussian communities in the late 19th century.[10,13] Based on this observation, the inference that being Protestant is a risk factor for suicide may well be wrong—that is, may result from an ecologic fallacy—as it is possible that most of the suicides within these communities are committed by Catholic individuals who, when in the minority (ie, when the proportion of Protestants is high), tend to be more socially isolated and therefore at a higher risk of suicide.

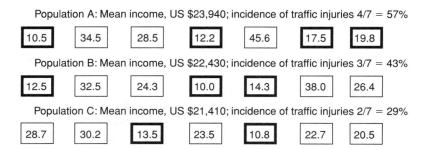

Figure 1–11 Schematic representation of a hypothetical study in which ecologic fallacy occurs. Boxes represent hypothetical individuals; thicker boxes represent incident cases of motor vehicle (MV) injuries; the numbers inside the boxes indicate individuals' annual incomes (in thousands of US dollars). Ecologically, the correlation is positive: population A has the highest values of both mean income and incidence of MV injuries; population B has intermediate values of both mean income and incidence of MV injuries; and population C has the lowest values of both mean income and incidence of MV injuries. In individuals, however, the relationship is negative: for all three populations combined, mean income is US $13,230 for cases and US $32,310 for noncases.

These examples demonstrate that the error associated with ecologic studies is a result of cross-level inference, which occurs when aggregate data are used to make inferences at the individual level.[10] The mistake in the example just discussed is to use the correlation between the proportion of Protestants (which is an aggregate measure) and suicide rate to infer that the risk of suicide is higher in Protestant than in Catholic *individuals*. However, if one were to make an inference at the population level, the conclusion that predominantly Protestant communities with Catholic minorities have higher rates of suicide would still be valid (provided that other biases and confounding factors were not present). Similarly, in the income/injuries example, the inference from the ecological analysis is only wrong if extended to individuals. If, on the other hand, the investigator's purpose is to understand the web of causality[2] involved in motor vehicle injuries, the ecological information may be valuable, as it may yield clues regarding the causes of motor vehicle injuries that are not provided by individual-level data. For example, higher mean population income may be associated with increased traffic volume. In addition, the inverse association between low individual-level income and motor vehicle injuries may be stronger in countries with high per capita income, that is, in the context of high traffic volume coupled with unsafe vehicles used by low-income individuals.

Because of the prevalent view that inference at the individual level is the "gold standard" when studying disease causation,[14] as well as the possibility of ecologic fallacy, ecologic studies are often merely considered as imperfect surrogates for studies in which individuals are the observation units. Essentially, ecologic studies are seen as preliminary studies that "can suggest avenues of research that may be promising in casting light on etiological relationships."[3(p170)] That this is often but not always true has been underscored by the examples discussed above. The following two situations illustrate the concept that an ecologic analysis may on occasion provide more accurate conclusions than an analysis using individual-level data (even if the level of inference in the ecologic study is at the individual level). The first situation is when the within-population variability of the exposure of interest is low but the between-population variability is high. For example, if salt intake of individuals in a given population were above the threshold needed to cause hypertension, a relationship between salt and hypertension might not be apparent in studies of individuals but could be seen in ecologic studies, including in populations with diverse dietary habits.[15] (A similar phenomenon has been postulated to explain why ecologic correlations, but not studies of individuals, have detected a relationship between fat intake and risk of breast cancer.[16]) The second situation is when, even if the intended level of inference is the individual, *the implications for prevention or intervention are at the population level*. Some examples of the latter situation are:

- In the classical studies on pellagra, Goldberger et al[17] assessed not only individual indicators of income but also food availability in the area markets. They found that, independently of individual socioeconomic indicators, food availability in local markets in the villages was strongly related to the occurrence of pellagra, leading them to conclude that

  the most potent factors influencing pellagra incidence in the villages studied were (a) low family income, and (b) unfavorable conditions regarding the availability of food supplies, suggesting that under conditions obtaining in some of these villages in the spring of 1916 many families were without sufficient income to enable them to procure an adequate diet, and that improvement in food availability (particularly of milk and fresh meat) is urgently needed in such localities.[17(p2712)]

It should be readily apparent in this example that an important (and potentially modifiable) link in the causal chain of pellagra occurrence—namely, food availability—would have been missed if the investigators had focused exclusively on individual income measures.

- Studies of risk factors for smoking initiation and/or smoking cessation may focus on regulations regarding advertisement or taxation of cigarettes at the population level. Although individual factors may influence the individual's predisposition to smoking (eg, psychological profile, smoking habits of relatives or friends), regulatory "ecological" factors may be strong determinants and modifiers of the individual behaviors. Thus, an investigator may choose to focus on these global factors rather than (or in addition to) individual behaviors.

- In studies of factors explaining the transmission of certain infectious diseases for which herd immunity is important, studies using individuals as observation units may be inappropriate. As discussed by Koopman and Longini,[18] ecological studies may be the only way to study these patterns and risk factors for transmissibility of infectious diseases.

Because ultimately all risk factors must operate at the individual level, the quintessential reductionist* approach would focus only on the causal pathways at the biochemical or intracellular level. For example, the study of the carcinogenic effects of tobacco smoking could focus on the effects of tobacco byproducts at the cellular level—that is, alteration of the cell's DNA. However, will that make the study of smoking habits irrelevant? Obviously not. Indeed, from a public health perspective, the use of a comprehensive theoretical model of causality—one that considers all factors influencing the occurrence of disease—often requires taking into account the role of ecological factors (including environmental, sociopolitical, and cultural) in the causal chain. As stated at the beginning of this chapter, the ultimate goal of epidemiology is to be effectively used as a tool to improve the health conditions of the public; in this context, the factors that operate at a global level may represent important links in the chain of

---

*Reductionism is a theory that postulates that all complex systems can be completely understood in terms of their components, basically ignoring interactions between these components.

causation, particularly when they are amenable to intervention (eg, improving access to fresh foods in villages or establishing laws that limit cigarette advertising). As a result, studies focusing on factors at the individual level may be insufficient in that they fail to address these ecologic links in the causal chain. This concept can be illustrated using the example of religion and suicide that was previously discussed. A study based on individuals would "correctly" find that the risk of suicide is higher in Catholics than in Protestants.[10] This finding would logically suggest explanations of why the suicide rate differs between these religious groups. For example, is the higher rate in Catholics due to Catholicism per se? Alternatively, is it because of some ethnic difference between Catholics and Protestants? If so, is it due to some genetic component that distinguishes these ethnic groups? The problem is that these questions, which attempt to characterize risk at the individual level, though important, are insufficient to fully explain the "web of causality,"[2] for they fail to consider the ecologic dimension of whether minority status explains and determines the increased risk of suicide. This example underscores the concept that both individual and ecological studies are necessary to study the complex causal determination not only of suicide but also of many other health and disease processes.[12] The combination of individual and ecologic levels of analysis poses analytical challenges for which statistical models (hierarchical models) have been developed. However, difficult conceptual challenges remain, such as the development of causal models that include all relevant risk factors operating from the social to the biological level and take into consideration their possible multilevel interaction.[12]

1.4 STUDIES BASED ON INDIVIDUALS AS OBSERVATION UNITS

There are three basic types of nonexperimental (observational) study designs in which individuals are the units of observation: the cohort or prospective study, the case-control study, and the cross-sectional study. In this section, key aspects of these study designs are reviewed. For a more comprehensive discussion of the operational and analytic issues related to these studies, the reader is referred to specialized texts.[19–23]

From a conceptual standpoint, the fundamental study design in observational epidemiology—that is, the design from which the others derive, and that can be considered as the "gold standard"—is the cohort or prospective study. Cohort data, if unbiased, reflect the "real-life" cause-effect temporal sequence of events, a sine qua non criterion to establish causality (see Hill[24]). From this point of view, the case-control and the cross-sectional designs are mere variations of the cohort study design and are primarily justified by logistical ease and efficiency, rather than by scientific desirability or intrinsic inferential logic.

1.4.1 Cohort Study

In a cohort study, a group of healthy people or *cohort** is identified and followed up for a certain time period to ascertain the occurrence of health-related events (Figure 1–12). The objective of a cohort study is usually to investigate whether the incidence of an event is related to a suspected exposure.

Study populations in cohort studies can be quite diverse and may include a sample of the general population of a certain geographical area (eg, the Framingham Study[25]); an occupational cohort, typically defined as a group of workers in a given occupation or industry who are classified according to exposure to agents thought to be occupational hazards; or a group of people who, because of certain characteristics, are at an unusually high risk of a given disease (eg, the cohort of homosexual men who are followed in the Multicenter AIDS Cohort Study [MACS]).[26] Alternatively, cohorts can be formed by "convenience" samples, or groups gathered because of their willingness to participate or because of other logistical advantages, such as ease of follow-up; examples include the Nurses Health Study cohort,[27] the Health Professionals Study cohort,[28] and the American Cancer Society cohort studies of volunteers.[29]

Once the cohort is defined and the participants are selected, a critical element in a cohort study is the ascertainment of events during the follow-up time (when the event of interest is a newly developed disease, prevalent cases are excluded from the cohort at baseline). This is the reason why these studies are also known as *prospective studies*.[30] A schematic depiction of a cohort of 1000 individuals is shown in Figure 1–13. In this hypothetical example, cohort members are followed up for a given time period during which four events such as incident disease cases or deaths (which appear in Figure 1–13 as "D" boxes) occur. In addition to these four events, seven individuals are lost to follow-up during the study period. These losses (represented in

---

*A definition of the term *cohort* broader than that found in the footnote in Section 1.2 is any designated group of individuals who are followed or traced over a given time period.[1]

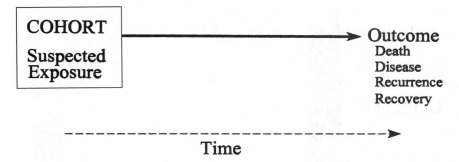

Figure 1–12 Basic components of a cohort study: exposure, time, and outcome.

the figure as arrows) are usually designated *censored observations* or *withdrawals*. As described in Chapter 2, these losses to follow-up need to be taken into account for the calculation of the incidence rates. Using the actuarial life-table approach as an example (see Section 2.2.1), incidence can be estimated as the number of events divided by the number of subjects in the cohort at baseline minus one half of the losses. Thus, for the hypothetical cohort in Figure 1–13, the incidence of D is $4/[1000 - (\frac{1}{2} \times 7)] = 4.01/1000$.

In the *cohort study's* most representative format, a defined population is identified, its subjects are classified according to exposure status, and the incidence of the disease (or any other health outcome of interest) is ascertained and compared across exposure categories (Figure 1–14). For example, based on the hypothetical cohort shown in Figure 1–13, and assuming that the prevalence of the exposure of interest is 50%, Figure 1–15 outlines the follow-up separately for exposed ($n = 500$) and unexposed ($n = 500$) individuals. Data analysis in this simple situation is straightforward, involving a comparison of the incidence of D between exposed and unexposed persons, using as the denominator the "population at risk," again taking into consideration the losses to follow-up (see Chapter 2). For example, using the actuarial life table approach as above, for the hypothetical cohort study depicted in Figure 1–15, the incidence of D in exposed individuals is $3/[500 - (\frac{1}{2} \times 4)] = 6.02/1000$, and in unexposed, $1/[500 - (\frac{1}{2} \times 3)] = 2.01/1000$. Based on these incidence estimates, the relative risk (see Chapter 3, Section 3.2.1) is estimated as $6.02/2.01 = 3.0$, thus suggesting that exposed individuals have a risk three times higher than that of unexposed individuals in the same cohort.

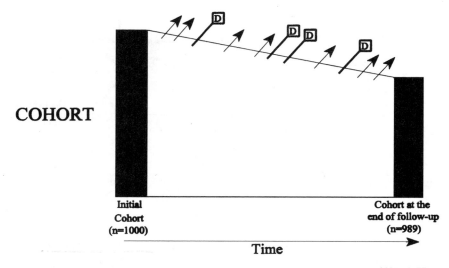

Figure 1–13 Diagram of a hypothetical cohort of 1000 subjects. During the follow-up, four disease events (D) and seven losses to follow-up (arrows) occur, so that the number of subjects under observation at the end of the follow-up is 989.

As discussed in Chapter 2, an important assumption for the calculation of incidence rates in a cohort study is that individuals who are lost to follow-up (the arrows in Figures 1–13 and 1–15) are similar to those who remain under observation with regard to characteristics affecting the outcome of interest. The reason is that even though techniques to "correct" the denominator for the number (and timing) of losses are available (see Chapter 2, Section 2.2), if the average risk of those who are lost differs from that of those remaining in the cohort, the incidence based on the latter will not represent accurately the true incidence in the initial cohort (see Chapter 2, Section 2.2.1). However, if the objective of the study is an *internal comparison* of the incidence between exposed and unexposed subjects, even if those lost to follow-up differ from the remaining cohort members, as long as the biases due to losses are similar in the exposed and the unexposed, they will cancel out when the relative risk is calculated (see Chapter 4, Section 4.2). Thus, a biased relative risk due to losses to follow-up is present only when losses are differential in exposed and unexposed subjects with regard to the characteristics influencing the outcome of interest—in other words, when losses are affected by both exposure and disease status.

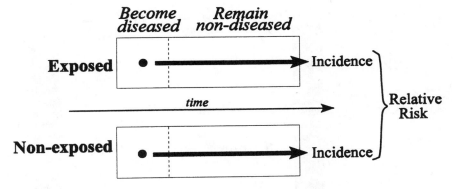

Figure 1–14 Basic analytical approach in a cohort study.

Cohort studies are defined as *concurrent*[3] (or truly "prospective"[30]) when the cohort is assembled at the present time—that is, the calendar time when the study starts—and is followed up toward the future (Figure 1–16). The main advantage of concurrent cohort studies is that the baseline exam and methods of follow-up and ascertainment of events are planned and implemented for the purposes of the study, thus best serving the study objectives; in addition, quality control measures can be implemented as needed (see Chapter 8). The disadvantages of concurrent studies relate to the amount of time needed to conduct them (results are available only after a sufficient number of events is accumulated) and their usually elevated costs. Alternatively, in *nonconcurrent* cohort studies (also known as *historical* or *retrospective* cohort studies), a cohort is identified and assembled in the past on the basis of existing records and is "followed up" to the present time—that is, the time when the study is conducted (Figure 1–16). An example of this type of design is a 1992 study in which the relationship between childhood weight and subsequent adult mortality was examined nonconcurrently on the basis of existing records of weight and height values obtained in 1933 through 1945 in school-age children.[31] The nonconcurrent design is also useful in occupational epidemiology, as occupational or census records can be linked to mortality or cancer registries: for example, a cohort of all electricians working in Norway in 1960 was followed up nonconcurrently through 1990 to study the relationship of electromagnetic radiation and cancer incidence.[32] *Mixed* designs with both nonconcurrent and concurrent follow-up components are also possible (Figure 1–16). Nonconcurrent cohort studies are obviously less expensive and can

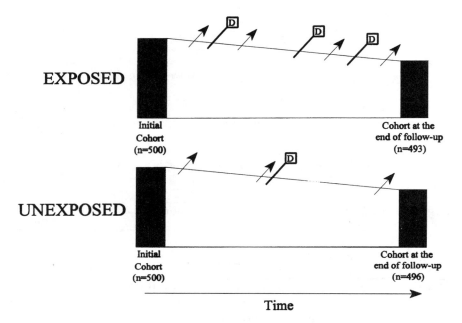

Figure 1–15 Same cohort study as in Figure 1–13, but the ascertainment of events and losses to follow-up is done separately among those exposed and unexposed.

be done more expeditiously than concurrent studies. Their main disadvantage is an obligatory reliance on available information; as a result, the quality of exposure or outcome data is sometimes less than ideal for fulfilling the study objectives. *can't measure unes perfed exposures*

1.4.2 Case-Control Study

As demonstrated by Cornfield[33] and discussed in basic epidemiology textbooks (eg, Gordis[3]), the case-control design is an alternative to the cohort study for investigating exposure-disease associations. In contrast to a cohort study, in which exposed and unexposed cohort participants are compared in relation to the disease incidence (or some other mean value for the outcome) (Figure 1–14), a case-control study usually compares the odds of past exposure to a suspected risk factor between cases (diseased individuals) and controls (usually nondiseased individuals). (Although the comparison of exposure odds is the typical analytic approach in case-control studies, other

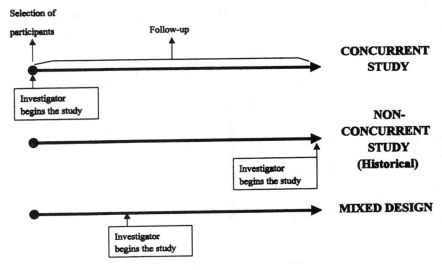

Figure 1–16 Types of cohort studies.

types of measurements can be compared between cases and controls, eg, mean blood pressure levels.) Thus, its main analytical strategy consists of the calculation of the exposure *odds ratio,* which is an estimate of the relative risk (Figure 1–17) (see Chapter 3, Section 3.2.1). The case-control study design has important advantages over the cohort design, particularly over the concurrent cohort study, as the need for a follow-up time is avoided, thus optimizing speed and efficiency.[3]

Case-Based Case-Control Study

In the simplest strategy for the selection of the groups in a case-control study, cases and noncases are identified at a given point in time among living individuals. An example of this strategy, sometimes called *case-based case-control study,* is a study in which cases are identified as the individuals in whom the disease of interest was diagnosed (eg, breast cancer) in a certain hospital or medical practice during a given year and controls are selected from among members of the community served by this hospital or practice who did not have a diagnosis of the disease of interest by the end of that same year. Note that although the study is carried out "cross-sectionally" (ie, cases and controls are identified at the same time), cases must necessarily occur

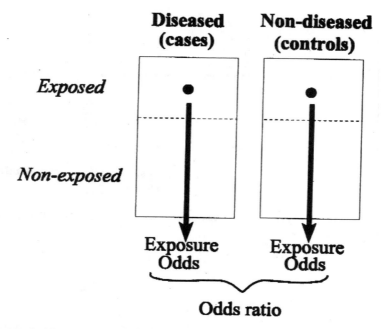

Figure 1–17 Basic analytical approach in a case-control study.

over a given time period prior to their inclusion in the study. Thus, it is necessary to assume that the cases who survive through the time when the study is done (Figure 1–18) are representative of all cases with regard to the exposure experience and that if exposure data are obtained through interviews, recall or other biases will not intrude (see Chapter 4). Furthermore, to validly compare cases and controls regarding their exposure status, it is necessary to assume that they originate from the same reference population—that is, from a more or less explicitly identified cohort, as depicted in Figure 1–18. In other words, for a case-control comparison to represent a valid alternative to a cohort study analysis, cases and controls are expected to belong to a common reference population (or to similar reference populations; see below). It is, however, frequently difficult to define the source cohort in a case-control study, as, for example, in a case-based study in which the cases are ascertained in a single hospital A but controls are selected from a population sample. In this example, it is important to consider the correspondence between the patient population of hospital A and the population of the geographic area from which controls are sampled. Thus, for example, if hospital A is the

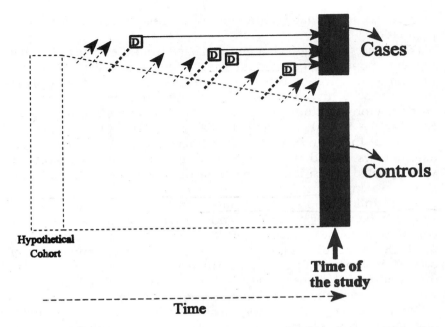

Figure 1–18 Hypothetical case-based case-control study, assuming that cases and controls are selected from a hypothetical cohort, as in Figure 1–13. The case group is assumed to include all cases that occurred in that hypothetical cohort up to the time when the study is conducted ("D" with horizontal arrows ending at the "case" bar): that is, they are assumed to be all alive and available to participate in the study; controls are selected from among those without the disease of interest (noncases) at the time when the cases are identified and assembled. Broken diagonal lines with arrows represent losses to follow-up.

only institution to which area residents can be admitted, and all cases are hospitalized, a sample of the same area population represents a valid control group. However, if residents use hospitals outside the area, alternative strategies have to be considered to select controls who are representative of the theoretical population from which cases originate (eg, random-digit dialing or matching by neighborhood).

The assumption that cases and controls originate from the same hypothetical source cohort is a critical issue affecting the validity of case-control data. Note that it is not strictly necessary that cases and controls be chosen from exactly the *same* reference population; however, they must originate from populations having *similar relevant characteristics.* Under these circumstances, the control group can be regarded as a reasonably representative sample of the case reference population.

When cases and controls are not selected from the same (or similar) reference population(s), *selection bias* may ensue, as discussed in detail in Chapter 4. Selection bias may occur even if cases and controls are from the same "hypothetical" cohort; this happens when losses occurring before the study groups are selected affect their comparability. For example, if losses among potential controls include a higher proportion of individuals with low socioeconomic status than losses among cases, biased associations may be found with socioeconomic status–related exposures. This example underscores the close relationship between selection bias in case-control studies and differential losses to follow-up in cohort studies. In this context, consider the similarity between Figures 1–18 and 1–13, in that the validity of the comparisons made in both cohort (Figure 1–13) and case-control (Figure 1–18) studies depends on whether the losses (represented by diagonal arrows in both figures) affect the representativeness of the baseline cohort (well defined in Figure 1–13, hypothetical in Figure 1–18) with regard to both exposure and outcome variables.

One particular type of (prior) "loss" that may affect comparability of cases and controls comprises *deaths* due to either other diseases or the disease of interest. For the type of design represented in Figure 1–18, characterized by cross-sectional ascertainment of study subjects, controls who die before they can be included in the study may have a different exposure experience compared with the rest of the source population. In addition, this design identifies primarily prevalent cases—that is, those with the the longest survival (Figure 1–19). These types of selection bias constitute generic problems affecting cross-sectional ascertainment of study participants; another problem is recall bias, which results from obtaining past exposure data long after disease onset. (For a detailed discussion of these and other biases in case-control studies, see Chapter 4.)

It should be emphasized that although cross-sectional ascertainment of cases and controls is often carried out, it is not a sine qua non feature of case-based case-control studies. An alternative strategy, which aims at minimizing selection and recall biases, and which should be used whenever possible, is to ascertain cases concurrently—that is, to identify (and obtain exposure information on) cases as soon as possible after disease onset. An example of this strategy is a study of risk factors for oral clefts conducted in Denmark.[34] In this study, case mothers were women who were hospitalized and gave birth to a liveborn child with cleft lip and/or palate (without other

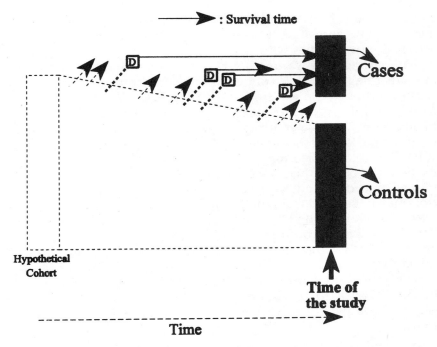

Figure 1-19 Survival bias in a case-based case-control study carried out "cross-sectionally": only cases with long survival after diagnosis (best prognosis) are included in the case group. In this hypothetical example, the horizontal lines starting in the cases' "D" boxes represent survival times; note that only two of the four cases are included in the study. Broken diagonal lines with arrows represent losses to follow-up.

malformations) between 1991 and 1994. Controls were the mothers of the two preceding births in the hospital where the case mother had given birth. Both case and control mothers were concurrently interviewed by trained nurses with regard to previous pregnancies, medications, smoking, diet, and other environmental and occupational exposures.

Case-Control Studies Within a Defined Cohort

When cases are identified within a well defined cohort, it is possible to carry out *nested case-control* or *case-cohort* studies. These designs have received considerable attention in recent years,[35-37] in part because of the increasing number of well-established large cohort studies that have been initiated and continued during the last few decades and in part because of recent methodological and analytic advances.

Case-control studies within a cohort are also known as *hybrid* or *ambidirectional designs*[35] because they combine some of the features and advantages of both cohort and case-control designs. In these studies, although the selection of the participants is carried out using a case-control approach (Figure 1–17), it takes place within a well-defined cohort. The case group consists of all (or a representative sample of) individuals with the outcome of interest occurring in the defined cohort over a specified follow-up period ("D" boxes in Figure 1–13). As discussed below, there are essentially two options for control selection when carrying out a case-control study within a cohort: (1) controls may be selected from the baseline cohort, or (2) controls may be selected from the individuals at risk at the time each case occurs. The first alternative has been labeled as a *case-cohort design,* and the second has been referred to as a *nested case-control design.*[36] It should be noted that regardless of the control selection strategy discussed next, because cases and controls are selected from the same source cohort in these studies, the likelihood of selection bias tends to be diminished in comparison with the traditional case-based case-control study.

Alternatives for the Selection of Controls in a Case-Control Study Within the Cohort. The first alternative for selection of controls is to make them a random sample of the total cohort at baseline. The term *case-cohort design* has been used when the sampling frame for the selection of controls is represented by the total cohort at baseline (Figure 1–20), thus allowing some cases that develop during follow-up to be part of both the case and the control groups ("D" boxes in Figure 1–20). It is somewhat peculiar, however, that although some of the cases are selected for inclusion in the cohort sample (the control group), others are not. Analytical techniques that take into account this special feature in the context of survival analyses have recently been developed (see Section 7.4.6).[37] An important advantage of case-cohort design is that the availability of a sample of the cohort (the control group) allows the estimation of risk factor distributions and prevalence rates needed for population attributable risk estimates (see Chapter 3, Section 3.2.2).

The second alternative is to make controls a random sample of the cohort selected at the time each case occurs. This study design is called a *nested case-control design* (Figure 1–21) and is based on a sampling approach known as *incidence density sampling*[35,38] or *risk-set sam-*

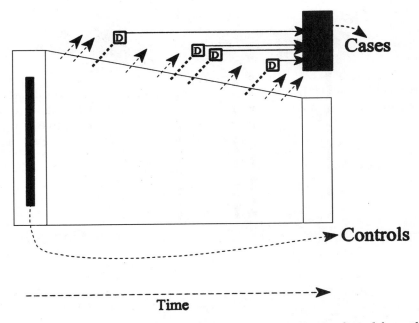

Figure 1–20 Case-control study in which the controls are selected from the baseline cohort (case-cohort study). Cases are represented by "D" boxes. Broken diagonal lines with arrows represent losses to follow-up.

pling.[20] The idea underlying this sampling scheme is that it allows the comparison of cases with a subset of the cohort members at risk of being cases at the time when each case occurs—that is, a "risk set" of all cohort members under observation at the time of each case's occurrence. By this strategy, cases occurring later in the follow-up are eligible to be controls for earlier cases. Incidence density sampling is the equivalent of matching cases and controls on duration of follow-up (see Section 1.4.5) and permits the use of straightforward statistical analysis techniques (eg, standard multiple regression procedures for the analysis of matched and survival data; see Chapter 7, Section 7.4.6).

Heretofore, the discussion has considered only case-control studies within the cohort in which cases are included in the sampling frame for the selection of controls; in this situation, it can be demonstrated that the estimated exposure odds ratio is a statistically unbiased estimate of the risk or rate ratio. If, however, cases are excluded from the

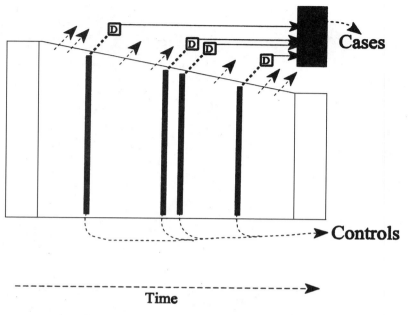

Figure 1–21 Nested case-control study in which the controls are selected at each time when a case occurs (incidence density sampling). Cases are represented by "D" boxes. Broken diagonal lines with arrows represent losses to follow-up.

potential control group, the analytic and inferential approaches are analogous to those of any case-control study: that is, the calculation of the exposure odds ratio yields an estimate of the disease odds ratio. A more detailed discussion of the influence of the sampling frame used for control selection on the parameter estimated by the exposure odds ratio is found in Chapter 3 (Section 3.4.1).

When Should a Case-Control Study Within a Cohort Be Done? In the above discussion, the terms *case-cohort study* and *nested case-control study* have been used to distinguish the selection of controls from either the baseline cohort (Figure 1–20) or risk sets (Figure 1–21), respectively. This terminology is probably the most commonly used in the field today.[37,39] Unfortunately, there is no consistency in the use of these terms. The expressions *nested case-control study* and *case-cohort study* are occasionally used to distinguish nested studies according to whether they exclude or include cases as potential controls (see above). Regardless of the terminology used, it is important to understand why it would be advantageous to compare cases and controls selected from a source cohort instead of analyzing data from the entire cohort (as in Figure 1–15). One reason is that case-control studies within a cohort represent an efficient approach when *additional information* that was not obtained or measured for the whole cohort is needed. A typical situation is a concurrent cohort study in which serum samples are collected at baseline and stored in freezers. Once a sufficient number of cases is accrued during the follow-up, the frozen serum samples for cases (or for a sample of cases) and for a sample of controls can be thawed and analyzed. This strategy not only reduces the cost that would have to be incurred if the analyte(s) of interest had been assayed in the whole cohort but in addition preserves serum samples for future analyses. A similar situation arises when the assessment of key exposures or confounding variables (see Chapter 5) requires labor-intensive data collection activities, such as data abstraction from medical or occupational records. Collecting this additional information in cases and a sample of the total cohort (or of the non-cases) is a cost-effective alternative to using the entire cohort. Some examples follow:

- A study was conducted to examine the relationship of military rank and radiation exposure to brain tumor risk within a cohort of male members of the US Air Force who had had at least 1 year of service between 1970 and 1989.[40] In this study, 230 cases of brain tumor were compared with 920 *noncases* (controls), matched on year of birth and race, who were still employed by the Air Force *at the time the case was diagnosed*. The reason for choosing a nested case-control design (ie, incidence density sampling; see Figure 1–21) instead of using the entire cohort of 880,000 US Air Force members in this study was that labor-intensive abstraction of occupational records was required to obtain accurate data on electromagnetic radiation exposure as well as other relevant information on potentially confounding variables. An alternative strategy would have been not to exclude cases from the eligible control sampling frame (see above). Yet another strategy would have been to use a case-cohort design whereby controls would have been sampled from among Air Force cohort members at the beginning of their employment (ie, at baseline; see Figure 1–20).
- An example of sampling controls from the total baseline cohort (ie, a case-cohort design; Figure 1–20) is given by a study conducted by Nieto et al[41] assessing the relationship between *Chlamydia pneumoniae* antibodies in serum collected at baseline and incident CHD in the Atherosclerosis Risk in Communities

(ARIC) study, a cohort study of approximately 15,800 men and women aged 45 to 64 years at the study's outset (1986–1989). During the follow-up of 3 to 5 years, 246 cases of incident CHD (myocardial infarctions or coronary deaths) were identified. The comparison group in this study consisted of a sample of 550 participants of the total baseline cohort, which actually included 10 of the 246 individuals who later developed CHD (incident cases), a fact that needs to be taken into account in the statistical analyses of these data (also see Section 7.4.6). For this study, instead of testing for the presence of *C. pneumoniae* IgG antibodies in the entire cohort, antibody levels were determined only in the sera of cases and in the cohort sample, that is, in approximately 800 individuals rather than in the almost 16,000 cohort participants. In addition to the estimation of risk ratios expressing the relationship between *C. pneumoniae* antibodies and incident CHD, the selection of a random cohort sample in Nieto et al's study allowed the estimation of the prevalence of relevant variables for the total cohort, which, as mentioned previously, can be used for the determination of population attributable risks (see Chapter 3).

1.4.3 Cross-Sectional Studies

In a cross-sectional study design, a sample of (or the total) reference population is examined at a given point in time. Like the case-control study, the cross-sectional study can be conceptualized as a way to analyze cohort data, albeit an often flawed one, in that it consists of taking a "snapshot" of a cohort by recording information on disease outcomes and exposures at a single point in time (Figure 1–22).* Accordingly, the case-based case-control study represented schematically in Figure 1–19 can also be regarded as a cross-sectional study, as it includes cross-sectionally ascertained prevalent cases and noncases (ie, cohort participants who survived long enough to be alive at the time of the study). It follows that when cross-sectional data are obtained for a defined reference population or cohort, the analytic approach may consist of either comparing point prevalence rates for the outcome of interest between exposed and unexposed individuals or using a "case-control" strategy, in which prevalent cases and non-

---

*Cross-sectional studies can also be done periodically for the purpose of monitoring disease or risk factor prevalence rates, as in the case of the US National Health Surveys.[42,43]

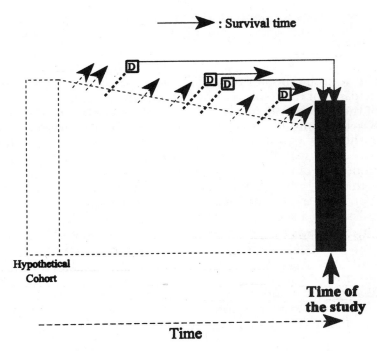

Figure 1–22 Schematic representation of a cross-sectional study, conceptually and methodologically analogous to the case-based case-control study represented in Figure 1–19, except that instead of explicitly selecting cases and controls, it selects a sample of the entire population. Broken diagonal lines with arrows represent losses to follow-up. Cases are represented by "D" boxes.

cases are compared with regard to odds of exposure (see Chapters 2 and 3).

Although cross-sectional morbidity surveys[44] offer an opportunity to examine exposure/outcome associations, cross-sectional analyses of baseline information in cohort studies are especially advantageous in that they allow confirmation when prospectively collected data become available. For example, in the ARIC study, cross-sectional associations were found at baseline between asymptomatic coronary artery atherosclerosis defined by B-mode ultrasound and both active and passive smoking.[45] These associations were subsequently confirmed by assessing data on progression of atherosclerosis in smokers and nonsmokers.[46]

The conditions influencing the validity of associations inferred from cross-sectional data are discussed in detail in Chapter 4 (Section 4.4.2).

1.4.4   Case-Crossover Design

Initially proposed by Maclure,[47] this design consists of comparing the exposure status of a case immediately before its occurrence with that of the same case at some other prior time (eg, during the previous year). It is especially appropriate to study acute (brief) exposures that produce a transient change in risk of an acute condition. For example, this design has been used to study acute triggers of myocardial infarction, such as episodes of anger[48] and sexual activity.[49] This design is a special type of matching (see next section) in that individuals serve as their own controls; thus, all fixed individual characteristics that could confound the association (eg, sex, genetic susceptibility) are controlled for. However, it assumes that the effects of exposure are not cumulative and that the disease does not have a preclinical stage that could inadvertently affect the exposure of interest. As in case-control studies, information on prior exposure relies on the cases' recall, thus being subject to recall bias (see Section 4.3.1).

1.4.5   Matching

In observational epidemiology, an important concern is that study groups may not be comparable with regard to characteristics that may distort ("confound") the associations of interest. The issue of *confounding* is key in epidemiological inference and practice and is discussed in detail in Chapter 5. Briefly, this issue arises when spurious factors (*confounding variables*) influence the direction and magnitude of the association of interest. For example, if a case-control study shows an association between hypertension (exposure) and coronary disease (outcome), it could be argued that this association may (at least in part) be due to the fact that coronary disease cases tend to be older than controls: because hypertension is more frequently seen in older people, age may spuriously produce the observed association (or distort its magnitude). Thus, if the question of interest is to assess the net relationship between hypertension and coronary disease (*independently* of age), it makes intuitive sense to select cases and controls with the same ages—that is, *matched* on age. Similarly, a putative association between serum markers of inflammation (eg, C-reactive protein) and the risk of CHD may result from confounding by smoking (ie, if smokers—who are at higher risk of coronary disease—tend to have higher levels of these markers due to, eg, chronic bronchitis). Recognizing this possibility, researchers did indeed match cases and controls according to smoking status (current, former, or never smoker) in a nested case-control study of the relationship between C-reactive protein and CHD.[50]

Matching in Case-Control and in Cohort Studies

The practice of matching is particularly prevalent and useful in the context of *case-control studies* when trying to make cases and controls as similar as possible with regard to potentially important confounding factors. Another example of matching, cited previously, is the study of risk factors for oral clefts,[34] in which cases and controls were matched according to place of birth (by selecting controls from the same hospital where the case mother had given birth) and time (by selecting the two preceding births). A special example of matching is the nested case-control study design based on incidence density sampling (see Section 1.4.2, Figure 1–21). As discussed previously, the application of this strategy results in matching cases and controls on follow-up time. In addition to time in the study, controls may be matched to cases according to other variables that could confound the association of interest. For example, in the US Air Force study of brain tumors mentioned earlier,[40] controls sampled from the risk sets at the time of occurrence of each case (and thus matched on follow-up time) were additionally matched on birth year and race.

In contrast, in cohort studies per se, matching on potentially confounding variables is not common. Cohort studies are often large and examine a multitude of exposure and outcomes. Thus, alternative means to control for confounding (eg, by adjustment; see Chapter 7) are usually chosen. Among the relatively rare instances in which matching is used in cohort studies are studies of prognostic factors for survival after cancer diagnosis in certain settings. For example, in a study examining age (the "exposure" of interest) as a prognostic factor in multiple myeloma patients following an autologous transplant,[51] older individuals (≥65 years old) were matched to younger individuals (<65 years old) with regard to other factors that affect prognosis and could thus confound the age-survival association (levels of β_2-microglobulin, albumin, creatinine, and C-reactive protein and the presence/absence of chromosomal abnormalities).

Types of Matching

Previous examples concerned studies in which cases and controls were *individually* matched: that is, for each case, one (or more) controls with the relevant characteristics matching the cases were selected from the pool of eligible individuals. Individual matching according to naturally categorical variables (eg, sex) is straightforward. When matching is conducted according to continuous variables (eg, age), a matching range is usually defined (eg, the matched control's age should be equal to the index case's age ± 5 years). In this situation, as well as when variables are arbitrarily categorized (eg, hypertensive/normotensive or current/former/never smoking), differences between cases and controls may remain, resulting in residual confounding (see Chapter 5, Section 5.4.3, and Chapter 7, Section 7.5).

Individual matching may be logistically difficult in certain situations, particularly when there is a limited number of potentially eligible controls and/or if matching is based on multiple variables. An alternative strategy is to carry out *frequency matching*, which consists of selecting a control group in such a way that its distribution of the matching variable (or variables) becomes similar to that of the cases, but without doing a case-by-case paired matching. To carry out frequency matching, advance knowledge of the distribution of the case group according to the matching variable(s) is usually needed so that the necessary sampling fractions within each stratum of the reference population for the selection of the control group can be estimated. For example, if matching is to be done according to sex and age (classified in two age groups, <45 years and ≥45 years), four strata would be defined: females younger than 45 years, females aged 45 years or older, males younger than 45 years, and males aged 45 years or older. Once the proportion of cases in each of these four groups is obtained, the number of controls to be selected from each sex-age stratum is chosen so that the proportion of controls in each stratum is the same as in the case group. If the controls are to be selected from a large population frame from which information on the matching variables is available, this can be easily done by stratified random sampling with the desirable stratum-specific sampling fractions. On the other hand, if this information is not available in advance (eg, when controls are chosen from among persons attending a certain outpatient clinic), the control selection can be done by systematic sampling and by successively adding the selected individuals to each stratum until they become full. Another strategy, if the distribution of cases according to matching variables is not known in advance, but the investigators wish to select and obtain information on cases and controls concurrently, is to obtain (and periodically update) provisional distributions of cases, thus allowing control selection to be carried out before all cases are identified.

An alternative method for matching on a large number of variables, including continuous variables, is the so-called *minimum Euclidean distance measure method*.[52] For example, in the study of age as a prognostic factor after transplantation in multiple myeloma patients described above,[51] older and younger individuals were matched according to five prognostic factors (four of them continuous variables). Matching according to categorical definitions of all those variables would have been rather cumbersome; furthermore, for some "exposed" individuals, it might have been difficult to find matches among "unexposed" persons. Thus, the authors of this study matched by the minimum Euclidean distance measure method, which is schematically illustrated in Figure 1–23. For the purpose of simplification, only two matching factors are considered in the figure. For each exposed case, the closest eligible person (eg, unexposed patient) in this bidimensional space defined by albumin and creatinine levels is chosen as a control. In Siegel et al's study,[51] the authors matched on more than two variables (levels of β_2-microglobulin, albumin, creatinine, and C-reactive protein and the presence/absence of chromosomal abnormalities) using this method. (However, the multidimensional space required when multiple variables are used in the matching is too difficult to represent in a diagram.) This method can also be used in the context of either case-based case-control studies and case-control studies within the cohort, as in the original application by Smith et al,[52] representing a convenient and efficient alternative form of matching when multiple and/or continuous variables need to be matched.

Advantages and Disadvantages of Matching

Although there is little doubt that matching is a useful strategy to control for confounding, it is far from being the only one. Chapter 7 is entirely devoted to describing some of the approaches that can be used at the analytical stage to address the problem of confounding—namely, stratification and adjustment. Whether investigators choose to deal with confounding prior to data collection by matching during the recruitment phase of the study rather than by stratification or adjustment at the analysis stage depends on a number of considerations.

Advantages of matching include the following:

1. In addition to being easy to understand and describe, matching may be the only way to guarantee some degree of control for

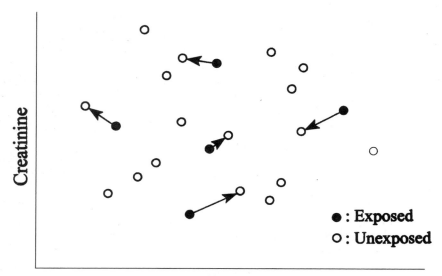

Figure 1–23 Matching according to minimal Euclidean distance measure method. Hypothetical example of a cohort study of survival after transplantation in multiple myeloma patients in which exposed individuals (eg, older individuals) are matched to unexposed (younger) patients according to two prognostic factors: serum albumin and creatinine levels. For each case, the closest unexposed individual in the bidimensional space defined by the two matching variables is chosen as control. *Source:* The authors, based on a study by DS Siegel et al, Age Is Not a Prognostic Variable with Autotransplants for Multiple Myeloma, *Blood,* Vol 93, pp 51–54, © 1999.

must match on variables to keep balance

confounding in certain situations. This may be particularly important in studies in which a potentially strong confounding variable may produce such an imbalance in the composition of the study groups that adjustment is difficult or outright impossible. For example, in a case-control study of risk factors for prostate cancer, it would make sense to match controls to cases according to age; at the very least, given that most prostate cancer cases are in the older age brackets, the investigator should *restrict* the eligibility of the control group to a certain age range. (Restriction is a somewhat "loose" form of matching.) Otherwise, if controls were to be sampled from the general population, the age range could be so broad that, particularly if the sample size were small, there might not be enough overlap with the restricted age range of cases (ie, not enough older subjects in the control sample) to allow for adjustment (see Chapter 5, Section 5.2.3).

2. If done according to strong confounders (variables that are related to both exposure and outcome; see Chapter 5), matching tends to increase the statistical power (efficiency) of the study.[53,54]

3. Matching (especially individual matching) is a logistically straightforward way to obtain a comparable control group when cases and controls are identified from a reference population for which there is no available sampling frame listing. For example, in a case-control study using cases of diabetes identified in an outpatient clinic, each case can be matched to the next control without diabetes with the same characteristics as the index case (eg, same age range, sex).

Disadvantages of matching should also be considered. They include the following:

1. In certain situations, it may be difficult or impossible to find a matched control (or matched controls, if the ratio of controls to cases is greater than 1:1) for a given case, particularly when sampling from a limited source population or when matching on multiple variables. Furthermore, even if matched controls are available, the process of identifying them may be cumbersome and may add costs to the study's recruitment phase.

2. When matching is done, the association between the matching variable(s) and the outcome cannot be assessed; the reason for this is that once matching on a certain variable is carried out, the study groups (eg, cases and controls) are set by design to be equal (or similar) with regard to this variable or set of variables.

3. It follows from (2) that it is not possible to assess additive interaction in matched case-control studies between the matching variable(s) and the exposure(s) of interest. As discussed in Chapter 6 (Section 6.4.2), the assessment of additive interaction in a typical case-control study relies on the formula for the joint expected effect of two variables A and Z, $RR_{A+Z+} = RR_{A+Z-} + RR_{A-Z+} - 1.0$ (using the odds ratios as estimates of the relative risks [RRs]). Assuming that A is the matching variable, its independent effect (RR_{A+Z-}) cannot be estimated, as it has been set to 1.0 by design (see (2) above). Therefore, the above formula cannot be applied.

4. Special statistical techniques for analyses of matched data need to be used, as detailed in Chapter 7 (Section 7.4.6).
5. Matching implies some kind of tailoring of the selection of the study groups to make them as comparable as possible; this increased "internal comparability" may, however, result in a lack of representativeness. For example, a control group that is made identical to the cases with regard to sociodemographic characteristics and confounding variables may no longer constitute a representative sample of the reference population. Thus, this control group may be of limited use for ancillary studies that could otherwise be conducted. For example, in studies that examine the association between novel risk factors and disease, a secondary, yet important, objective may be to study the distribution or correlates of these factors in the reference population. If controls are matched to cases, it may be a complicated task to use the observed distributions in the control group to make inferences to the population at large (complex weighted analyses taking into account the sampling fractions associated with the matching process are required). On the other hand, if a random sample of the reference population is chosen (as is done in case-cohort studies), it will be appropriate to generalize the distributions of risk factors in the control group to the reference population. Obtaining these distributions (eg, the prevalence of exposure in the population) is particularly important for the estimation of the population attributable risk (see Chapter 3, Section 3.2.2). In addition, a control group that is selected as a random sample of the source population can be used as a comparison group for another case group selected from the same cohort or reference population. For example, in the case-cohort study that assessed the relationship between *C. pneumoniae* and incident CHD,[41] the control group (*n* = 550) was selected as a random sample of the baseline cohort; serum antibodies for *C. pneumoniae* were compared between these controls and the 246 individuals who became CHD cases during follow-up. The same control group can be used for the assessment of the role of *C. pneumoniae* for a different outcome, such as strokes. Thus, as follow-up time in this cohort study is extended, and once a sufficient number of stroke cases develop, a subsequent case-cohort analysis evaluating the association between *C. pneumoniae* antibodies and stroke can be conducted by carrying out the antibody measurements only in the stroke cases, and again using as comparison the same data obtained in the control group.

[handwritten margin notes: interested in the effect of sss don't overadjust match based on a covariate variable i.e. race ... wash out the variable of interest]

6. Because when matching is done, it cannot be "undone," it is important that the matching variables not be strongly correlated with the variable of interest; otherwise, the phenomenon of "overmatching" may ensue. For example, matching cases and controls on race may to a great extent make them very similar with regard to variables of interest related to socioeconomic status. For further discussion of this topic and additional examples, see Chapter 5 (Section 5.2.3).

7. Finally, no statistical power is gained if the matching variables are weak confounders. If the matching variables are weakly related to exposure, even if these variables are related to the outcome, the gain in efficiency may be very small. Moreover, if the matching variables are weakly or not related to the outcome of interest, matching can result in a loss of power.[53,54]

[handwritten margin note: no power in weak confounders]

When matching is conducted according to categorical definitions of continuous variables, residual differences between cases and controls may remain (*residual confounding;* see Chapter 5, Section 5.4.3, and Chapter 7, Section 7.5). In these situations, it may be necessary to adjust for the variable in question in the analyses to eliminate variation within the matching categories. For example, in a study on the relationship between cytomegolovirus (CMV) antibodies in serum samples collected in 1974 (and retrospectively analyzed) and the presence of carotid atherosclerosis measured by B-mode ultrasound of the carotid arteries as part of the baseline ARIC study examination (1987–1989),[55] 150 controls (selected among individuals with normal carotid arteries) were frequency matched to 150 carotid atherosclerosis cases according to sex and two relatively broad age groups (45–54 years, 55–64 years). Thus, by design, both the case and control groups had identical number of individuals in all four sex-age groups; however, cases in this study were 58.3 years of age on the average, whereas the average age in controls was 56.7 years. Therefore, even though the study groups were matched on two age categories, the residual age difference prompted the authors to adjust for age *as a continuous variable* in the multivariate logistic regression analyses (see Chapter 7, Section 7.4.3).

The same residual differences may remain even in individually matched studies if the matching categories are broadly categorized. The reason for this phenomenon is illustrated in Figure 1–24. Even though the cases and controls are equally represented in both age groups, within each age group, cases tend to be older, thus resulting in an overall difference.

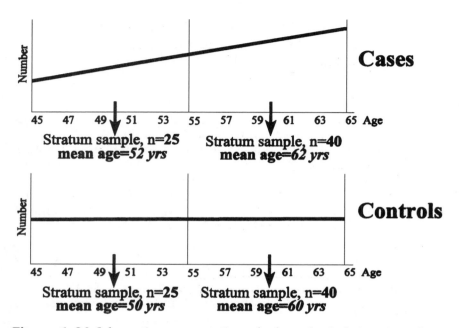

Figure 1–24 Schematic representation of a hypothetical situation where matching cases and controls according to broad age categories (45–54 years; 55–64 years) results in a residual mean age difference (residual confounding). Cases are skewed toward older ages, but the age distribution of controls is flat. As a result, the mean age within each age group is higher in cases than in controls, resulting in an overall mean age of 58.2 years in cases and 56.2 years in controls.

In summary, investigators should always consider carefully whether to match or not. Unlike post hoc means to control for confounding (stratification and adjustment), matching is irreversible once implemented. Although it may be the strategy of choice in studies with limited sample size and a clear-cut set of objectives, it should be avoided in most situations in which a reasonable overlap on potential confounding variables is expected to exist (thus allowing adjustment) or in which secondary hypotheses are being studied.

REFERENCES

1. Last JM. *A Dictionary of Epidemiology*. 3rd ed. New York, NY: Oxford University Press; 1995.

2. MacMahon B, Pugh TF. *Epidemiology: Principles and Methods.* Boston, Mass: Little, Brown and Co; 1970.

3. Gordis L. *Epidemiology.* Philadelphia, Pa: WB Saunders; 1996.

4. Strong JP, McGill HC. The pediatric aspects of atherosclerosis. *J Atheroscl Res.* 1969;9:251–265.

5. Frost WH. The age-selection of tuberculosis mortality in successive decades. *Am J Hyg.* 1939;30:91–96.

6. López-Abente G, Pollán M, Vergara A, et al. Age-period-cohort modeling of colorectal cancer incidence and mortality in Spain. *Cancer Epidemiol Biomarkers Prev.* 1997;6:999–1005.

7. Rocca WA, Cha RH, Waring SC, Kokmen E. Incidence of dementia and Alzheimer's disease: a reanalysis of the Rochester, Minnesota 1975-1984 data. *Am J Epidemiol.* 1998;148:51–62.

8. Newschaffer CJ, Bush TL, Hale WE. Aging and total cholesterol levels: cohort, period, and survivorship effects. *Am J Epidemiol.* 1992;136:23–34.

9. Keys A. *Seven Countries: A Multivariate Analysis of Death and Coronary Heart Disease.* Cambridge, Mass: Harvard University Press; 1980.

10. Morgenstern H. Ecological studies in epidemiology: concepts, principles, and methods. *Ann Rev Public Health.* 1995;16:61–81.

11. Diez-Roux AV, Nieto FJ, Muntaner C, et al. Neighborhood environments and coronary heart disease: a multilevel analysis. *Am J Epidemiol.* 1997;146:48–63.

12. Diez-Roux AV. Bringing context back into epidemiology: variables and fallacies in multilevel analysis. *Am J Public Health.* 1998;88:216–222.

13. Durkheim E. *Suicide: A Study in Sociology.* New York, NY: Free Press; 1951.

14. Piantadosi S, Byar DP, Green SB. The ecological fallacy. *Am J Epidemiol.* 1988; 127:893–903.

15. Elliott P. Design and analysis of multicentre epidemiological studies: the INTER-SALT study. In: Marmot M, Elliot P, eds. *Coronary Heart Disease Epidemiology: From Aetiology to Public Health.* Oxford, England: Oxford University Press; 1992:166–178.

16. Wynder EL, Cohen LA, Muscat JE, et al. Breast cancer: weighing the evidence for a promoting role of dietary fat. *J Natl Cancer Inst.* 1997;89:766–775.

17. Goldberger J, Wheeler GA, Sydenstrycker E. A study of the relation of family income and other economic factors to pellagra incidence in seven cotton mill villages of South Carolina in 1916. *Public Health Rep.* 1916;35:2673–2714.

18. Koopman JS, Longini IM. The ecological effects of individual exposures and nonlinear disease dynamics in populations. *Am J Public Health.* 1994;84:836–842.

19. Breslow NE, Day NE. *Statistical Methods in Cancer Research. Vol 1. The Analysis of Case-Control Studies.* Lyon, France: IARC Scientific Publications; 1980.

20. Breslow NE, Day NE. *Statistical Methods in Cancer Research. Vol 2. The Design and Analysis of Cohort Studies.* Lyon, France: IARC Scientific Publications; 1987.

21. Samet J, Muñoz A, eds. Cohort studies. *Epidemiol Rev.* 1998;20(1).

22. Schlesselman JJ. Case Control Studies. New York, NY: Oxford University Press; 1982.

23. Armenian H, ed. Applications of the case-control method. *Epidemiol Rev.* 1994; 16(1):1–164.

24. Hill AB. The environment and disease: association or causation? *Proc Royal Soc Med.* 1965;58:295–300.

25. Dawber TR. *The Framingham Study: The Epidemiology of Atherosclerotic Disease.* Cambridge, Mass: Harvard University Press; 1980.

26. Kaslow RA, Ostrow DG, Detels R, et al. The Multicenter AIDS Cohort Study: rationale, organization, and selected characteristics of the participants. *Am J Epidemiol.* 1987;126:310–318.

27. Stampfer MJ, Willett WC, Colditz GA, et al. A prospective study of postmenopausal estrogen therapy and coronary heart disease. *N Engl J Med.* 1985;313:1044–1049.

28. Ascherio A, Rimm EB, Stampfer MJ, et al. Dietary intake of marine n-3 fatty acids, fish intake, and the risk of coronary disease among men. *N Engl J Med.* 1995;332: 977–982.

29. Garfinkel L. Selection, follow-up, and analysis in the American Cancer Society prospective studies. *Natl Cancer Inst Monogr.* 1985;67:49–52.

30. Vandenbroucke JP. Prospective or retrospective: what's in a name? *Br Med J.* 1991;302:249–250.

31. Nieto FJ, Szklo M, Comstock GW. Childhood weight and growth as predictors of adult mortality. *Am J Epidemiol.* 1992;136:201–213.

32. Tynes T, Andersen A, Langmark F. Incidence of cancer in Norwegian workers potentially exposed to electromagnetic fields. *Am J Epidemiol.* 1992;136:81–88.

33. Cornfield J. A method of estimating comparative rates from clinical data: applications to cancer of the lung, breast and cervix. *J Natl Cancer Inst.* 1951;11: 1269–1275.

34. Christensen K, Olsen J, Nørgaard-Pedersen B, et al. Oral clefts, transforming growth factor alpha gene variants, and maternal smoking: a population-based case-control study in Denmark, 1991-1994. *Am J Epidemiol.* 1999;149:248–255.

35. Kleinbaum DG, Kupper LL, Morgentern H. (1982). *Epidemiologic Research: Principles and Quantitative Methods.* Belmont, Calif: Lifetime Learning Publications.

36. Langholz B, Thomas DC. Nested case-control and case-cohort methods of sampling from a cohort: a critical comparison. *Am J Epidemiol.* 1990:131;169–176.

37. Thomas D. New techniques for the analysis of cohort studies. *Epidemiol Rev.* 1998;20:122–134.

38. Checkoway H, Pearce NE, Crawford-Brown DJ. *Research Methods in Occupational Epidemiology.* New York, NY: Oxford University Press; 1989.

39. Rothman KJ, Greenland S. *Modern Epidemiology.* 2nd ed. Philadelphia, Pa: Lippincott-Raven Publishers; 1998.

40. Grayson JK. Radiation exposure, socioeconomic status, and brain tumor risk in the US Air Force: a nested case-control study. *Am J Epidemiol.* 1996;143:480–486.

41. Nieto FJ, Folsom AR, Sorlie P, et al. *Chlamydia pneumoniae* infection and incident coronary heart disease: the Atherosclerosis Risk in Communities (ARIC) Study. *Am J Epidemiol.* 1999; 150:149–156.

42. Flegal KM, Carroll MD, Kuczmarski RJ, et al. Overweight and obesity in the United States: prevalence and trends, 1960-1994. *Int J Obes Relat Metab Disord.* 1998; 22:39–47.

43. Hickman TB, Briefel RR, Carroll MD, et al. Distributions and trends of serum lipid levels among United States children and adolescents ages 4-19 years: data from the

Third National Health and Nutrition Examination Survey. *Prev Med.* 1998;27:
879–890.

44. Lister SM, Jorm LR. Parental smoking and respiratory disease in Australian children aged 0-4 years: ABS 1989-90 National Health Survey results. *Aust NZ J Public Health.* 1998;22:781–786.

45. Howard G, Burke GL, Szklo M, et al. Active and passive smoking are associated with increased carotid wall thickness: the Atherosclerosis Risk in Communities study. *Arch Intern Med.* 1994;154:1277–1282.

46. Howard G, Wagenknecht LE, Burke GL, et al. Cigarette smoking and progression of atherosclerosis: the Atherosclerosis Risk in Communities (ARIC) study. *JAMA.* 1998;279:119–124.

47. Maclure M. The case-crossover design: a method for studying transient effects on the risk of acute events. *Am J Epidemiol.* 1991;133:144–153.

48. Mittleman MA, Maclure M, Sherwood JB, et al. Triggering of acute myocardial infarction onset by episodes of anger: Determinants of Myocardial Infarction Onset Study Investigators. *Circulation.* 1995;92:1720–1725.

49. Muller JE, Mittleman MA, Maclure M, et al. Triggering of acute myocardial infarction by sexual activity: low absolute risk and prevention by regular physical exertion. Determinants of Myocardial Infarction Onset Study Investigators. *JAMA* 1996;275:1405–1409.

50. Ridker PM, Cushman M, Stampfer MJ, et al. Inflammation, aspirin, and the risk of cardiovascular disease in apparently healthy men. *N Engl J Med.* 1997;336:973–979.

51. Siegel DS, Desikan KR, Mehta J, et al. Age is not a prognostic variable with auto-transplants for multiple myeloma. *Blood.* 1999;93:51–54.

52. Smith AH, Kark JD, Cassel JC, Spears GFS. Analysis of prospective epidemiologic studies by minimum distance case-control matching. *Am J Epidemiol.* 1977;105:567–574.

53. Samuels ML. Matching and design efficiency in epidemiological studies. *Biometrika.* 1981;68:577–588.

54. Thompson WD, Kelsey JL, Walter SD. Cost and efficiency in the choice of matched and unmatched case-control study designs. *Am J Epidemiol.* 1982;116:840–851.

55. Nieto FJ, Adam E, Sorlie P, et al. Cohort study of cytomegalovirus infection as a risk factor for carotid intimal-medial thickening, a measure of subclinical atherosclerosis. *Circulation.* 1996;94:922–927.

PART II

Measures of Disease Occurrence and Association

CHAPTER 2

Measuring Disease Occurrence

2.1 INTRODUCTION: BASIC ELEMENTS OF EPIDEMIOLOGIC INFERENCE—DEFINING AND COUNTING DISEASE OUTCOMES

The outcomes of epidemiologic research have been traditionally defined in terms of disease, although the growing application of epidemiology to public health and preventive medicine increasingly requires the use of outcomes measuring health indicators in general (eg, outcome measures of functional status in epidemiologic studies related to aging). Outcomes can be expressed as either discrete (eg, disease occurrence or severity) or continuous variables.

Continuous variables, such as blood pressure and glucose levels, are commonly used as outcomes in epidemiology. The main statistical tools used to deal with these types of outcomes are the correlation coefficients, analysis of variance, and linear regression analysis, which are discussed in numerous statistical textbooks. Linear regression is briefly reviewed in Chapter 7 (Section 7.4.1) as a background for the introduction to multivariate regression analysis techniques in epidemiology. Other methodological issues regarding the use of continuous variables in epidemiology, covered in Chapter 8, relate to quality control and reliability of measurements.

Most of the present chapter deals with *categorical* dichotomous outcome variables, which are the most often used in epidemiologic studies. The frequency of this type of outcome can be generically defined as the number of individuals with the outcome (the numerator) divided by the number of individuals at risk for that outcome (the denominator). There are two types of absolute measures of outcome frequency: incidence and prevalence (Table 2–1).

outcome
at risk

55

Table 2–1 Absolute Measures of Disease Frequency

Measure	Expresses	Types of Events
Incidence	Frequency of a new event	Newly developed disease Death in the total population at risk (mortality) Death in patients (case fatality) Recurrence of a disease Development of a side effect of a drug
Prevalence	Frequency of an existing event	Point prevalence: cases at a given point in time Period prevalence: cases during a given period (eg, 1 year) Cumulative (lifetime) prevalence: cases at any time in the past

Although the term *incidence* has been traditionally used to indicate a proportion of newly developed (incident) disease, in fact it encompasses the frequency of any new health- or disease-related event and thus also includes death, recurrent disease among patients, disease remission, menopause, and so forth. Incidence is particularly important for analytic epidemiologic research, as it allows the estimation of risk necessary to assess causal associations.

Prevalence, on the other hand, measures the frequency of an existing outcome either at one point in time—point prevalence—or during a given period—period prevalence. A special type of period prevalence is the lifetime prevalence, which measures the cumulative lifetime frequency of an outcome up to the present time (ie, the proportion of people who have had the event at any time in the past).

For both prevalence and incidence, it is necessary to have a clear definition of the outcome as an *event* (a "noteworthy happening" as defined in an English dictionary[1]). In epidemiology, an event is defined as the occurrence of any phenomenon of disease or health that can be discretely characterized. For incidence (see Section 2.2), this characterization needs to include a precise definition of the time of occurrence of the event in question. Some events are easily defined and located in time, such as "birth," "death," "surgery," and "acute myocardial infarction." Others are not easily defined and require some more or less arbitrary operational definition for study, such as "menopause," "recovery," "dementia," and cytomegalovirus (CMV) disease (Table 2–2). An example of the complexity of defining certain clinical events is given by the widely adopted definition of a case of acquired immunodeficiency syndrome (AIDS), which uses a number of clinical and laboratory criteria.[6]

The next two sections of this chapter describe the different alternatives for the calculation of <u>incidence</u> and <u>prevalence</u>. The last section describes the *odds*, an alternative measure of disease frequency that is the basis for analytical tools often used in epidemiology, particularly in case-control studies (Chapter 1, Section 1.4.2)—namely, the relative odds (Chapter 3, Section 3.4.1) and logistic regression (Chapter 7, Section 7.4.3).

Table 2–2 Examples of Operational Definitions of Events in Epidemiologic Studies

Event	Definition	Reference
Menopause	Date of last menstrual period after a woman has stopped menstruating for 12 months	Bromberger et al[2]
Remission of diarrhea	Two days diarrhea free (diarrhea = passage of ≥3 liquid or semisolid stools in a day)	Mirza et al[3]
Dementia	A hospital discharge, institutionalization, or admission to a day care center in a nursing home or psychiatric hospital with a diagnosis of dementia (ICD-9-CM codes 290.0–290.4, 294.0, 294.1, 331.0–331.2)	Breteler et al[4]
CMV disease	Evidence of CMV infection (CMV antigen on white blood cells, CMV culture, or seroconversion) accompanied by otherwise unexplained spiking fever over 48 hours and either malaise or a fall in neutrophil count over 3 consecutive days	Gane et al[5]

2.2   MEASURES OF INCIDENCE

Incidence is best understood in the context of prospective (cohort) studies (Chapter 1, Section 1.4.1). The basic structure of any incidence indicator is represented by the number of events occurring in a defined population over a specific period of time (numerator), divided by the population at risk for that event over that time (denominator). There are two types of measures of incidence defined by the type of denominator: (1) incidence measures based on persons at risk and (2) incidence measures based on person-time units at risk.

2.2.1   Incidence Based on Individuals at Risk

This is an index defined in terms of the probability of the event, also known as *cumulative incidence*, which is the basis for the statistical techniques collectively known as *survival analysis*.

If follow-up is complete on every individual in the cohort, the estimation of the cumulative incidence is simply the number of events occurring during the follow-up time divided by the initial population. Often in epidemiologic studies, however, the follow-up is incomplete for many or all individuals in the study. In a typical cohort study, there are individuals lost to follow-up, those dying from causes other than the outcome of interest, and those whose follow-up is shorter because they are recruited later in the accrual period for the study; these are all called *censored observations* and require special analytical approaches. The traditional techniques for the estimation of cumulative incidence (or its complement, *cumulative survival* or *survival function*) in the presence of censored observations are the life table of the actuarial type (interchangeably referred to in this chapter as the *classical, actuarial, or interval-based life table*) and the Kaplan-Meier method.[7]

As an example, Figure 2–1 provides a schematic representation of a study for which the outcome of interest is death, in which 10 individuals are followed for up to 2 years (1996–1997). Each horizontal line in the figure represents the follow-up time of a unique individual. Follow-up can be terminated either by the event (D) or by withdrawal from the study (C, referred to as *censored observation*, as mentioned above). Note that individuals are recruited at different points in time and also leave the study (because of either death or censoring) at different times. For example, individual no. 1 is recruited in November 1996 and dies in December 1996, after only 1 month of follow-up, and individual no. 5 lives throughout the entire follow-up period

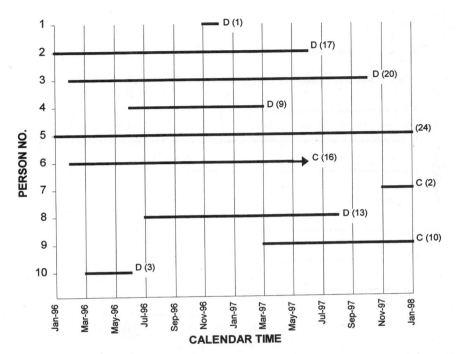

Figure 2–1 Hypothetical cohort of 10 persons followed for up to 24 months between January 1996 and December 1997. D, death; C, censored observation; ( ), duration of follow-up in months (all assumed to be exact whole numbers).

(2 years). Figure 2–2 shows a reorganization of the data in Figure 2–1, where the time scale has been transformed to follow-up time rather than calendar time. Thus, time 0 now represents the beginning of the follow-up in each individual (regardless of the actual date of the start of follow-up). Much of the discussion of incidence indexes that follows is based on Figure 2–2.

Cumulative Incidence Based on the <u>Life Table Interval</u> Approach (Classical Life Table)

The cumulative probability of the event during a given interval (beginning at time x and lasting m units of time) is the proportion of new events during that period of time (with events noted as $_md_x$), in which the denominator is the initial population (l_x) corrected for losses ($_mc_x$). In the classical life table, this measure corresponds to the

$$\frac{new}{population - losses}$$

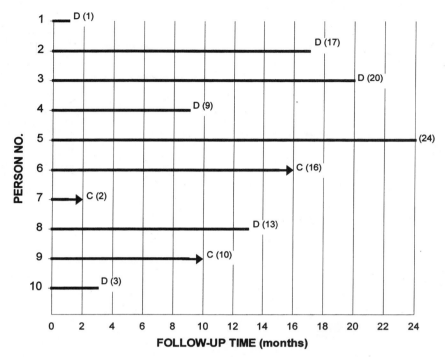

Figure 2–2 Same cohort as in Figure 2–1, with person-time represented according to time since the beginning of the study. D, death; C, censored observation; ( ), duration of follow-up in months (all assumed to be exact whole numbers).

interval-based probability of the event $_mq_x$.[8] Its calculation is straight-forward. As seen in Figure 2–2, 6 deaths occurred among the 10 individuals who were alive at the beginning of the follow-up. If no individual had been lost to observation, $_2q_0$ (with times specified in years) would be simply the number of deaths over this 2-year interval ($_2d_0$) divided by the number of individuals at the beginning of the interval (l_0): that is, 6/10 = 0.60 or 60%. However, because the three individuals lost to observation (censored, $_2c_0$) were not at risk during the entire duration of the follow-up, their limited participation must be accounted for in the denominator of the cumulative probability. By convention, half of these individuals are subtracted from the denominator, and the probability estimate is then calculated as

[Equation 2.1]

$$_2q_0 = \frac{_2d_0}{l_0 - 0.5\,(_2c_0)} = \frac{6}{10 - 0.5\,(3)} = 0.71$$

The conventional approach of subtracting one half of the total number of censored observations from the denominator is based on the assumption that the censoring occurred uniformly throughout that period and thus, that on the average, these individuals were at risk for only half of the follow-up period.

The complement of this cumulative probability of the event is the cumulative probability of survival: that is,

$$_2p_0 = 1 - _2q_0 = 0.29$$

It is important to note that the cumulative probability of an event (or the cumulative survival) has no time period intrinsically attached to it: time must be specified. Thus, in this example, one has to describe q as the "*2-year* cumulative probability of death." Usually, the classical life table uses multiple intervals—for example, five intervals of 2 years for a total follow-up of 10 years. A cumulative probability of survival over more than one interval—for example, a 4-year follow-up with two 2-year intervals—is obtained by calculating the joint probability of not having the event (survival): that is, the probability of surviving through the first interval multiplied by the "conditional probability" of surviving through the second one (ie, the probability of surviving through the second interval given that one survived through the first interval, as those who did not survive through the first interval will not have the opportunity to enter the second interval). In this example,

$$_4p_0 = (_2p_0)\,(_2p_2)$$

The cumulative probability of having the event is the complement of this joint probability of survival:

[Equation 2.2]

$$_4q_0 = 1 - _4p_0 = 1 - (_2p_0)\,(_2p_2)$$

This is analogous to the calculation of the cumulative survival function using the Kaplan-Meier method illustrated in the section that follows.

Note that it is not necessary that the intervals in a classical (interval-based) life table be of the same duration. The length of the interval should be determined by the pace at which incidence changes over time. For example, to study survival after an acute myocardial infarction, the intervals should be very short, soon after onset of symptoms when the probability of death is very high and rapidly changing. However, subsequent intervals could be longer, as the probability of recurrent events and death tends to stabilize.

Examples of the use of the actuarial life table method can be found in reports from classical epidemiologic studies (eg, Pooling Project Research Group[9]). More details and additional examples can be found in other epidemiology textbooks (eg, Gordis[10] and Kahn and Sempos[11]).

Cumulative Incidence Based on the Kaplan-Meier (Exact Event Times) Approach

The Kaplan-Meier approach involves the calculation of the probability of each event at the time it occurs. The denominator for this calculation is the population at risk at the time of each event's occurrence.[7] As for the actuarial life table, these are "conditional probabilities": in other words, they are conditioned on being at risk (alive and not censored) at each event time. If each event (first, second, etc) is designated by its time of occurrence i, then the formula for the conditional probability is simply

$$q_i = \frac{d_i}{n_i}$$

where d_i is the number of deaths (or other types of events) occurring at time i (a number that is always 1 if there are no ties) and n_i is the number of individuals still under observation (ie, at risk of the event) at time i.

For example, in Figure 2–2, when the first death occurs exactly at the end of the first month (person no. 1), there are 10 individuals at risk; the conditional probability is then

$$q_1 = \frac{1}{10}$$

When the second death occurs after 3 months of follow-up (person no. 10), there are only 8 persons at risk; this is because, in addition to the one previous death, one individual had been lost to observation (c) after 2 months (person no. 7) and therefore was not at risk when the second death occurred. Thus, the conditional probability at the time of the second death is estimated as

$$q_3 = \frac{1}{8} = 0.125$$

Table 2–3 (column 4) shows the calculation of these conditional probabilities for each event time. Note that the previously censored observations are skipped in these calculations (they do not represent an identified event) ~~but are accounted for in the denominator~~ for each event probability in which the event occurred before the loss to follow-up. This represents the most efficient use of the available information.[7]

Column 5 in Table 2–3 shows the complements of the conditional probabilities of the event at each time—that is, the conditional probabilities of survival (p_i), which, as in the classical life table method, represent the probability of surviving beyond time *i* among those who were still under observation at that time (ie, conditioned on having survived up to time *i*). Column 6, also shown graphically in Figure 2–3, presents the cumulative probabilities of survival—that is, the so-called Kaplan-Meier *survival function* (usually notated as S_i). This represents the probability of surviving from the beginning of the follow-up up to beyond time *i*, calculated as the product of all conditional survival probabilities up to time *i*. For example, the cumulative probability of surviving through the end of the follow-up period of 2 years (S_i, where $i = 24$ months) is

$$S_{24} = \frac{9}{10} \times \frac{7}{8} \times \frac{6}{7} \times \frac{4}{5} \times \frac{2}{3} \times \frac{1}{2} = 0.180$$

cum. probability of not getting the disease

Thus, the estimate of the cumulative probability of the event $(1 - S_i)$ is

$$1 - S_{24} = 1 - 0.18 = 0.82$$

As for the cumulative probability based on the actuarial life table approach (Equation 2.2), the time interval for the cumulative probability using the Kaplan-Meier approach also needs to be specified (in

---

Table 2–3 Calculation of Kaplan-Meier Survival Estimates for the Example in Figure 2–2

Time (Months) (1) *i*	Individuals at Risk (2) n_i	Number of Events (3) d_i	Conditional Probability of the Event (4) $q_i = d_i/n_i$	Conditional Probability of Survival (5) $p_i = 1 - q_i$	Cumulative Probability of Survival (6) S_i
1	10	1	1/10 = 0.100	9/10 = 0.900	0.900
3	8	1	1/8 = 0.125	7/8 = 0.875	0.788
9	7	1	1/7 = 0.143	6/7 = 0.857	0.675
13	5	1	1/5 = 0.200	4/5 = 0.800	0.540
17	3	1	1/3 = 0.333	2/3 = 0.667	0.360
20	2	1	1/2 = 0.500	1/2 = 0.500	0.180

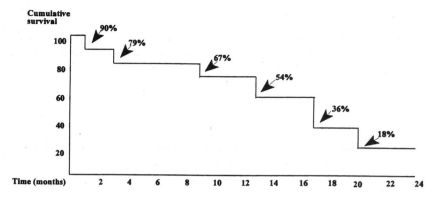

Figure 2–3 Kaplan-Meier curve corresponding to the data in Table 2–3, column 6.

---

this example, 24 months or 2 years). For methods to estimate confidence limits of cumulative survival probabilities, see Appendix A, Section A.1.

Regardless of the method used in the calculation (actuarial or Kaplan-Meier), the cumulative incidence is a proportion in the strict sense of the term. It is unitless, and its values can range from 0 to 1 (or 100%).

Assumptions in the Estimation of Cumulative Incidence Based on Survival Analysis

Uniformity of Events and Losses Within Each Interval (Classical Life Table). Implicit in the classical life table calculation (see above) is the generic assumption that events and losses are approximately uniform during each defined interval. If risk increases or decreases too rapidly within a given interval (ie, if the interval is too long vis-à-vis the risk changes that take place within it), then calculating an average risk over the interval is not fully informative. The application of the correction for losses (ie, subtracting one half of the losses from the denominator, Equation 2.1) also depends on the uniformity assumption as applied to losses. The assumption of uniformity of events and losses within a given interval is entirely related to the way the life table is defined and can be met by adjusting the interval definitions to appropriately uniform risk intervals—for example, by shortening them. Furthermore, this assumption does not apply to the Kaplan-Meier calculation, where intervals are not defined a priori.

interval based assumption - only for life table method
Kap Meier - no set interval

Whereas this interval-based assumption applies only to classical life table estimates, the two following assumptions apply to both classical life table and Kaplan-Meier estimates and are key to survival analysis techniques and analyses of cohort data in general: (1) independence of censoring and survival and (2) lack of secular trends during the study's accrual period.

Independence Between Censoring and Survival. For the calculations of the conditional and cumulative incidences using the above methods, censored individuals are included in the denominator during the entire time when they are under observation; once censored, they are ignored in subsequent calculations. Thus, if one wants to infer that the estimated overall cumulative survival (eg, $S_{24} = 18\%$, as in Figure 2.3) is generalizable to the entire population present at the study's outset (at time 0), one needs to assume that *the censored observations have the same probability of the event (after censoring) as those remaining under observation.* In other words, censoring needs to be independent of survival; otherwise, bias will ensue. For example, if the risk were higher for censored than for noncensored observations (eg, study subjects withdrew because they were sicker), over time the study population would include a progressively greater proportion of lower risk subjects; as a result, the (true) overall cumulative incidence would be underestimated (ie, survival would be overestimated). The opposite bias would occur if censored observations tended to include healthier individuals. The likely direction of the bias according to the reason why censoring occurred is summarized in Table 2–4. With regard to censored observations due to *death from other causes* in cause-specific outcome studies, if the disease of interest shares risk factors with other diseases that are associated with mortality, censoring may not be independent of survival. An example is a study in which the outcome is lung cancer death, and participants dying from other causes, including coronary heart disease deaths, are censored at the time of their death (as they are no longer at risk of dying from a lung cancer!). Because lung cancer and coronary heart disease share an important risk factor, smoking, it is possible that individuals dying from coronary heart disease would have had a higher risk of lung cancer if they had not died from heart disease, resulting in a violation of the assumption of independence between censoring and survival.

Other frequent reasons for censoring include refusal of study participants to allow subsequent follow-up contacts (in a study where assessment of the outcome events depends on such contacts) and loss of contact due to migration out of the area of the study. Individuals

Table 2–4 Relationship Between Reason for Censoring and the Assumption of Independence Between Censoring and Survival in Survival Analysis

Type of Censoring	May Violate Assumption of Independence of Censoring/Survival	If Assumption Is Violated, Likely Direction of Bias on the Cumulative Incidence Estimate
Deaths from other causes when there are common risk factors*	Yes	Underestimation
Refusal to follow up contacts	Yes	Underestimation
Migration	Yes	Variable
Administrative censoring	Unlikely†	Variable

*In cause-specific incidence or mortality studies.
†More likely in studies with a prolonged accrual period in the presence of secular trends.

who refuse follow-up contacts may have a less healthy lifestyle than individuals who are more compliant with the demands of a prospective study; if that is the case, censoring for this reason may lead to an underestimation of the cumulative incidence. The direction of the bias resulting from the loss to follow-up of individuals due to *migration* is a function of the sociodemographic context in which the migration occurs—for example, whether the individuals who migrate are of higher or lower socioeconomic status (SES). For example, if losses occurred mainly among those in the upper SES, who tend to be healthier, those remaining in the study would tend to have a poorer survival. On the other hand, if the losses occurred primarily among individuals with a lower SES, and thus poorer health, the survival of those remaining in the study would be inflated.

For the so-called *administrative* losses, defined as those that occur because the follow-up ends (eg, persons no. 7 and 9 in Figure 2–1), the assumption of independence between censoring and survival is regarded as more justified, as these losses are usually thought to be independent of the characteristics of the individuals per se. (However, administrative losses are amenable to temporal changes occurring during the accrual period; see below under "Lack of Secular Trends.")

In summary, the key *assumption* of independence between censoring and survival for the calculation of cumulative incidence/survival estimates depends on the reasons why censoring occurred (Table 2–4). This assumption is particularly relevant when the magnitude of the absolute incidence estimate is the focus of the study; it may be less important if the investigator is primarily interested in a relative estimate (eg, when comparing incidence/survival in two groups defined by exposure levels in a cohort study), provided that biases resulting from losses are reasonably similar in the groups being compared. (For a discussion of a related bias, see "Selection Bias" in Chapter 4, Section 4.2.) Finally, note that this assumption can be often verified. For example, it is usually possible to compare baseline characteristics related to the outcome of interest between individuals lost and those not lost to observation. It is possible to use the National Death Index to compare the mortality experience of those lost and those not lost to follow-up.   ⟶ ex: insulin, AIDS

Lack of Secular Trends. In studies in which the accrual time covers an extended period, the decision to pool all individuals at time 0 (as in Figure 2–2) assumes lack of secular trends with regard to the type and characteristics of these individuals that affect the outcome of interest. This, however, may not be the case in the presence of *birth cohort* and *period* (calendar time) effects (see Chapter 1, Section 1.2). Changes over time in the characteristics of recruited participants as well as significant secular changes in relevant exposures and/or treatments may introduce bias in the cumulative incidence/survival estimates, with direction and magnitude dependent on the characteristics of these cohort or period effects. Thus, for example, it would not have been appropriate to estimate survival from diagnosis of all patients identified with insulin-dependent diabetes from 1915 through 1935 as a single group, as this extended accrual period would inappropriately combine two very heterogeneous patient cohorts: those diagnosed before and those diagnosed after the introduction of insulin. Similarly, it would not be appropriate to carry out a survival analysis pooling at time 0 all HIV-seropositive individuals recruited into a cohort accrued between 1995 and 1999—that is, both before and after a new effective treatment (protease inhibitors) became available.

2.2.2 Incidence Rate Based on Person-Time

Rather than individuals, the denominator for this type of incidence measure is formed by time units (t) contributed to the follow-up period by the individuals at risk (n). For example, consider a hypothetical cohort in which 12 events occur and the total amount of follow-up time for all individuals is 500 days. The incidence rate in this example is $12/500 = 0.024$ per person-day or 2.4 per 100 person-days. Note that the number of individuals in the group is not provided; thus, the "person-time" estimate in the example could have originated from 50 individuals seen during 10 days each (50×10), 5 individuals observed for 100 days (5×100), and so on.

Incidence rates are *not* proportions. They are measured in units of time^{-1} and can range from 0 to infinity, depending on the units of time that are used. For example, the incidence rate above could be expressed in a number of ways: 12/500 person-days = 12/1.37 person-years = 8.76 per person-year (or 876 per 100 person-years). The latter value exceeds 1 (or 100%) only because of the arbitrary choice of the time unit used in the denominator. Thus, the actual value of the incidence rate depends on the choice of the unit for the person-time denominator. If a person has the event of interest after a follow-up of 6 months and the investigator chooses to express the rate per person-years, the rate will be 1/0.5 or 200 per 100 person-years.

The time unit used is at the discretion of the investigator and is usually selected on the basis of the frequency of the event under study. The main reason why many epidemiologic studies use *person-years* as the unit of analysis is because it is a convenient way to express rare events. On the other hand, when one is studying more or less frequent health or disease events, it may be more convenient to use some other unit of time (Table 2–5). The choice is entirely arbitrary and will not affect the inferences derived from the study.

Rather than a unitless proportion of the individuals who had the event out of the total who were at risk (see cumulative incidence

---

Table 2–5 Examples of Person-Time Units According to the Frequency of Events under Investigation

Population	Event Studied	Person-Time Unit Typically Used
General	Incident breast cancer	Person-years
General	Incident myocardial infarction	Person-years
Malnourished children	Incident diarrhea	Person-months
Lung cancer cases	Death	Person-months
Influenza epidemic	Incident influenza	Person-weeks
Children with acute diarrhea	Recovery	Person-days

above), the incidence rate estimate expresses the "rate" at which the events occur in the population at risk at any given point in time. This type of rate is also called *incidence density*, a concept analogous to that of velocity: the instantaneous rate of change or the "speed" at which individuals develop the event (disease, death, etc) in the population. This concept is the basis for some of the mathematical modeling techniques used for the analysis of incidence rates (eg, Poisson regression models; see Chapter 7, Section 7.4.5). However, because the instantaneous rate for each individual cannot be directly calculated, the average incidence over a period of time for a population is usually used as a proxy. The average incidence can be calculated based on individual or aggregate follow-up data, as will be discussed below. For practical purposes, the terms *rate* and *density* are used interchangeably; however, in the discussion that follows, the term *rate* will be primarily used in the context of grouped data, whereas *density* will denote a rate based on data obtained from each individual in the study.

Incidence Rate Based on Aggregate Data

This type of incidence is typically obtained for a geographic location by using as the denominator the average population estimated for a certain time period. Provided that this period is not excessively long and that the population and its demographic composition in the area of interest are relatively stable, the average population can be estimated as the population at the middle of the period (eg, July 1 for a 1-year period). In a cohort study, the average of the population at the beginning and at the end of the period can be obtained for a given follow-up interval. Thus, for a given time interval,

$$\text{Incidence rate} = \frac{\text{Number of events}}{\text{Average population}}$$

In Figure 2–2 for example, 10 individuals are alive and present in the study at the beginning of the follow-up period ("point zero"). Only one person is alive and present in the study when the 2-year follow-up ends. Thus, the average population (n) for the total 2-year follow-up period is

$$n = \frac{10 + 1}{2} = 5.5$$

The average population n can be also calculated by subtracting one half of the events (*d*) and losses (*c*) from the initial population:

$$n = 10 - 1/2 \ (6 + 3) = 5.5$$

As is the case with all mean values, the underlying assumption when using this approach is that, on the average, there were 5.5 persons for the duration of the study (2 years). For this assumption to be met, events and withdrawals must occur uniformly throughout the follow-up period. The rate of new events in relation to the average population is then calculated as

$$\text{Incidence rate} = \frac{6}{5.5} = 1.09 \text{ per person–2 years}$$

Note that in this example, the rate is based on a time unit of 2 years and not on the number of individuals (see below). The assumption underlying the use of the average population is that 5.5 individuals were followed for the entire 2-year period, during which 6 events were observed. This example again highlights the fact that this type of rate is not a proportion and thus is not bound to be below 1 (or 100%). In this particular example, the seemingly counterintuitive rate of 109 per 100 person-time obviously resulted from the fact that "2 years" is being used as the time unit; if a "person-year" unit had been used instead, the rate would have been 1.09/2 years = 0.545 per person-year (or 54.5 per 100 person-years).

The above example illustrates the estimation of the incidence rate using the average population of a defined cohort (ie, the hypothetical cohort represented in Figure 2–2). However, this is not its usual application. Instead, the calculation of incidence based on grouped data is typically used to estimate mortality based on vital statistics information, or incidence of newly diagnosed disease based on population-based registries (eg, cancer): in other words, when incidence needs to be estimated for aggregate of individuals, defined by their residence in a given geographic area over some time period. These aggregates are called open or dynamic cohorts because they include individuals who are added or withdrawn from the pool of the population at risk as they migrate in or out of the area (ie, a situation more clearly represented by the diagram in Figure 2–1 than that in Figure 2–2).

Incidence Density Based on Individual Data

This type of incidence can be estimated when relatively precise data on the timing of events or losses are available for each individual from a defined cohort. The total person-time for the study period is simply the sum of the person-time contributed to by each individual. The average incidence density is then calculated as

$$\text{Incidence density} = \frac{\text{Number of events}}{\text{Total person-time}}$$

For each individual in the example shown in Figures 2–1 and 2–2, the length of the horizontal line represents the length of time between the beginning of the follow-up and the point when the individual either died (*d*) or was lost to observation (*c*). For example, for individual no. 1, death occurred exactly after 1 month. Thus, this individual's contribution to the total number of person-years in the first follow-up year (see Figure 2–2) would be 1/12 = 0.083; obviously, this person made no contribution to the follow-up during the second year. On the other hand, individual no. 2 died after remaining in the study for 17 months, or 1 year and 5 months. Thus, his or her contribution to the first follow-up year was 12/12 and to the second year was 5/12, for a total of 1.417 person-years.

The contribution of censored individuals is calculated in an identical fashion. For example, the contribution of individual no. 6 to the total number of person-years was equivalent to 16 months, or 1 full person-year in the first year and 4/12 in the second year, for a total of 1.333 person-years. The calculation of person-years for all 10 study participants is shown in Table 2–6. In this example, the incidence density applicable to the total follow-up period is, therefore, 6/9.583 = 0.63 per person-year (or 63 per 100 person-years). Alternatively, the incidence density could be expressed as 6/(9.583 × 12 months) = 0.052 per person-months (5.2 per 100 person-months). For a method to estimate confidence limits of incidence rates, see Appendix A, Section A.2.

Assumptions in the Estimation of Incidence Rates Based on Person-Time

The assumptions of independence between censoring and survival and of lack of secular trends discussed in Section 2.2.1 are also relevant in the context of person-time analysis. These assumptions have to do with lack of selection bias and apply to any type of statistical analysis of a cohort study. Furthermore, as for incidence based on the actuarial life table (Equation 2.1) (Section 2.2.1), an important assumption when using the person-time approach is that the risk of the event remains approximately constant over time during the interval of interest, or, in other words, that the estimated risk should apply equally to *any time unit within the interval*. This means that *n* persons followed during *t* units of time are equivalent to *t* persons observed during *n* units of time: for example, the risk of an individual living five units of time within the interval is equivalent to that of five individuals living one unit each (Figure 2–4). When individuals are exposed to a given risk factor, another interpretation of this assumption

must have $n \cdot t = t \cdot n$

Table 2–6 Calculation of the Number of Person-Years Based on Figure 2–2

Person No.	Total Follow-Up (in Months)	Contribution to the Total Number of Person-Years by Participants In:		
		1st Year of Follow-Up	2nd Year of Follow-Up	Total Follow-Up Period
1	1	1/12 = 0.083	0	0.083
2	17	12/12 = 1.000	5/12 = 0.417	1.417
3	20	12/12 = 1.000	8/12 = 0.667	1.667
4	9	9/12 = 0.750	0	0.750
5	24	12/12 = 1.000	12/12 = 1.000	2.000
6	16	12/12 = 1.000	4/12 = 0.333	1.333
7	2	2/12 = 0.167	0	0.167
8	13	12/12 = 1.000	1/12 = 0.083	1.083
9	10	10/12 = 0.833	0	0.833
10	3	3/12 = 0.250	0	0.250
Total	115 months	7.083 years	2.500 years	9.583 years

is that the effect resulting from the exposure is not cumulative within the follow-up interval of interest. Often this assumption is difficult to accept, as, for example, when doing studies of risk of chronic respiratory disease in smokers: the risk of chronic bronchitis for 1 smoker followed for 10 years is certainly not the same as that of 10 smokers followed for 1 year, in view of the strong cumulative effect of smoking. To decrease the dependency of the person-time approach on this assumption, the follow-up period can be divided in smaller intervals and densities calculated for each interval. For example, using data from Table 2–6 and from Figure 2–2, it is possible to calculate densities separately for the first and the second years of follow-up, as follows:

First follow-up year: 3/7.083 = 42.4/100 person-years (or 3/85 = 3.6/100 person-months)

Second follow-up year: 3/2.500 = 120/100 person-years (or 3/30 = 10/100 person-months)

Relationship Between Density (Based on Individual Data) and Rate (Based on Grouped Data)

It is of practical interest that when withdrawals (or additions in an open population or dynamic cohort) and events occur uniformly, rate (grouped data) and density (individual data) are virtually the same,

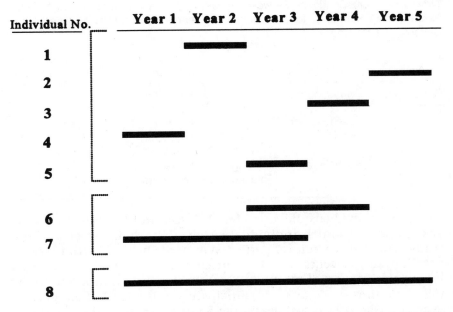

Figure 2–4 Follow-up time for eight individuals in a hypothetical study. It is assumed that the sum of the person-time units for individuals no. 1 to 5 (with a short follow-up time of 1 year each) is equivalent to the sum for individuals no. 6 and 7 (with follow-up times of 2 and 3 years, respectively) and to the total time for individual no. 8 (who has the longest follow-up time, 5 years). For each group of individuals (no. 1–5, 6 and 7, and 8), the total number of person-years of observation is 5.

and the density per person-time corresponds to a rate per average population, averaged for the corresponding time unit (eg, yearly).

$$\text{Rate} = \frac{\dfrac{\text{No. events } (x)}{\text{average population } (n)}}{\text{time } (t)} = \frac{x}{n \times t} = \text{Density}$$

This idea can be understood intuitively. For a given time unit, such as 1 year, the denominator of the rate (the average population) is analogous to the total number of time units lived by all the individuals in the population in that given time period. An example is given in Table 2–7, based on data for four persons followed up for a maximum of 4 years. One individual is lost to follow-up (censored) after 1

Table 2–7 Correspondence Between Density and Rate in a Study in which Four Persons Are Followed up for a Maximum of 2 Years and Events and Losses Are Uniformly Distributed

Individual No.	Outcome	Timing of Event/Loss	No. of Person-Years
1	Death	At 0.5 years (6 months)	0.5
2	Loss to observation	At 1 year	1.0
3	Death	At 1.5 years (18 months)	1.5
4	Administrative censoring	At 2 years	2.0
		Total no. of person-years:	5.0

year; two individuals die, one after 1/2 year and the other after 1.5 years; and the fourth individual survives through the end of the study. There is, therefore, perfect symmetry in the distribution of withdrawals or events, which occurred after 0.5, 1, 1.5, and 2 years following the onset of the study. Summing up the contribution to the follow-up time made by each participant yields a total of 5.0 person-years. Density is thus two deaths per 5 person-years, or 0.40.

The average population (n) in this example can be estimated as (initial population + final population)/2, or $(4 + 1)/2 = 2.5$. The rate for the total time (t) = 2 years is then 2/2.5. The average yearly rate is thus equivalent to the density using person-time as the denominator:

$$\text{Yearly Rate} = \frac{\frac{x}{n}}{t} = \frac{x}{n \times t} = \frac{x}{\text{person years}}$$

$$= \text{Density} = \frac{2}{2.5 \times 2} = \frac{2}{5} = 0.40$$

On the other hand, when losses and events do not occur in an approximate uniform fashion, the incidence rate based on the average study population and the incidence density based on the same population may be discrepant over the corresponding follow-up period. For example, based on the data in Figure 2–2, the estimate of the mean yearly incidence based on the average population was 54.5/100 person-years, whereas that based on the incidence density was 63/100 person-years. The hypothetical example schematically illustrated in Figures 2–1 and 2–2 is based on a very small sample size, and thus the lack of uniformity may be due to sampling variability. When the sample size is large, and provided that the interval is reasonably short, the assumption of uniformity of events/losses is more likely to be held.

The notion that the average population is equivalent to the total number of person-time when events and withdrawals are uniform is analogous to the assumption regarding withdrawals in the actuarial life table (see Section 2.2.1, Equation 2.1). When it is not known exactly when the events occurred in a given time period, each person who either suffers the event or withdraws from the study is assumed to contribute one half the follow-up time of a given time unit. (It is expected that this will be the average across a large number of individuals entering/exiting at different times throughout each unit of time.)

In an open (dynamic) cohort, in addition to losses due to events and withdrawals, individuals are added (eg, by immigration). These additions are also captured by using the average population, which corresponds to the person-time that these added individuals contribute, provided that they entered the population uniformly throughout the time period. The correspondence between rate (based on grouped data) and density (based on individual person-time) makes it possible to compare an average yearly rate based on an average population—which, in vital statistics, is usually the midpoint, or July 1, population estimate—to a density based on person-years. It is, for example, a common practice in occupational epidemiology studies to obtain an expected number of events needed for the calculation of the standardized mortality ratio by applying population vital statistics age-specific rates to the age-specific number of person-years accumulated by an exposed cohort (see Chapter 7, Section 7.3.2).

Stratifying Person-Time and Rates According to Follow-up Time and Covariates

The calculation of person-time lived by a given population or group is simply the sum of the person-time lived by each individual in the group during the follow-up period. In most analytical prospective studies relevant to epidemiology, the risk of the event changes with time. For example, the incidence of fatal or nonfatal events may increase with time, as when healthy individuals are followed up as they age. In other situations, risk diminishes as follow-up progresses, as in a study of complications after surgery or of case fatality after an acute myocardial infarction. Because calculating an overall average rate over a long time period when the incidence is not uniform does not make a lot of sense, it is necessary to estimate the event rate for time intervals within which homogeneity of risk can be assumed. Thus, as discussed above, it is often important to stratify the follow-up time and calculate the incidence rate for each time stratum (eg, Table 2–6). In a cohort study, one may additionally wish to control for potentially confounding variables. Time and confounders can be taken into account by stratifying the follow-up time for each individual according to other time variables (eg, age) and categories of the confounder(s) and then adding up the person-time within each stratum.

The following examples illustrate the calculation of person-time and the corresponding incidence rates based on the data shown in Table 2–8, based on a hypothetical study of four postmenopausal women followed for mortality after breast cancer surgery (1980–1990). Table 2–8 provides the dates of surgery ("entry"), the date of the event (death or censoring), ages at surgery and at menopause, and smoking status.

One Time Scale. Based on the data from Table 2–8, the follow-up of these four women is displayed in Figure 2–5. The top panel of Figure 2–5 displays the follow-up according to calendar time for each of the four women; the bottom panel displays the follow-up time after surgery. Note that in Figure 2–5, top, as the precise date of surgery and events is not known, it is assumed that these occur in the middle of the corresponding year (see above).

If it could be assumed that the risk of the event was approximately uniform within 5-year intervals, we would be justified in calculating the person-time separately for the first and the second 5-year calendar period (Figure 2–5, top); the calculation of the rates is shown in Table 2–9. Note that individuals whose follow-up starts or ends sometime during a given year are assigned one half person-year: for example, a contribution of 0.5 person-year is made by woman no. 1 in 1983, as her surgery was carried out at some time in 1983. Thus, the total

---

Table 2–8 Hypothetical Data for Four Postmenopausal Women Followed for Mortality after Breast Cancer Surgery

	Woman No. 1	Woman No. 2	Woman No. 3	Woman No. 4
Date of surgery	1983	1985	1980	1982
Age at surgery	58	50	48	54
Age at menopause	54	46	47	48
Smoking at time of surgery	Yes	No	Yes	No
Change in smoking status (year)	Quits (1986)	No	No	Starts (1983)
Event	Death	Loss	Withdrawal alive	Death
Date of event	1989	1988	1990	1984

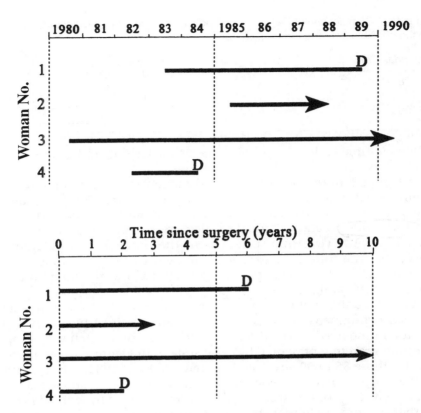

Figure 2–5 Schematic representation of person-time for the hypothetical data in Table 2–8, according to one time scale: calendar time (top) and follow-up time (bottom) (censored observations are shown with arrows).

person-time for the period 1980 to 1984 is 1.5 years (woman no. 1) + 4.5 years (woman no. 3) + 2 years (woman no. 4) = 8 person-years.

Alternatively, one might be interested in examining the rates in this study according to follow-up time, as shown in Table 2–10. For example, because woman no. 1 was followed from 1983.5 to 1989.5, she can be assumed to have a full 6-year follow-up (Figure 2–5, bottom).

Two or More Time Scales. Epidemiologic cohorts are usually constituted by free-living individuals who interact and are the subject of multiple and varying biological and environmental circumstances. Thus, it is frequently important to take into consideration more than one time scale; the choice of time scales used for the stratification of

Table 2–9 Stratification of Person-Time and Rates According to Calendar Time, Based on Table 2–8 and Figure 2–5, Top

Calendar Time	Person-Years	Events	Rate
1980–84	8	1	0.125
1985–89	12.5	1	0.080
(1990–94)	(0.5)	(0)	(0)

follow-up time varies according to the characteristics and goals of the study (Table 2–11).

In Figure 2–6, the person-time and outcomes of the four women from Table 2–8 are represented according to two time scales, age and calendar time. In this type of graphical representation (known as a *Lexis diagram*), each individual's trajectory is represented by diagonals across the two time scales. As in the previous example, and given that the time data are approximate (in whole years), it is assumed that entry and event (or censoring) occur at the midpoint of the 1-year interval.

Table 2–12 shows the corresponding estimates of total person-time in each two-dimensional stratum. These are obtained by adding up the total time lived by the individuals in the study in each age/calendar time stratum represented by eight squares in Figure 2–6: for example, for those 55 to 59 years old between 1980 and 1984, it is the sum of the 1.5 years lived by woman no. 4 (between age 55 and age 56.5, the assumed age of her death) and the 1.5 years lived by woman no. 1 in that stratum. Note that the events are also assigned to each corresponding stratum, thus allowing the calculation of calendar- and age-specific incidence rates, also shown in Table 2–12.

Other time scales may be of interest. In occupational epidemiology, for example, it may be of interest to obtain incidence rates of certain outcomes, taking into account three time scales simultaneously: for example, age (if the incidence depends on age), calendar time (if there have been secular changes in exposure doses), and time since

Table 2–10 Stratification of Person-Time and Rates According to Follow-up Time (Time since Surgery), Based on Table 2–8 and Figure 2–5, Bottom

Time since Surgery	Person-Years	Events	Rate
0–4 years	15	1	0.0667
5–9 years	6	1	0.1667

Table 2–11 Examples of Time Scales Frequently Relevant in the Context of Cohort Studies

Time Scale	Type of Study
Follow-up time (time since recruitment)	All studies
Age	All studies
Calendar	All studies (if recruitment is done over an extended period)
Time since employment	Occupational studies
Time since menarche	Studies of reproductive outcomes
Time since seroconversion	Follow-up of patients with HIV infection

employment (since this may influence cumulative doses). For this situation, one could picture a tridimensional analogue to Figure 2–6: cubes defined by strata of the three time scales and each individual's person-time going across the tridimensional diagonals.

The layout for the calculation of person-time and associated incidence rates described above can be used for the internal or external comparison of stratified rates using standardized mortality or incidence ratios (see Chapter 7, Section 7.3.2).

Time and Fixed and Time-Dependent Covariates. In certain cases, it may be appropriate to stratify by specific covariates in addition to time. For example, Figure 2–7 displays the person-time and events for the four women in Table 2–8 according to three time scales: age, calendar time, and time since menopause changes (arbitrarily defined as a dichotomous variable), in addition to smoking status at baseline (the time of surgery). Note that in Figure 2–7, woman no. 1 shifts diagrams as her status regarding time since menopause changes (when she turns 59.5—i.e., 1 year into the study—she becomes a woman who is "≥5 years since menopause"). Similarly, woman no. 3 (who entered the study in 1980—or rather, 1980.5—when she was 1 year postmenopausal) shifts from the "menopause <5 years" to the "≥5 years since menopause" stratum 4 years after initiation of follow-up (ie, at some time in 1984, or in 1984.5).

Note that in Figure 2–7, smoking is used as a fixed covariate, as only baseline status is considered; however, information on smoking status change is available on the hypothetical study data shown in Table 2–8. Changes in exposure status for certain covariates can easily be taken into account when using the person-time strategy. For example, using the information at baseline and change in smoking status

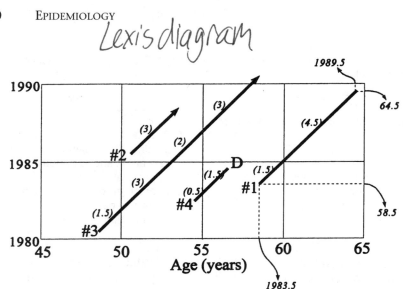

Figure 2–6 Schematic representation of person-time for the four women in Table 2–8 according to two time scales, age and calendar time, categorized in 5-year intervals. Because time data are given in whole years, entry, events, and withdrawals are assumed to occur exactly at the middle of the year. Censored observations are represented by an arrow. The total time within each time stratum for all four women is shown in parentheses. The entry and exit times for woman no. 1 are given in italics.

shown in Table 2–8, assignment of person-time according to smoking as a time-dependent covariate can be represented as illustrated in Figure 2–8. Using this approach, each event is assigned to the exposure status at the time of the event. Thus, the death occurring in woman no. 1 is assigned to the "nonsmoking" group, whereas that of woman no. 4 is assigned to the "smoking" group. (Note that the latter assignments are opposite to those based on smoking status at baseline—Figure 2–7.)

To use the person-time approach to take into account changing exposures involves an assumption akin to that used in crossover clinical trials: that once the exposure status changes, so does the associated risk. This is merely another way to state that there is no cumulation of risk and thus that the effect of a given exposure is "instantaneous." Whether this assumption is valid depends on the specific exposure or outcome being considered. For example, for smoking, the assumption may be reasonable when studying thromboembolic events likely to result from the acute effects of smoking (eg, those leading to sudden cardiac death). On the other hand, given the well-known latency and

Table 2–12 Stratification of Person-Time and Rates According to Calendar Time and Age (See Figure 2–6)

Calendar Time	Age (Years)	Person-Years	Events	Rate
1980–84	45–49	1.5	0	0
	50–54	3.5	0	0
	55–59	3	1	0.3333
	60–64	0	–	–
1985–89	45–49	0	–	–
	50–54	5	0	0
	55–59	3	0	0
	60–64	4.5	1	0.2222

cumulative effects leading to smoking-related lung cancer, the assumption of an "instantaneous" effect would be unwarranted. (The cumulative effect of smoking on lung cancer risk can be easily inferred from the fact that the risk in smokers who quit never becomes equivalent to that in never smokers.) If there is cumulative effect, the approach illustrated in Figure 2–8 (eg, assigning the event in woman no. 1 to the nonsmoking category) will result in misclassification.

The cumulative effects of exposure can be taken into account with more complex exposure definitions: for example, total pack-years of smoking could be considered even among noncurrent smokers. Moreover, lag or latency times could also be introduced in the definition of person-time in relation to events, a frequent practice in occupational or environmental epidemiology studies.[12(pp150–155)] Obviously, stratification according to more than one time scale and several covariates may make it cumbersome to calculate person-time and rates for each multidimensional stratum. Fortunately, computer programs are available to facilitate this procedure.[13–15]

2.2.3 Comparison Between Measures of Incidence

For the estimation of the various incidence measures, the numerator (number of deaths) is constant; the differentiation between the measures is given by the way the denominator is calculated. The main features that distinguish cumulative probability on the one hand and density or rate on the other are shown in Exhibit 2–1. As discussed previously, the upper limit of values for a rate or a density may exceed 100%, whereas values for probabilities cannot be greater than 100%.

Smoker at baseline

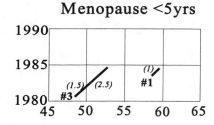

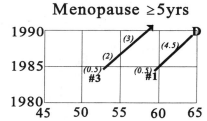

Non smokers at baseline

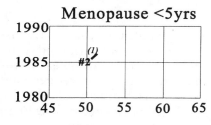

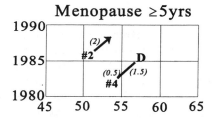

Figure 2–7 Person-time according to calendar time, age, time since menopause, and smoking at the time of surgery for the women in Table 2–8.

Rates are often calculated to as *yearly average rates* or *rates per 100 person-years*, the latter implying a rate per 100 persons per year, which underscores the correspondence between vital statistics–derived rate and a rate per person-time as discussed in the previous section—in this case, correspondence between a "yearly rate" and a "rate per person-year(s)." On the other hand, no time unit whatsoever is attached to a cumulative incidence (a probability), which must always be specified (eg, "the cumulative probability *for the initial 3 years of follow-up*").

Finally, another difference between the person-time and the cumulative incidence approach of practical relevance is that, as implied by these terms, it is not possible to obtain an overall cumulative *rate* over several time intervals (using an average population or a person-time approach), analogous to a cumulative incidence calculated by means of the survival analysis techniques; this is, of course, a consequence of the "instantaneous" character of rate estimates.

With regard to assumptions, all methods for the calculation of incidence rates share the fundamental assumptions in the analysis of cohort data that were discussed in previous sections and are summa-

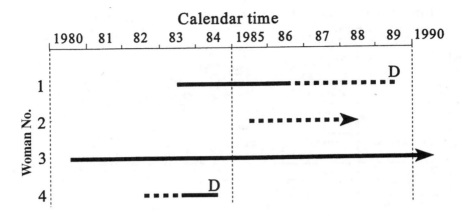

Figure 2–8 Schematic representation of person-time for the four women in Table 2–8, according to time-dependent smoking status. Solid lines represent smoking status; broken lines represent nonsmoking status.

rized in Exhibit 2–2: independence between censoring and survival and lack of secular trends. Additional assumptions are needed depending on the specific requirements of the method (eg, uniformity of risk across defined interval in classical life table and/or person-time–based analyses).

Experienced epidemiologists have learned that whereas each approach has advantages and disadvantages, the ultimate choice on how to present incidence data is dictated by pragmatism (and/or personal preference). Thus, in a cohort study without an "internal" unexposed group—as is often the case in occupational epidemiology research—estimation of densities, rather than probabilities, allows using available population rates as control rates. On the other hand, probabilities are typically estimated in studies with a focus on the temporal behavior of a disease—as in studies of survival after diagnosis of disease.

2.2.4 The Hazard Rate

An alternative definition of an instantaneous incidence rate is the so-called *hazard rate* or instantaneous conditional incidence or *force of morbidity (or mortality)*. In the context of a cohort study, the hazard rate is defined as each individual's instantaneous probability of the event at precisely time t (or at a small interval $[t, t + \Delta t]$), given that

Hazard Rate-

Exhibit 2-1 Comparing Measures of Incidence: Cumulative Incidence Versus Incidence Rate

	Cumulative Incidence		Incidence Rate	
	If Follow-up Is Complete	If Follow-up Is Incomplete	Individual Data (Cohort)	Grouped Data (Area)
Numerator	Number of cases	Classical life table	Number of cases	Number of cases
Denominator	Initial population	Kaplan-Meier	Person-time	Average population*
Units	Unitless		Time^{-1}	
Range	0 to 1		0 to infinity	
Synonyms	Proportion Probability		Incidence density†	

*Equivalent to person-time when events and losses (or additions) are homogeneously distributed over the time interval of interest.
†In the text, the term *density* is used to refer to the situation in which the exact follow-up time for each individual is available; in real life, however, the terms *rate* and *density* are often used interchangeably.

(or "conditioned" on the fact that) the individual was at risk at time *t*. The hazard rate is defined for each particular point in time during the follow-up. In mathematical terms, this is defined for a small time interval (Δt close to zero) as follows:

$$h(t) = \frac{P \text{ (event in interval between } t \text{ and } [t + \Delta t] \mid \text{alive at } t)}{\Delta t}$$

The hazard is also a rate measured in units of time^{-1}. The hazard rate is a useful concept for anyone trying to understand some of the statistical techniques used in survival analysis, particularly the methodology known as proportional hazards regression methods (see Chapter 7, Section 7.4.4). Despite its theoretical importance, however, the hazard rate cannot be directly obtained in epidemiologic studies. It is out of the scope of this textbook to discuss the mathematical properties of the hazard rate, which are complex and properly addressed in statistical textbooks.[16] It is analogous, however, to the conditional probability of the event that is calculated at each event time using Kaplan-Meier's approach (Table 2-3). In addition, average hazard for a certain time period in the classical life table can be estimated. Furthermore, the hazard *function* can be estimated using parametric survival analysis techniques (the interested reader should consult specialized texts, such as Collett's[16]).

Exhibit 2–2 Assumptions Necessary for Survival and Person-Time Analyses

	Survival Analysis	*Person-Time*
If there are losses to follow-up:	Censored observations have an outcome probability that is similar to that of individuals remaining under observation.	
If intervals are used, and there are losses during a given interval:	Losses are uniform over the interval.	
If risk is calculated over intervals:	Risk is uniform during the interval.	N individuals followed for T units of time have the same risks as T individuals followed for N units of time.
If accrual of study subjects is done over a relatively long time period:	There are no secular trends over the calendar period covered by the accrual.	

2.3 MEASURES OF PREVALENCE

Prevalence is defined as the frequency of existing cases, both old and new (with recent onset). There are two kinds of prevalence, point prevalence and period prevalence (Table 2–1). *Point prevalence* is the frequency of a disease or condition at a point in time; it is the measure estimated in the so-called prevalence or cross-sectional surveys, such as the National Health, Nutrition and Examination Surveys (NHANES) conducted by the US National Center for Health Statistics. *Period prevalence* is less commonly used and is defined as the frequency of an existing disease or condition during a defined time period, such as 1 year. A special type of period prevalence is the *cumulative lifetime prevalence*, which provides an estimate of the occurrence of a condition at any time during an individual's past. In general, when the term *prevalence* is not specified, it can be taken to mean *point prevalence*. Although prevalence is an extremely useful index of the magnitude of current health problems, this measure is less useful than incidence in etiologic studies because it is simultaneously a function of incidence and duration of the disease after its onset. (Duration is, in turn, determined by either survival for fatal or recovery for nonfatal diseases.)

Although the dependence of point prevalence on a disease's duration makes it less than ideal for assessing associations between risk factors and disease outcomes, its relationship to incidence allows its use as a proxy of "risk," which can be appropriate if its limitations are well understood.

Limitations of point prevalence can be appreciated by observation of the formula defining its connection with incidence and duration of the disease:*

[Equation 2.3]

$$\left(\frac{\text{Point Prevalence}}{1 - \text{Point Prevalence}}\right) = \text{Incidence} \times \text{duration}$$

Note that the term Point Prevalence/(1 − Point Prevalence) is the odds of point prevalence (see Section 2.4).

In this equation and those derived from it, the time unit for incidence and duration should be the same: that is, if incidence is given as a yearly average, duration should be given using year(s) or fraction thereof. In addition, it is assumed that incidence and duration of disease have remained relatively stable over the years. Equation 2.3 can be rewritten as

---

*The derivation of this formula is fairly straightforward. The main assumption is that the disease is in steady state, which means that the incidence and the number of existing cases at any given point (eg, X) are approximately constant. For an incurable disease, this implies that the number of *new cases* during any given time period is approximately equal to the *number of deaths* among the cases. If N is the population size, I is the incidence, and F is the case fatality rate, the number of new cases can be estimated by multiplying the incidence times the number of potentially "susceptible" ($N - X$); in turn, the number of deaths can be estimated by multiplying the case fatality rate times the number of prevalent cases. Thus, the above assumption can be formulated as follows: $I \times (N - X) \approx F \times X$. If there is no immigration, the case fatality rate is the inverse of the duration (D).[17] Thus, after a little arithmetical manipulation, and dividing numerator and denominator of the right-hand side term by N:

$$I \times D \approx \frac{X}{(N - X)} = \frac{\text{Prevalence}}{(1 - \text{Prevalence})}$$

Analogous reasoning can be applied to nonfatal diseases, for which F is the proportion cured.

[Equation 2.4]

Point Prevalence = Incidence $\times$ duration $\times$ (1 − Point Prevalence)

As will be discussed in Chapters 3 and 4, Equation 2.4 underscores the two elements of a disease that are responsible for the difference between incidence and point prevalence: its duration and the magnitude of its point prevalence. When the point prevalence is low—for example, 0.05 or less—the term (1 − Point Prevalence) is almost equal to 1.0, and the following well-known formula defining the relationship between prevalence and incidence is obtained:

Point Prevalence $\approx$ Incidence $\times$ duration

For example, if the incidence of a disease that has remained stable over the years (eg, diabetes) is 1% per year, and its approximate duration (survival after diagnosis) is 15 years, its point prevalence will be approximately 15%.

2.4 ODDS

Odds is the ratio of the probability of the event of interest to that of the nonevent. This can be defined both for incidence and for prevalence. For example, when dealing with incidence probabilities, the odds is

$$\text{Odds} = \frac{q}{1 - q}$$

(Alternatively, knowing the odds allows the calculation of probability: $q = \text{Odds}/[1 + \text{Odds}]$.)

The prevalence odds is as follows (see also Equation 2.3):

$$\frac{\text{Point Prevalence}}{1 - \text{Point Prevalence}}$$

Both odds and proportions can be used to express "frequency" of the disease. An odds approximates a proportion when the latter is small, eg, less than 0.1. For example,

Proportion = 0.05

Odds = 0.05/(1 − 0.05) = 0.05/0.95 = 0.0526

It is easier to grasp the intuitive meaning of the proportion than that of the odds, perhaps because in a description of odds the nature of the latter as a ratio is often not clearly conveyed. For example, if the proportion of smokers in a population is 0.20, the odds is

$$\text{Odds} = \frac{\text{proportion of smokers}}{1 - \text{proportion of smokers}} = \frac{\text{proportion of smokers}}{\text{proportion of nonsmokers}}$$

or $0.20/(1 - 0.20) = 0.20/0.80 = 1:4 = 0.25$.

There are two alternative ways to describe an odds estimate: either as an isolated number, 0.25, implying that the reader understands that it intrinsically expresses a ratio, 0.25:1.0, or as a ratio—in the example, 1:4—clearly conveying the message that, in the study population, for every smoker there are four nonsmokers.

The odds as an isolated absolute measure of occurrence is rarely if ever used by epidemiologists. However, the ratio of two odds (the odds ratio) is an extremely popular measure of association both because the logistic regression adjustment method is widely used, and because the odds ratio allows the estimation of the easier-to-grasp relative risk in case-control studies (see Chapter 1, Section 1.4.2; Chapter 3, Section 3.2.1; and Chapter 7, Section 7.4.3).

REFERENCES

1. *Webster's Ninth New Collegiate Dictionary.* Springfield, Mass: Miriam-Webster Inc; 1988.
2. Bromberger JT, Matthews KA, Kuller LH, et al. Prospective study of the determinants of age at menopause. *Am J Epidemiol.* 1997;145:124–133.
3. Mirza NM, Caufield LE, Black RE, et al. Risk factors for diarrheal duration. *Am J Epidemiol.* 1997;146:776–785.
4. Breteler MMB, de Groot RRM, van Romunde LKJ, Hofman A. Risk of dementia in patients with Parkinson's disease, epilepsy, and severe head trauma: a register-based follow-up study. *Am J Epidemiol.* 1995;142:1300–1305.
5. Gane E, Saliba F, Garcia Valdecasas JC, et al. Randomised trial of efficacy and safety of oral ganciclovir in the prevention of cytomegalovirus disease in liver-transplant recipients. *Lancet.* 1997;350:1729–1733.
6. Centers for Disease Control. Revision of the CDC surveillance case definition for acquired immunodeficiency syndrome. *JAMA.* 1987;258:1143–1145.
7. Kaplan EL, Meier P. Nonparametric estimation from incomplete observations. *J Am Stat Assoc.* 1958;53:457–481.
8. Reed LJ, Merrell M. A short method for constructing an abridged life table. *Am J Hyg.* 1939;30:33–62.
9. Pooling Project Research Group. Relationship of blood pressure, serum cholesterol, smoking habit, relative weight and ECG abnormalities to incidence of major coronary events: final report of the Pooling Project. *J Chron Dis.* 1978;31:201–306.
10. Gordis L. *Epidemiology.* Philadelphia, Pa: WB Saunders Co; 1996.

11. Kahn HA, Sempos CT. *Statistical Methods in Epidemiology.* New York, NY: Oxford University Press; 1989.

12. Checkoway H, Pearce NE, Crawford-Brown DJ. *Research Methods in Occupational Epidemiology.* New York, NY: Oxford University Press; 1989.

13. Monson RR. Analysis of relative survival and proportional mortality. *Comput Biomed Res.* 1978;7:324–332.

14. Macaluso M. Exact stratification of person-years. *Epidemiology.* 1992;3:441–448.

15. Pearce N, Checkoway H. A simple computer program for generating person-time data in cohort studies involving time-related factors. *Am J Epidemiol.* 1987;125:1085–1091.

16. Collett D. *Modelling Survival Data in Medical Research.* London, England: Chapman & Hall; 1994.

17. Rothman KJ, Greenland S. *Modern Epidemiology.* 2nd ed. Philadelphia, Pa: Lippincott-Raven Publishers; 1998.

CHAPTER 3

Measuring Associations Between Exposures and Outcomes

3.1 INTRODUCTION

Epidemiologists are often interested in assessing the presence of associations expressed by differences between measures of disease frequency. Measures of association can be based on either *absolute differences* between groups being compared (eg, exposed versus unexposed) or *relative differences* or ratios (Table 3–1). Measures based on absolute differences are often preferred when public health or preventive activities are contemplated, as their main goal is often an absolute reduction in the risk of an undesirable outcome. Furthermore, when the outcome of interest is continuous, the assessment of mean absolute differences between exposed and unexposed individuals may be an appropriate method for the determination of an association.

Relative differences, which can be assessed for discrete outcomes, are commonly used by epidemiologists to assess causal associations (Table 3–1).

3.2 MEASURING ASSOCIATIONS IN A COHORT STUDY

In traditional prospective or cohort studies, study participants are selected in one of two ways: (1) a defined population or population sample is included in the study and classified according to level of exposure, or (2) exposed and unexposed individuals are specifically identified and included in the study. These individuals are then followed concurrently or nonconcurrently[1,2] for ascertainment of the

Table 3-1 Types of Measures of Association Used in Analytic Epidemiologic Studies

Type	Examples	Usual application
Absolute difference	Attributable risk in exposed	Primary prevention impact; search for causes
	Population attributable risk	Primary prevention impact
	Efficacy	Impact of intervention on recurrences, case fatality, etc
	Mean differences (continuous outcomes)	Search for determinants
Relative difference	Relative risk/rate	Search for causes
	Relative odds	Search for causes

outcome(s), allowing for the estimation of an incidence measure in each group (see also Chapters 1 and 2).

So as to simplify the concepts described in this chapter, only two levels of exposure are considered in most of the examples that follow—exposed and unexposed. Furthermore, length of follow-up is assumed to be complete in all individuals in the cohort (ie, no censoring occurs). (However, the discussion that follows also generally applies to risk and rate estimates that take into account incomplete follow-up and censoring, described in the previous chapter, Section 2.2.) For simplification purposes, this chapter will focus almost exclusively on the ratio of two probabilities or odds (ie, the relative risk and the odds ratio) or on the absolute difference between two probabilities (ie, the attributable risk). However, concepts described in relation to these measures also apply to a great extent to the other related association measures, such as the rate ratio, and the hazard ratio. Last, for the purposes of describing measures of association, it is generally assumed that the estimates are not affected by either confounding or bias.

3.2.1 Relative Risk (Risk Ratio) and Odds Ratio

A classical two-by-two cross-tabulation of exposure and disease in a cohort study is shown in Table 3–2. Of a total of $(a + b)$ exposed and $(c + d)$ unexposed individuals, a exposed and c unexposed develop the disease of interest during the follow-up time. The corresponding risk and odds estimates are shown in the last two columns of Table 3–2. Note that the probability odds of the disease (the ratio of the probability of disease to the probability of no disease) arithmetically reduces to the ratio of the number of diseased cases divided by the

Table 3–2 Cross-Tabulation of Exposure and Disease in a Cohort Study

Exposure	Diseased	Nondiseased	Disease Incidence (Risk)	Probability Odds of Disease		
Present	a	b	$q_+ = \dfrac{a}{a + b}$	$\dfrac{q_+}{1 - q_+} = \dfrac{\dfrac{a}{a+b}}{1 - \left(\dfrac{a}{a+b}\right)} = \dfrac{a}{b}$		
Absent	c	d	$q_- = \dfrac{c}{c + d}$	$\dfrac{q_-}{1 - q_-} = \dfrac{\dfrac{c}{c+d}}{1 - \left(\dfrac{c}{c+d}\right)} = \dfrac{c}{d}$		

number of individuals who do not develop the disease for each exposure category.

The *relative risk* of developing the disease is expressed as the ratio of the risk (incidence) in exposed individuals (q_+) to that in unexposed (q_-):

[Equation 3.1]

$$\text{Relative risk (RR)} = \frac{q_+}{q_-} = \frac{\dfrac{a}{a+b}}{\dfrac{c}{c+d}}$$

For methods on estimating confidence limits and p-values for a relative risk, see Appendix A, Section A.3.

The *odds ratio* of disease development is the ratio of the odds of developing the disease; because, in this example, it is based on the incidence risks or probabilities, it is occasionally designated *risk relative odds* or *probability relative odds*. Note that the ratio of the probability odds of disease is equivalent to the *cross-product ratio, ($a \times d$)/($b \times c$),* using the notation in Table 3–2:

$$\text{Probability odds ratio (OR)} = \frac{\dfrac{q_+}{1 - q_+}}{\dfrac{q_-}{1 - q_-}} = \frac{\dfrac{\dfrac{a}{a+b}}{1 - \left(\dfrac{a}{a+b}\right)}}{\dfrac{\dfrac{c}{c+d}}{1 - \left(\dfrac{c}{c+d}\right)}} = \frac{\dfrac{\dfrac{a}{a+b}}{\dfrac{b}{a+b}}}{\dfrac{\dfrac{c}{c+d}}{\dfrac{d}{c+d}}} = \frac{\left(\dfrac{a}{b}\right)}{\left(\dfrac{c}{d}\right)}$$

Thus,

[Equation 3.2]

$$OR = \frac{a \times d}{b \times c}$$

For methods on obtaining confidence limits and p-values for an odds ratio, see Appendix A, Section A.4.

In the hypothetical example shown in Table 3–3, severe hypertension and acute myocardial infarction are the exposure and the outcome of interest, respectively. The sample size for each level of exposure was arbitrarily set at 10,000 to facilitate the calculations. For these data, because the probability (risk) of myocardial infarction is low for both the exposed and the unexposed groups, the probability odds of developing the disease approximate the probabilities (Table 3–3); as a result, the probability odds ratio of disease (exposed vs unexposed) approximates the relative risk:

$$RR = \frac{\dfrac{180}{10{,}000}}{\dfrac{30}{10{,}000}} = \frac{0.0180}{0.0030} = 6.00$$

$$\text{Probability OR} = \frac{\dfrac{180}{9820}}{\dfrac{30}{9970}} = \frac{0.01833}{0.00301} = 6.09$$

A different situation emerges when the probabilities of developing the outcome are high in exposed and unexposed individuals. For example, Seltser et al[3] examined the incidence of local reactions in individuals assigned randomly to either an injectable influenza vaccine or a placebo group. Table 3–4, based on this study, shows that as the probability (incidence) of local reactions is high, the probability odds estimates of local reactions do not approximate the probabilities, and thus that the probability odds ratio of local reactions (vaccine vs placebo) is fairly different from the relative risk:

$$RR = \frac{\dfrac{650}{2570}}{\dfrac{170}{2410}} = \frac{0.2529}{0.0705} = 3.59 \qquad OR = \frac{\dfrac{650}{1920}}{\dfrac{170}{2240}} = \frac{0.3385}{0.0759} = 4.46$$

When the condition has a high incidence and when prospective data are available, as was the case in this vaccination trial, it is usually

Table 3–3 Hypothetical Cohort Study of the 1-Year Incidence of Acute Myocardial Infarction in Individuals with Severe Systolic Hypertension ($\geq$ 180 mm Hg) and Normal Systolic Blood Pressure (<120 mm Hg)

Blood Pressure Status	Number	Myocardial Infarction Present	Absent	Probability	Probability $Odds_{dis}$
Severe hypertension	10,000	180	9820	180/10,000 = 0.0180	180/(10,000 − 180) = 180/9820 = 0.01833
Normal	10,000	30	9970	30/10,000 = 0.0030	30/(10,000 − 30) = 30/9970 = 0.00301

better to report the relative risk because it is a more easily understood measure of association between the risk factor and the outcome.

Although the odds ratio is a valid measure of association in its own right (see below), it is often used as an approximation of the relative risk. Use of the odds ratio *as an estimate of the relative risk* biases it in a direction opposite to the null hypothesis: that is, it tends to exaggerate the magnitude of the association. When the disease is relatively rare, this "built-in" bias is negligible, as in the example from Table 3–3 above. However, when the incidence is high, as in the vaccine trial example (Table 3–4), the bias can be substantial.

An expression of the mathematical relationship between the OR on the one hand and the relative risk on the other can be derived as follows. Assume that q_+ is the incidence (probability) in exposed (eg, vaccinated) and q_- the incidence in unexposed individuals. The odds ratio is then

[Equation 3.3]

$$OR = \frac{\left(\dfrac{q_+}{1 - q_+}\right)}{\left(\dfrac{q_-}{1 - q_-}\right)} = \frac{q_+}{1 - q_+} \times \frac{1 - q_-}{q_-}$$

$$= \frac{q_+}{q_-} \times \left(\frac{1 - q_-}{1 - q_+}\right)$$

Notice that the term q_+/q_- in Equation 3.3 is the relative risk. Thus, the term

$$\left(\frac{1 - q_-}{1 - q_+}\right)$$

Table 3–4 Incidence of Local Reactions in the Vaccinated and Placebo Groups, Influenza Vaccination Trial

| | | Local Reaction | | | |
Group	Number	Present	Absent	Probability	Probability Odds$_{dis}$
Vaccine	2570	650	1920	650/2570 = 0.2529	650/(2570 − 650) = 650/1920 = 0.3385
Placebo	2410	170	2240	170/2410 = 0.0705	170/(2410 − 170) = 170/2240 = 0.0759

Note: Based on data for individuals 40 years old or older in Seltser et al.[3] To avoid rounding ambiguities in subsequent examples based on these data (Figure 3–4, Tables 3–7 and 3–9), the original sample sizes in Seltzer et al's study (257 vaccinees and 241 placebo recipients) were multiplied by 10.

Source: Data from R Seltser, PE Sartwell, and JA Bell, A Controlled Test of Asian Influenza Vaccine in Population of Families, *American Journal of Hygiene,* Vol 75, pp 112–135, © 1962.

defines the *bias* responsible for the discrepancy between the relative risk and the odds ratio estimates (*built-in bias*). If the association between the exposure and the outcome is positive, $q_- < q_+$, thus $(1 - q_-) > (1 - q_+)$. The bias term will therefore be greater than 1.0, leading to an overestimation of the relative risk by the odds ratio. By analogy, if the factor is protective, the opposite occurs—that is, $(1 - q_-) < (1 - q_+)$—and the odds ratio will again overestimate the strength of the association. In general, the odds ratio tends to yield an estimate further away from 1.0 than the relative risk on both sides of the scale (above or below 1.0).

In the hypertension/myocardial infarction example (Table 3–3), the bias factor is of a small magnitude, and the odds ratio estimate, albeit a bit more distant from 1.0, still approximates the relative risk; using Equation 3.3:

$$OR = RR \times \text{"built-in bias"} = 6.0 \times \frac{1 - 0.0030}{1 - 0.0180} = 6.0 \times 1.015 = 6.09$$

However, in the example of local reactions to the influenza vaccine (Table 3–4), there is a considerable bias when using the odds ratio to estimate the relative risk:

$$OR = 3.59 \times \frac{1 - 0.0705}{1 - 0.2529} = 3.59 \times 1.244 = 4.46$$

Regardless of whether the odds ratio can properly estimate the relative risk, it is, as mentioned previously, a bona fide measure of association. It is especially valuable because it can be measured in case-control (case-noncase) studies and because it is directly derived from logistic regression models (see Chapter 7, Section 7.4.3). In addition, unlike the relative risk, the odds ratio of an event is the exact reciprocal of the odds ratio of the nonevent. For example, in the study of local reactions to the influenza vaccine discussed above,[3] the odds ratio of a local reaction,

$$OR_{\text{local reaction (+)}} = \frac{\left(\dfrac{650}{1920}\right)}{\left(\dfrac{170}{2240}\right)} = 4.46$$

is the exact reciprocal of the odds ratio of not having a local reaction,

$$\text{Probability } OR_{\text{local reaction (-)}} = \frac{\left(\dfrac{1920}{650}\right)}{\left(\dfrac{2240}{170}\right)} = 0.22 = \frac{1}{4.46}$$

This feature is not shared by the relative risk: using the same example,

$$RR_{\text{local reaction (+)}} = \frac{\dfrac{650}{2570}}{\dfrac{170}{2410}} = 3.59$$

and

$$RR_{\text{local reaction (-)}} = \frac{\left(\dfrac{1920}{2570}\right)}{\left(\dfrac{2240}{2410}\right)} = 0.8 \neq \frac{1}{3.59}$$

This seemingly paradoxical finding results from the sensitivity of the relative risk to the magnitude of an outcome: that is, the relative risk of a common endpoint approaches 1.0. This is easily appreciated when studying the complement of rare outcomes. For example, if the case fatality rates of patients undergoing surgery using a standard surgical technique and a new technique were, respectively, 0.02 and 0.01, the relative risk for the relatively rare outcome "death" would be 0.02/0.01 = 2.0. However, the relative risk for survival would be 0.98/0.99, which is virtually equal to 1.0, suggesting that the new surgical technique did not affect survival. On the other hand, the odds ratio of death would be

$$OR_{death} = \frac{\dfrac{0.02}{1.0 - 0.02}}{\dfrac{0.01}{1.0 - 0.01}} = 2.02$$

and that of survival would be

$$OR_{survival} = \frac{\dfrac{0.98}{1.0 - 0.98}}{\dfrac{0.99}{1.0 - 0.99}} = 0.495 = \frac{1.0}{2.02}$$

3.2.2   Attributable Risk

The *attributable risk* (AR) is a measure of association based on the absolute difference between two risk estimates. Thus, the AR estimates the absolute excess risk associated with a given exposure. Because the AR is often used to imply a cause-effect relationship, it should be interpreted as a true *etiologic fraction* only when there is reasonable certainty of a causal connection between the exposure and the outcome.[4,5] The term *excess fraction* has been suggested as an alternative to attributable risk or etiologic fraction when causality has not been firmly established.[4] It should also be noted that, although the formulas and examples in this section generally refer to attributable *risks,* they are also applicable to attributable rates or densities, ie, if incidence data based on person-time are used, an attributable rate among the exposed (see below) can be calculated in units of rate per person-time.

As extensively discussed by Gordis,[2] the AR assumes different formats, including the following.

Attributable Risk in Exposed Individuals (AR_{exp})

The AR_{exp} is merely the difference between the risk estimates of different exposure levels and a reference exposure level; the latter is usually formed by the unexposed category. Assuming a binary exposure, and letting risk in exposed equal q_+ and risk in unexposed equal q_-, the AR_{exp} is simply,

[Equation 3.4]

$$AR_{exp} = q_+ - q_-$$

The AR_{exp} measures the excess risk for a given exposure category associated with the exposure. For example, based on the example in Table 3–3, the cumulative incidence of myocardial infarction among the hypertensive individuals (q_+) is 0.018 (or 1.8%), and that for normotensives (reference or unexposed category) (q_-) is 0.003 (or 0.3%); thus the excess risk associated with exposure to hypertension is 0.018 − 0.003 = 0.015 (or 1.5%). That is, assuming a causal association (and thus, no confounding or bias—see Chapters 4 and 5), and if the excess incidence were completely reversible, <u>the cessation of the exposure (severe systolic hypertension) would lower the risk in the exposed group from 0.018 to 0.003.</u> In Figure 3–1, the two bars represent the cumulative incidence in exposed and nonexposed individuals; thus, the AR_{exp} (Equation 3.4) is the difference in height of these bars. (The graphical analogue for the relative risk [Equation 3–1] is how many times taller is the bar for the exposed compared to the bar for the unexposed in Figure 3–1.) Note that the AR_{exp}—the difference between two incidence measures—is also an incidence magnitude and therefore is measured using the same units. The estimated AR_{exp} of 1.5% in the above example represents the absolute excess incidence that would be prevented by eliminating severe hypertension.

Because <u>most exposure effects are cumulative, cessation of exposure</u> (even if causally related to the disease) <u>usually does not reduce the risk in exposed individuals to the level found in those who were never exposed.</u> Thus, the maximum risk reduction is usually achieved only through prevention of exposure rather than its cessation.

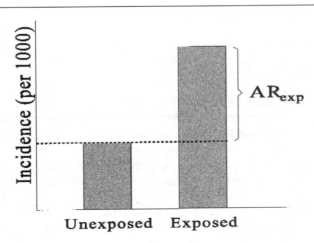

Figure 3–1 Attributable risk in the exposed.

Percent AR_exp

A percent AR_{exp} ($\%AR_{exp}$) is merely the AR_{exp} expressed as a percentage of the q_+—the excess associated with the exposure as a percentage of the total q_+. For a binary exposure variable, it is:

[Equation 3.5]

$$\%AR_{exp} = \left(\frac{q_+ - q_-}{q_+}\right) \times 100$$

In the example above, the $\%AR_{exp}$ is

$$\%AR_{exp} = \frac{0.018 - 0.003}{0.018} \times 100 = 83.3\%$$

If causality has been established, the percent AR_{exp} can be interpreted as the percentage of the total risk in the exposed attributable to the exposure. It may be useful to express Equation 3.5 above in terms of the relative risk:

$$\%AR_{exp} = \left(\frac{q_+ - q_-}{q_+}\right) \times 100 = \left(1 - \frac{1}{RR}\right) \times 100 = \left(\frac{RR - 1.0}{RR}\right) \times 100$$

Thus, in the above example, using the relative risk ($0.018/0.003 = 6.0$) in this formula produces the same result as when applying Equation 3.5:

$$\%AR_{exp} = \left(\frac{6.0 - 1.0}{6.0}\right) \times 100 = 83.3\%$$

The obvious advantage of the formula

[Equation 3.6]

$$\%AR_{exp} = \left(\frac{RR - 1.0}{RR}\right) \times 100$$

is that it can be used in case-control studies, in which incidence data (ie, q_+ or q_-) are unavailable, but the odds ratio can be used as an estimate of the relative risk if the disease is relatively rare (see Section 3.2.1).

Note that the $\%AR_{exp}$ is analogous to percent efficacy when assessing an intervention such as a vaccine. The usual formula for efficacy is equivalent to the formula for $\%AR_{exp}$ (Equation 3.5) when q_+ is replaced by q_{cont} (risk in control group, eg, the group receiving placebo) and q_- is replaced by q_{interv} (risk in those undergoing intervention):

[Equation 3.7]

$$\text{Efficacy} = (\frac{q_{cont} - q_{interv}}{q_{cont}}) \times 100$$

For example, in a randomized trial to evaluate the efficacy of a vaccine, the risks in persons receiving the vaccine and the placebo are, respectively, 5% and 15%. Using Equation 3.7, efficacy is found to be 66.7%:

$$\text{Efficacy} = \left(\frac{15\% - 5\%}{15\%}\right) \times 100 = 66.7\%$$

Alternatively, Equation 3.6 can be used to estimate efficacy. In the example above, the relative risk (placebo/vaccine) is, 15% ÷ 5% = 3.0. Thus,

$$\text{Efficacy} = \left(\frac{3.0 - 1.0}{3.0}\right) \times 100 = 66.7\%$$

Note that the use of Equation 3.6 for the calculation of efficacy requires that when calculating the relative risk, the group not receiving the intervention (eg, placebo) be labeled "exposed," and the group receiving the active intervention (eg, vaccine) be labeled as "unexposed." A mathematically equivalent approach would consist of first obtaining the relative risk, but this time with the risk of those receiving the active intervention (eg, vaccine) in the numerator and those not receiving it in the denominator (eg, placebo). In this case, efficacy is calculated as the complement of the relative risk, ie, $(1.0 - RR) \times 100$. In the above example, using this approach, the vaccine efficacy would be,

$$\text{Efficacy} = \left[1.0 - \left(\frac{5\%}{15\%}\right)\right] \times 100 = 66.7\%$$

As for percent AR, the correspondence between the relative risk and the odds ratio in most practical situations allows the estimation of efficacy in case-control studies using Equation 3.6.

Levin's Population Attributable Risk

Levin's population attributable risk (Pop AR) estimates the proportion of the disease risk in the total population associated with the exposure.[6] For example, let the exposure prevalence in the target population (p_e) be 0.40 (and, thus prevalence of *nonexposure*, $(1 - p_e)$ be 0.60), and the risks in exposed and unexposed be, respectively, $q_+ = 0.20$ and $q_- = 0.15$. Thus, the risk in the total population (q_{pop}) is a weighted sum of the risks in the exposed and unexposed individuals in the population:

[Equation 3.8]

$$q_{pop} = [q_+ \times p_e] + [q_- \times (1 - p_e)]$$

In the example:

$$q_{pop} = (0.20 \times 0.40) + (0.15 \times 0.60) = 0.17$$

The Pop AR is the difference between the risk in the total population and that in unexposed subjects, or $0.17 - 0.15 = 0.02$, representing the excess in total population risk associated with the exposure. That is, if the relationship were causal, and if the effect of the exposure were completely reversible, exposure cessation would be expected to result in a decrease in total population risk (q_{pop}) from 0.17 to 0.15, ie, to the level of risk of the unexposed group. The Pop AR is usually expressed as the percentage population attributable risk, %Pop AR. In the example above, the %Pop AR is $(0.02/0.17) \times 100$, or approximately 12%.

Mathematically, the %Pop AR can be expressed as follows:

[Equation 3.9]

$$\%Pop\ AR = [(q_{pop} - q_-)/q_{pop}] \times 100$$

As seen in Equation 3.8, the incidence in the total population is the sum of the incidence in the exposed and that in the unexposed, weighted for the proportions of exposed and unexposed individuals in the population. Thus, when the exposure prevalence is low, the population incidence will be closer to the incidence among the unexposed (Figure 3–2A). Similarly, if the exposure is highly prevalent (Figure 3–2B), the population incidence will be closer to the incidence among the exposed. As a result, the Pop AR approximates the AR_{exp} when exposure prevalence is high.

After simple arithmetical manipulation*, Equation 3.9 can be expressed as a function of the prevalence of exposure in the population

------

*Using Equation 3.8, Equation 3.9 can be rewritten as a function of the prevalence of exposure (p_e) and the incidence in exposed (q_+) individuals, as follows:

$$\%Pop\ AR = \frac{[q_+ \times p_e] + [q_- \times (1 - p_e)] - q_-}{[q_+ \times p_e] + [q_- \times (1 - p_e)]} \times 100$$

$$= \frac{[q_+ \times p_e] - [q_- \times p_e]}{[q_+ \times p_e] - [q_- \times p_e] + q_-} \times 100$$

This expression can be further simplified by dividing all the terms in numerator and denominator by q_-

$$\%Pop\ AR = \frac{\dfrac{q_+}{q_-} \times p_e - p_e}{\dfrac{q_+}{q_-} \times p_e - p_e + 1} \times 100 = \frac{p_e \times \left(\dfrac{q_+}{q_-} - 1\right)}{p_e \times \left(\dfrac{q_+}{q_-} - 1\right) + 1} \times 100$$

$$= \frac{p_e \times (RR - 1)}{p_e \times (RR - 1) + 1} \times 100$$

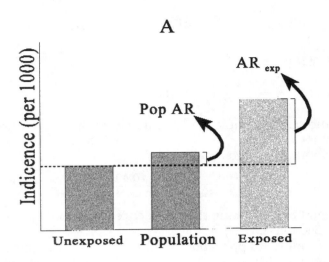

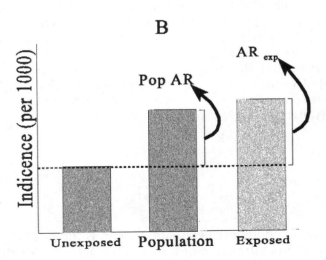

Figure 3–2 Population attributable risk and its dependence on the population prevalence of the exposure. As the population is composed of exposed and unexposed individuals, the incidence in the population is similar to the incidence in the unexposed when the exposure is rare **(A)** and is closer to that in the exposed when the exposure is common **(B)**. Thus, for a fixed relative risk (eg, RR ≈ 2 in the figure) the population attributable risk is heavily dependent on the prevalence of exposure.

and the relative risk in the following formula, first described by Levin:[6]

[Equation 3.10]

$$\%\text{Pop AR} = \frac{p_e \times (\text{RR} - 1)}{p_e \times (\text{RR} - 1) + 1} \times 100$$

Using the same example of a population with an exposure prevalence of 0.40 and a RR = 0.20/0.15 = 1.33, Equation 3.10 yields the same %Pop AR estimated above:

$$\%\text{Pop} = \frac{0.40 \times (1.33 - 1)}{0.40 \times (1.33 - 1) + 1} = \frac{0.40 \times 0.33}{0.40 \times 0.33 + 1} = 12\%$$

For a method of calculating the confidence limits for Pop AR, see Appendix A, Section A.5.

Levin's formula is applicable to case-control studies (by replacing the relative risk with the odds ratio value) when the exposure prevalence in the reference population is known. This underscores the importance of the two critical elements contributing to the magnitude of the population attributable risk: the relative risk and the prevalence of exposure. The dependence of the population AR on the exposure prevalence is further illustrated in Figure 3–3, which shows that for all values of the relative risk, the population AR increases markedly as the exposure prevalence increases.

All the preceding discussion relates to a binary exposure variable (ie, exposed vs unexposed). When exposure is defined with more than just two categories, an extension of Levin's formula has been derived by Walter.[7]

$$\% \text{Pop Ar} = \frac{\sum\limits_{i=0}^{k} p_i \times (\text{RR}_i - 1)}{1 + \sum\limits_{i=0}^{k} p_i \times (\text{RR}_i - 1)} \times 100 =$$

$$= \left[1.0 - \frac{1.0}{\sum\limits_{i=0}^{k} (p_i \times \text{RR}_i)} \right] \times 100$$

The subscript i denotes each exposure level; p_i is the proportion of the study population in the exposure level i; and "RR_i" is the unadjusted RR for the exposure level i compared to the unexposed (reference) level.

It is important to emphasize that Levin's formula and Walter's extension for multilevel exposures assume there is no confounding (see Chapter 5). If confounding is present, it is not correct to calculate the adjusted relative risk (using any of the approaches described in Chapter 7) and plug it into Levin's or Walter's formulas in order to obtain an adjusted Pop AR.[8] The correct approach to calculate the adjusted Pop AR has been described elsewhere.

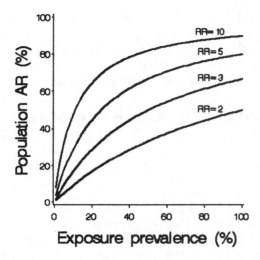

Figure 3–3 Population attributable risk: dependence on prevalence of exposure and relative risk.

3.3 CROSS-SECTIONAL STUDIES: POINT PREVALENCE RATE RATIO

When cross-sectional data are available, often associations are assessed using the point prevalence rate ratio (PRR). The PRR's ability to estimate the relative risk is a function of the relationship between incidence and point prevalence, as discussed previously in Chapter 2 (Section 2.3, Equation 2.4):

Point Prevalence = Incidence × Duration × (1 − Point Prevalence)

Using the notations "Prev" for point prevalence, "q" for incidence, and "Dur" for duration, and denoting presence or absence of a given exposure by "+" or "−", the relationship between the PRR and the incidence ratio is

$$\text{PRR} = \frac{\text{Prev}_+}{\text{Prev}_-} = \frac{q_+ \times \text{Dur}_+ \times [1.0 - \text{Prev}_+]}{q_- \times \text{Dur}_- \times [1.0 - \text{Prev}_-]}$$

As the incidence ratio is the relative risk, this formula can be written as

[Equation 3.11]

$$\text{PRR} = \text{RR} \times \left(\frac{\text{Dur}_+}{\text{Dur}_-}\right) \times \left(\frac{1 - \text{Prev}_+}{1 - \text{Prev}_-}\right)$$

Thus, the two bias factors that differentiate the PRR from the relative risk are the ratio of the disease durations, (Dur_+/Dur_-), and the ratio of the complements of the point prevalence estimates $(1 - Prev_+/1 - Prev_-)$ in the exposed and unexposed groups. Chapter 4 (Section 4.4.2) provides a discussion and examples of these biases.

3.4 MEASURING ASSOCIATIONS IN CASE-CONTROL STUDIES

3.4.1 Odds Ratio

One of the major advances in risk estimation in epidemiology occurred in 1951 when Cornfield[9] pointed out that the odds ratio of disease (OR_{dis}) and the odds ratio of exposure (OR_{exp}) are mathematically equivalent. This simple yet key concept allows calculating the odds ratio of disease in case-control studies, as it is algebraically identical to the odds ratio of exposure.

As seen previously in Equation 3.2, the ratio of the odds of disease development in exposed and unexposed individuals results in the *cross-product ratio*, $(a \times d)/(b \times c)$. Using the *prospective* data shown in Table 3–3, now reorganized as shown in Table 3–5, and assuming that the cells in the table represent the distribution of the cohort participants during a 1-year follow-up, it is possible to carry out a case-control analysis comparing the 210 individuals who developed a myocardial infarction (cases) with the 19,790 individuals who remained free of clinical coronary heart disease during the follow-up. The *absolute* odds of exposure ($Odds_{exp}$) among cases and the analogous odds of exposure among controls is estimated as the ratio of the proportion of individuals exposed to the proportion of individuals unexposed:

$$Odds_{exp/cases} = \frac{\dfrac{a}{a+c}}{1 - \left(\dfrac{a}{a+c}\right)} = \frac{a}{c}$$

$$Odds_{exp/controls} = \frac{\dfrac{b}{b+d}}{1 - \left(\dfrac{b}{b+d}\right)} = \frac{b}{d}$$

The following derivation demonstrates that the odds ratio of exposure (OR_{exp}) is identical to the odds ratio of disease (OR_{dis}; Equation 3.2):

Table 3–5 Hypothetical Case-Control Study of Myocardial Infarction in Relation to Systolic Hypertension, Based on a 1-Year Complete Follow-up of the Study Population from Table 3–3

	Myocardial Infarction			
Systolic Blood Pressure Status*	Present		Absent	
Severe hypertension	180	(a)	9820	(b)
Normal	30	(c)	9970	(d)
Total	210	(a + c)	19790	(b + d)

*Severe systolic hypertension ≥180 mm Hg, and normal systolic blood pressure < 120 mm Hg.

[Equation 3.12]

$$OR_{exp} = \frac{\frac{a}{c}}{\frac{b}{d}} = \frac{a \times d}{b \times c} = \frac{\frac{a}{b}}{\frac{c}{d}} = OR_{dis}$$

For the example shown in Table 3–5, the OR_{exp} is

$$OR_{exp} = \frac{\frac{180}{30}}{\frac{9820}{9970}} = \frac{180 \times 9970}{9820 \times 30} = 6.09 = OR_{dis}$$

In this example based on prospective data, all cases and noncases (controls) have been used for the estimation of the odds ratio (assuming a complete 1-year follow-up for all 20,000 individuals). However, case-control studies are typically based on samples. If the total number of cases is small, as in the example shown in Table 3–5, the investigator may attempt including all cases and a sample of controls. For example, if 100% of cases and a sample of approximately 10% of the noncases were studied (Table 3–6), assuming no random variability, results would be identical to those obtained when including all noncases, as in Table 3–5:

$$OR_{exp} = \frac{\frac{180}{30}}{\frac{982}{997}} = \frac{180 \times 997}{982 \times 30} = 6.09 = OR_{dis}$$

Table 3–6 Case-Control Study of the Relationship of Myocardial Infarction to Presence of Severe Systolic Hypertension Including All Cases and a 10% Sample of Noncases from Table 3–5

Systolic Blood Pressure Status*	Myocardial Infarction			
	Present		Absent	
Severe hypertension	180	(a)	982	(b)
Normal	30	(c)	997	(d)
Total	210	(a + c)	1979	(b + d)

*Severe systolic hypertension ≥180 mm Hg, and normal systolic blood pressure < 120 mm Hg.

This example underscores the notion that the sampling fractions do not have to be the same in cases and controls. However, to obtain unbiased estimates of the absolute odds of exposure for cases and controls, sampling fractions must be independent of exposure: that is, they should apply equally to cells (a) and (c) for cases and cells (b) and (d) for controls. (For exceptions to this rule, see Chapter 4, Section 4.2.)

In the example of local reactions to vaccination (Table 3–4), a case-control study could have been carried out including, for example, 80% of the cases who had local reactions and 50% of the controls. Assuming no random variability, data would be obtained as outlined in Figure 3–4 and shown in Table 3–7. Note that the investigator samples cases and noncases and hopes that the sampling fraction will apply equally to exposed (vaccinated) and unexposed (unvaccinated) cases and controls. The results are again identical to those seen in the total population, in which the (true) odds ratio is 4.46:

$$\text{OR}_{\text{exp}} = \frac{\left(\dfrac{520}{136}\right)}{\left(\dfrac{960}{1120}\right)} = 4.46 = \text{OR}_{\text{dis}}$$

The fact that the OR_{exp} is identical to the OR_{dis} explains why the interpretation of the odds ratio in case-control studies is "prospective." Thus, in the example above based on a case-control strategy (and assuming that the study is unbiased and free of confounding), the interpretation of results is that for individuals who received the vaccine the odds of developing local reactions is 4.46 times greater than the odds for those who received the placebo.

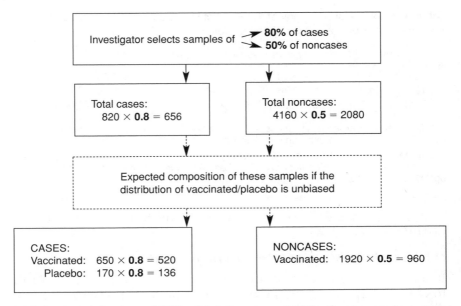

Figure 3–4 Selection of 80% of total cases and 50% of noncases in a case-control study from the study population shown in Table 3–4. Expected composition is assuming no random variability. *Source:* Data from R Seltser, PE Sartwell, and JA Bell, A Controlled Test of Asian Influenza Vaccine in a Population of Families, *American Journal of Hygiene*, Vol 75, pp 112–135, © 1962.

Note that the use of the ratio of the $Odds_{exp}$ for cases to that for controls,

$$OR_{exp} = \frac{Odds_{exp\ cases}}{Odds_{exp\ controls}}$$

is strongly recommended as the first step for the calculation of the OR_{exp}, rather than the cross-products ratio, so as to avoid confusion over different arrangements of the table, as, for example, when placing control data on the left and case data on the right:

Exposure	Controls	Cases
Yes	"a"	"b"
No	"c"	"d"

In this example, the mechanical application of the cross-product ratio, $(a \times b)/(c \times d)$, results in an estimate of the odds ratio that is the inverse of the true relative odds. On the other hand, dividing the ex-

Table 3-7 Case-Control Study of the Relationship Between Occurrence of Local Reaction and Previous Influenza Immunization

Vaccination	Cases of Local Reaction	Controls Without Local Reaction
Yes	520	960
No	136	1120
Total	$820 \times 0.8 = 656$	$4160 \times 0.5 = 2080$

Note: Based on a perfectly representative sample of 80% of the cases and 50% of the controls from the study population shown in Table 3-4 (see Figure 3-4).

Source: Data from R Seltser, PE Sartwell, and JA Bell, A Controlled Test of Asian Influenza Vaccine in a Population of Families, *American Journal of Hygiene*, Vol 75, pp 112-135, © 1962.

posure odds of cases by that in controls results in the correct odds ratio, $(b/d) \div (a/c)$.

Odds Ratio in Matched Case-Control Studies

In a matched paired case-control study in which the ratio of controls to cases is 1:1, an unbiased estimate of the odds ratio is obtained by dividing the number of pairs in which the case, but not the matched control, is exposed (case[+], control[−]), by the number of pairs in which the control, but not the case, is exposed (case[−], control[+]). The underlying intuitive logic for this calculation and an example of this approach are discussed in Chapter 7, Section 7.3.3.

Odds Ratio as an Estimate of the Relative Risk: The Rarity Assumption

In a case-control study, the use of the odds ratio to estimate the relative risk is based on the assumption that the disease under study has a low incidence, thus resulting in a small built-in bias (Equation 3.3), as discussed previously in Section 3.2.1. When the incidence of the disease is high, this bias can be substantial, as was shown in the example of the relationship between influenza vaccination and local reactions.

As in prospective studies (see Section 3.2.1), the rare-disease assumption *applies only to situations in which the odds ratio is used to estimate the relative risk.* When the odds ratio is used as a measure of association in itself, this assumption is obviously not needed. In addition, the rare-disease assumption does not apply to situations in which the control group is a sample of the total population,[10] which is the usual strategy in case-control studies within a defined cohort (Chapter 1, Section 1.4.2).

The irrelevance of the rare-disease assumption when controls compose a sample of the total reference population can be demonstrated by comparing the calculation of the odds ratio using different types of control groups. Referring to the cross-tabulation including all cases and all noncases in a defined population shown in Table 3–8, when noncases are used as the control group, as seen previously (Equation 3.12), the OR_{exp} is used to estimate the OR_{dis} by dividing the $Odds_{exp}$ in cases by that in controls:

$$OR_{exp} = \frac{Odds_{exp\ cases}}{Odds_{exp\ noncases}} = \frac{\frac{a}{c}}{\frac{b}{d}} = OR_{dis}$$

Another option is to use as a control group the total study population at baseline, rather than only the noncases. If this is done in the context of a cohort study, the case-control study is usually called a *case-cohort study* (Chapter 1, Section 1.4.2), and the division of the $Odds_{exp}$ in cases by the $Odds_{exp}$ in controls (total population) yields the relative risk:

[Equation 3.13]

$$OR_{exp} = \frac{Odds_{exp\ cases}}{Odds_{exp\ total\ population}} = \frac{\left(\frac{a}{c}\right)}{\left(\frac{a+b}{c+d}\right)} = \frac{\left(\frac{a}{a+b}\right)}{\left(\frac{c}{c+d}\right)} = RR$$

Using again the local reaction/influenza vaccination investigation as an example (Table 3–4), a case-cohort study could be conducted using all cases and the total study population as the control group. The ratio of the exposure odds in cases ($Odds_{exp\ cases}$) to the exposure odds in the total study population ($Odds_{exp\ pop}$) yields the relative risk:

Table 3–8 Cross-Tabulation of a Defined Population by Exposure and Disease Development

Exposure	Cases	Noncases	Total Population (Cases + Noncases)
Present	a	b	a + b
Absent	c	d	c + d

$$OR_{exp} = \frac{Odds_{exp\ cases}}{Odds_{exp\ pop}} = \frac{\left(\dfrac{650}{170}\right)}{\left(\dfrac{2570}{2410}\right)} = \frac{\left(\dfrac{650}{2570}\right)}{\left(\dfrac{170}{2410}\right)} = \frac{q_+}{q_-} = 3.59 = RR$$

where q_+ is the incidence in exposed and q_- the incidence in unexposed individuals.

In the estimation of the relative risk above, all cases and the total study population were included. However, because unbiased sample estimates of the $Odds_{exp\ cases}$ and the $Odds_{exp\ pop}$ provide an unbiased estimate of the relative risk, a sample of cases and a sample of the total population can be compared in a case-cohort study. For example, assuming no random variability, unbiased samples of 40% of the cases and 20% of the total population would produce the results shown in Table 3–9; the product of the division of the $Odds_{exp\ case}$ by the $Odds_{exp\ pop}$ can be shown to be identical to the relative risk obtained prospectively for the total cohort, as follows:

$$OR_{exp} = \frac{\dfrac{260}{68}}{\dfrac{514}{482}} = 3.59 = RR$$

Again, more commonly, because of the small number of cases relative to the population size, case-cohort studies try to include all cases and a sample of the reference population.

One of the advantages of the case-cohort approach is that it allows direct estimation of the relative risk and thus does not have to rely on

---

Table 3–9 Case-Cohort Study of the Relationship of Previous Vaccination to Local Reaction

Previous Vaccination	Cases of Local Reaction	Cohort Sample
Yes	260	514
No	68	482
Total	328	996

Note: Based on a random sample of the study population in Table 3–4, with sampling fractions of 40% for the cases and 20% for the cohort.

Source: Data from R Seltser, PE Sartwell, and JA Bell, A Controlled Test of Asian Influenza Vaccine in a Population of Families, *American Journal of Hygiene,* Vol 75, pp 112–135, © 1962.

the rarity assumption. Another advantage is that because the control group is a sample of the total reference population, an unbiased estimate of the exposure prevalence (or distribution) needed for the estimation of Levin's Pop AR (Equation 3.10) can be obtained. A control group formed by an unbiased sample of the cohort also allows the assessment of relationships between different exposures, or even between exposures and outcomes other than the outome of interest in the cohort sample.

Furthermore, there are occasions in which excluding cases from the control group is logistically difficult and can add costs and participants' burden. For example, in diseases with a high proportion of a subclinical phase (eg, chronic cholecystitis, prostate cancer), excluding cases from the pool of eligible controls (eg, apparently healthy individuals) would require conducting more or less invasive examinations (eg, contrasted X-rays, rectal exam). Thus, in these instances, a case-cohort approach might be indicated: selecting "controls" from the general population irrespective of (ie, ignoring) the possible presence of the disease (clinical or subclinical).

In general, however, it is appropriate to conduct a case-cohort study only when a defined population from which the study cases originated can be identified, as when dealing with a defined cohort in the context of a prospective study. On the other hand, conducting case-cohort studies when dealing with "open" cohorts or populations at large requires assuming that these represented the source populations from which the cases originated (see Chapter 1, Section 1.4.2).

It should be emphasized that when the disease is rare, the strategy of ignoring disease status when selecting controls would most likely result in few, if any, cases being actually included in the control group; thus, in practice, Equation 3.13 will be almost identical to Equation 3.12 because $(a + b) \approx b$ and $(c + d) \approx d$. For example, in the myocardial infarction/hypertension example shown in Table 3–3, the "case-cohort" strategy (selecting a 50% sample of cases and a 10% sample of controls) would result in the following estimate of the odds ratio:

$$\text{OR}_{\text{exp}} = \frac{\text{Odds}_{\text{exp cases}}}{\text{Odds}_{\text{exp pop}}} = \frac{\left(\dfrac{90}{15}\right)}{\left(\dfrac{1000}{1000}\right)} = 6.00 = \text{RR}$$

In this same example, a case-"noncase" strategy would result in the following estimate:

$$OR_{exp} = \frac{Odds_{exp\ cases}}{Odds_{exp\ noncases}} = \frac{\left(\dfrac{90}{15}\right)}{\left(\dfrac{982}{997}\right)} = 6.09 = OR_{dis}$$

In other words, this situation is analogous to the situation discussed in Section 3.2.1 with regard to the similarity of the odds ratio and the relative risk when the disease is rare.

It is also worth noting that, fortunately for us (both as epidemiologists and as human beings at risk), most disease outcomes are relatively rare. Common outcomes (eg, frequencies of 10% or higher) are seen in clinical trials, such as the vaccine-local reactions trial described previously or clinical studies of prognosis after cancer diagnosis. Generally, for most diseases, incidence in population-based studies is below 5%. In these instances, as already discussed, the odds ratio is usually a good approximation to the relative risk. It follows that from the viewpoint of the measure of association, a case-cohort strategy is practically equivalent to a traditional case-control study in which controls are noncases.

Influence of the Sampling Frame for Control Selection on the Parameter Estimated by the Odds Ratio of Exposure: Cumulative Incidence Versus Density Sampling

In addition to considering whether controls are selected from either noncases or the total study population, it is important to further specify the sampling frame for control selection. As discussed in Chapter 1 (Section 1.4.2), when one is selecting controls from a defined total cohort, sampling frames may consist of either (1) the baseline cohort or (2) individuals at risk when cases occur during the follow-up period (density sampling). The first alternative (exemplified by the "local reaction/influenza vaccination" analysis discussed above) has been designated *case-cohort design* and the latter, *nested case-control design*.[11] As demonstrated next, the case-cohort and nested designs allow the estimation of the relative risk and the rate ratio, respectively. An intuitive way to conceptualize which of these two parameters is being estimated by the OR_{exp} (ie, relative risk or rate ratio) is to think of cases as the "numerator" and controls as the "denominator" of the absolute measure of disease frequency to which the parameter relates (see Chapter 2).

Selecting Controls from the Cohort at Baseline: The Case-Cohort Design. As described previously (Section 1.4.2), when the case-cohort design is used, the case group is composed of cases identified during the follow-up period, and the controls compose a sample of the total cohort at baseline (Figure 1–20). The cases and the sampling frame for controls can be regarded, respectively, as the type of numerator and denominator that would have been selected to calculate a probability based on the initial population, q. Thus, when one is selecting these controls, the OR_{exp} yields a ratio of the probability in exposed (q_+) to that in unexposed (q_-) individuals: that is, the cumulative incidence ratio or relative risk. Because the distribution of follow-up times in the sample of the initial cohort—which by definition includes those not lost as well as those subsequently lost to observation during follow-up—will be different from that of cases (whose "risk set"* by definition does not include previous losses), it is necessary to correct for losses that occur during the follow-up in a case-cohort study using survival analysis techniques (see Section 2.2.1).

It is also possible to exclude cases from the control group when sampling the cohort at baseline: that is, the sampling frame for controls would be formed by individuals who have remained disease-free through the duration of the follow-up. These are the persons who would have been selected as the denominator of the *odds based on the initial population:*

$$\left(\frac{q}{1-q}\right)$$

Thus, the calculation of the OR_{exp} when carrying out this strategy yields an estimate of the OR_{dis}, comparing the odds of developing the disease during the follow-up between exposed and unexposed at baseline.

Density Sampling: The Nested Case-Control Design. The nested case-control design is based on incidence density sampling and is also described in Chapter 1 (Section 1.4.2). It consists of selecting a control group that represents the sum of the subsamples of the cohort selected during the follow-up at the approximate times when cases occur (*risk set*) (Figure 1–21). These controls can be also regarded as a population sample "averaged" over all points in time when the events happen (see Chapter 2, Section 2.2.2). Therefore, the OR_{exp} thus obtained estimates the rate or density ratio (or relative rate or relative density). This strategy explicitly recognizes that there are

---

*Defined as the subset of the cohort members under observation at the time of each case's occurrence (see Section 1.4.2, Figure 1–21).

losses (censored observations) during the follow-up of the cohort, in that cases and controls are chosen from the same reference populations excluding previous losses, thus matching cases and controls on duration of follow-up. When cases are excluded from the sampling frame of controls, the OR_{exp} estimates the density odds ratio.

A summary of the effect of the specific sampling frame for control selection on the parameter estimated by the OR_{exp} is shown in Table 3–10.

Calculation of the Odds Ratio When There Are More Than Two Exposure Categories

Although the examples given so far in this chapter have referred to only two exposure categories, often more than two levels of exposure are assessed. Among the advantages of studying multiple exposure categories is the assessment of different exposure dimensions (eg, "past" vs "current") and of graded ("dose-response") patterns.

In the example shown in Table 3–11, children with craniosynostosis undergoing craniectomy were compared with normal children in regard to maternal age.[12] To calculate the odds ratio for the different maternal age categories, the youngest maternal age was chosen as the reference category. Next, for cases and controls separately, the odds for each maternal age category (vis-à-vis the reference category) were calculated (columns 4 and 5). The odds ratio is calculated as the ratio of the odds of each maternal age category in cases to the odds

---

Table 3–10 Summary of the Influence of Control Selection on the Parameter Estimated by the Odds Ratio of Exposure in Case-Control Studies Within a Defined Cohort

Design	Population Frame for Control Selection	Exposure Odds Ratio Estimates
Case-cohort	Total cohort at baseline	Cumulative incidence ratio (relative risk)
	(Total cohort at baseline minus cases that develop during follow-up)	(Probability odds ratio)
Nested case-control	Population at approximate times when cases occur during follow-up	Rate (density) ratio
	(Population during follow-up minus cases)	(Density odds ratio)

Table 3–11 Distribution of Cases of Craniosynostosis and Normal Controls According to Maternal Age

Maternal Age (Years) (1)	Cases (2)	Controls (3)	Odds of Specified Maternal Age vs Reference in Cases (4)	Odds of Specified Maternal Age vs Reference in Controls (5)	Odds Ratio (6) = (4)/(5)
<20*	12	89	12/12	89/89	1.00*
20–24	47	242	47/12	242/89	1.44
25–29	56	255	56/12	255/89	1.63
>29	58	173	58/12	173/89	2.49

*Reference category.

Source: Data from BW Alderman et al, An Epidemiologic Study of Craniosynostosis: Risk Indicators for the Occurrence of Craniosynostosis in Colorado, *American Journal of Epidemiology,* Vol 128, pp 431–438, © 1988, The Johns Hopkins University School of Hygiene & Public Health.

in controls (column 6). In this study, a graded and positive (direct) relationship was observed between maternal age and the odds of craniosynostosis.

When the multilevel exposure variable is ordinal (eg, age categories in Table 3–11), it may be of interest to perform a trend test (see Appendix B).

3.4.2 Attributable Risk in Case-Control Studies

As noted previously (Section 3.2.2), percent AR in the exposed can be obtained in case-control (case-noncase) studies when the odds ratio is a reasonable estimate of the relative risk by replacing its corresponding value in equation 3.6:

[Equation 3.14]

$$\%AR_{exp} = \left(\frac{OR - 1.0}{OR}\right) \times 100$$

In studies dealing with preventive interventions, the measure analogous to the $\%AR_{exp}$ is efficacy (see Section 3.2.2, Equation 3.7). The fact that the odds ratio is usually a good estimate of the relative risk makes it possible to use equation 3.14 in case-control studies of the efficacy of an intervention such as screening.[13]

The same reasoning applies to the use of case-control studies to estimate the population attributable risk using a variation of Levin's formula:

[Equation 3.15]

$$\%\text{Pop AR} = \frac{b \times (\text{OR} - 1.0)}{b \times (\text{OR} - 1.0) + 1.0}$$

In Equation 3.15, the proportion of exposed subjects in the reference population, b, can be estimated by the exposure prevalence in controls as long as the disease is rare and the control group is reasonably representative of all noncases in the population.[13] Obviously, if a case-cohort study is conducted, the rarity assumption is not needed (Section 3.4.1), as both the relative risk and the exposure prevalence can be directly estimated.

As shown by Levin and Bertell,[14] if the odds ratio is used as the relative risk estimate, Equation 3.15 reduces to a simpler equation:

$$\% \text{ Pop AR} = \frac{b_{\text{case}} - b_{\text{cont}}}{1.0 - b_{\text{cont}}}$$

where b_{case} represents the prevalence of exposure among cases—that is, $a/(a + c)$ in Table 3–8—and b_{cont} represents the prevalence of exposure among controls—that is, $b/(b + d)$ in Table 3–8.

3.5   ASSESSING THE STRENGTH OF ASSOCIATIONS

The values of the measures of association discussed in this chapter are often used to rank the relative importance of risk factors. However, because risk factors vary in terms of their physiologic modus operandi, as well as their exposure levels and units, such comparisons are unwarranted. Consider, for example, the absurdity of saying that systolic blood pressure is a more important risk factor for myocardial infarction than total cholesterol, based on comparing the odds ratio associated with a 50–mmHg increase in systolic blood pressure with that associated with a 1-mg/dl increase in total serum cholesterol. In addition, regardless of the size of the units used, it is hard to compare association strengths, given the unique nature of different risk factors.

An alternative way to assess the strength of the association of a given risk factor with an outcome is to estimate the exposure intensity necessary for that factor to produce an association of the same magnitude as that of well-established risk factors or vice-versa. For example, in a recent study, Tverdal et al[15] evaluated the level of expo-

Exhibit 3–1 A Possible Way To Describe the Strength of an Association Between a Risk Factor and an Outcome

A relative risk of 2.2 for coronary heart disease mortality comparing men drinking 9+ cups of coffee/day vs <1 cup/day corresponds to:

Smoking: 4.3 cigarettes/day
Systolic blood pressure: 6.9 mm/Hg
Total serum cholesterol: 0.47 mmol/L
Serum high-density lipoprotein: −0.24 mmol/L

Source: Data from A Tverdal et al, Coffee Consumption and Death from Coronary Heart Disease in Middle-Aged Norwegian Men and Women, *British Medical Journal,* Vol 300, pp 566–569, © 1990.

sure of four well-known risk factors for coronary heart disease mortality necessary to replicate the relative risk of 2.2 associated with a coffee intake of nine or more cups per day. As seen in Exhibit 3–1, a relative risk of 2.2 corresponds to smoking about 4.3 cigarettes per day or having an increase in systolic blood pressure of about 6.9 mm Hg, and so on.

Exhibit 3–2 Cross-Sectionally Determined Mean Wall (Intima Plus Media) Thickness (IMT) of the Carotid Arteries (mm) by Passive Smoking Status in Never-Active Smokers, the Atherosclerosis Risk in Communities (ARIC) Study, 1987 to 1989

	Passive Smoking Status in Never-Active Smokers		Estimated Increase by Year of Age
	Absent (*n* = 1,774)	Present (*n* = 3,358)	
Mean IMT (mm) →	0.700	0.711	0.011

Age-equivalent excess attributable to passive smoking:
(0.711 − 0.700)/0.011 = 1 year

Source: Data from G Howard et al, Active and Passive Smoking Are Associated with Increased Carotid Wall Thickness. The Atherosclerosis Risk in Communities Study, *Archives of Internal Medicine,* Vol 154, pp 1277–1282, © 1994, American Medical Association.

Another example comes from a study by Howard et al,[16] who evaluated the cross-sectional association between passive smoking and subclinical atherosclerosis measured by B-mode ultrasound-determined thickness (intima plus media) of the carotid artery walls. Because passive smoking had not been studied previously in connection with directly visualized atherosclerosis, its importance as a risk factor was contrasted with that of a known atherosclerosis determinant, age (Exhibit 3–2). As seen in the exhibit, the cross-sectional association between passive smoking and atherosclerosis is equivalent to an age difference of 1 year. That is, assuming that the cross-sectional association adequately represents the prospective relationship between age and atherosclerosis and that the data are valid, precise, and free of confounding, the average thickness of the carotid arteries of passive smokers looks like that of never smokers who are 1 year older. This inference was extended by Kawachi and Colditz,[17] who, on the basis of data from Howard et al's study, estimated that the change in wall thickness related to passive smoking would result in an increase in the risk of clinical cardiovascular events equivalent to an increment of 7 mm Hg of systolic blood pressure, or 0.7 mmol/L of total cholesterol—thus, not negligible.

REFERENCES

1. Lilienfeld DE, Stolley PD. *Foundations of Epidemiology.* 3rd ed. New York, NY: Oxford University Press; 1994.
2. Gordis L. *Epidemiology.* Philadelphia, Pa: WB Saunders; 1996.
3. Seltser R, Sartwell PE, Bell JA. A controlled test of Asian influenza vaccine in a population of families. *Am J Hyg.* 1962;75:112–135.
4. Greenland S, Robins JM. Conceptual problems in the definition and interpretation of attributable fractions. *Am J Epidemiol.* 1988;128:1185–1197.
5. Rothman KJ, Greenland S. *Modern Epidemiology.* 2nd ed. Philadelphia, Pa: Lippincott-Raven Publishers; 1998.
6. Levin ML. The occurrence of lung cancer in man. *Acta Un Intern Cancer.* 1953;9: 531–541.
7. Walter SD. The estimation and interpretation of attributable fraction in health research. *Biometrics.* 1976;32:829–849.
8. Rockhill B, Newman B, Weinberg C. Use and misuse of population attributable fractions. *Am J Public Health.* 1998;88:15–19.
9. Cornfield J. A method of estimating comparable rates from clinical data: applications to cancer of the lung, breast, and cervix. *J Natl Cancer Inst.* 1951;11: 1269–1275.
10. Prentice RL. A case-cohort design for epidemiologic cohort studies and disease prevention trials. *Biometrika.* 1986;73:1–11.

11. Langholz B, Thomas DC. Nested case-control and case-cohort methods of sampling from a cohort: a critical comparison. *Am J Epidemiol.* 1990;131:169–176.
12. Alderman BW, Lammer EJ, Joshua SC, et al. An epidemiologic study of craniosynostosis: risk indicators for the occurrence of craniosynostosis in Colorado. *Am J Epidemiol.* 1988;128:431–438.
13. Coughlin SS, Benichou J, Weed DL. Attributable risk estimation in case-control studies. *Epidemiol Rev.* 1994;16:51–64.
14. Levin ML, Bertell SR. Re: "Simple estimation of population attributable risk from case-control studies." *Am J Epidemiol.* 1978;108:78–79.
15. Tverdal A, Stensvold I, Solvoll K, et al. Coffee consumption and death from coronary heart disease in middle aged Norwegian men and women. *Br Med J.* 1990;300:566–569.
16. Howard G, Burke GL, Szklo M, et al. Active and passive smoking are associated with increased carotid wall thickness: the Atherosclerosis Risk in Communities study. *Arch Intern Med.* 1994;154:1277–1282.
17. Kawachi I, Colditz GA. Confounding, measurement error, and publication bias in studies of passive smoking. *Am J Epidemiol.* 1996;144:909–915.

PART III

Threats to Validity and Issues of Interpretation

CHAPTER 4

Understanding Lack of Validity: Bias

4.1 OVERVIEW

Bias can be defined as the result of a *systematic* error in the design or conduct of a study. This systematic error results from flaws either in the method of selection of study participants or in the procedures for gathering relevant exposure and/or disease information; as a consequence, the observed study results will *tend* to be different from the true results. This *tendency* toward erroneous results is called bias. As will be discussed in this chapter, many types of bias can affect the study results. Bias, in addition to confounding (see Chapter 5) is an important consideration and is often a major problem in observational epidemiologic studies. Systematic error (bias) needs to be distinguished from error due to random variability (sampling error), which results from the use of a population sample to estimate the study parameters in the reference population. The sample estimates may differ substantially from the true parameters because of random error, especially when the study sample is small.

Note that the definition of bias relates to the process—that is, the design and procedures—of the study and not the results of any particular study. If the design and procedures of a study are unbiased, the study is considered to be *valid* because its results will (on average) be correct. A faulty study design is considered to be biased (or *invalid*) because it will produce an erroneous result *on average*. However, because of sampling variability, a given study using "biased" methods can produce a result close to the truth (Figure 4–1).

Bias is said to exist when, *on the average*, the results of an infinite number of studies (related to a specific association and reference population) differ from the true result—for example, when the average relative odds of a large (theoretically infinite) number of case-control

studies is 2.0 but in fact there is no association (Figure 4–1). This definition of bias, however, is of little use to the epidemiologist who must
infer from results of his or her only study. Even when the epidemiologist carries out an overview or meta-analysis, the available published
studies are but a fraction of what, by any definition, can be regarded
as "an infinite number of studies." (A related problem is publication
bias—namely, the tendency to publish studies in which results are
"positive"; see Section 4.5.) Bias, therefore, has to be assessed in the
context of a careful evaluation of the specific study design, methods,
and procedures. Prevention and control of bias are accomplished on
two levels: (1) ensuring that the study design is appropriate for addressing the study hypotheses and (2) establishing and carefully monitoring procedures of data collection that are valid and reliable. The
latter is the subject of Chapter 8, which discusses the quality assurance and control procedures used in epidemiologic studies.

Many types of bias have been described in the epidemiologic literature (see, eg, Sackett[1]). However, most biases related to the study design and procedures can be classified in two basic categories: *selection*
and *information.*

Selection bias is present when individuals have different probabilities of being included in the study sample according to relevant study
characteristics: namely, the exposure and the outcome of interest. Fig-

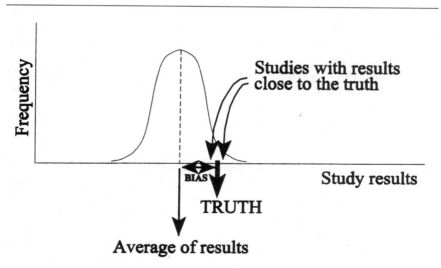

Figure 4–1 Hypothetical distribution of results from a biased study design.

ure 4–2 illustrates a general situation where exposed cases have a higher probability of being selected for the study than other categories of individuals. An instance of this type of bias is *medical surveillance bias*, which one might encounter, for example, when conducting a case-control study to examine the relationship of the use of oral contraceptives to any disease with an important subclinical component—such as diabetes. Because oral contraceptive use is likely to be related to a higher average frequency of medical encounters, any subclinical disease is more likely to be diagnosed in these women than in other women. As a result, in a study comparing cases of diabetes and controls without diabetes, a spurious association with oral contraceptive use may ensue. The effect of selection bias on the direction of the measure of association is, of course, a function of which cell(s) in a $n \times k$ table (eg, a 2×2 table such as that shown in Figure 4–2) is/are subject to a spuriously higher or lower probability of selection.

Information bias results from a systematic tendency for individuals selected for inclusion in the study to be erroneously placed in different exposure/outcome categories, thus leading to *misclassification*. The classical example of information bias leading to misclassification is *recall bias*, in which the ability to recall past exposure is dependent

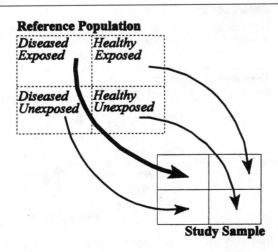

Figure 4–2 Selection bias: one relevant group in the population (exposed cases in the example) has a higher probability of being included in the study sample.

on case-control status. In the hypothetical example sketched in Figure 4–3, cases are more likely than controls to overstate past exposure.

What follows is a discussion of the most common selection and information biases affecting exposure-outcome associations in observational epidemiologic studies. Inevitably, because different types of bias overlap, any attempt to classify bias entails some duplication; as will be readily noted, some types of bias may be categorized as either selection or information bias (or as both). The classification of the different types of biases discussed in the following sections is thus mainly set up for didactic purposes and is by no means intended to be a rigid and mutually exclusive taxonomy.

4.2   SELECTION BIAS

Selection bias occurs when a systematic error in the ascertainment of study subjects—cases or controls in case-control studies, or exposed or unexposed subjects in cohort studies—results in a tendency toward distorting the measure expressing the association between exposure and outcome. Selection bias is often referred to as *Berksonian bias*, par-

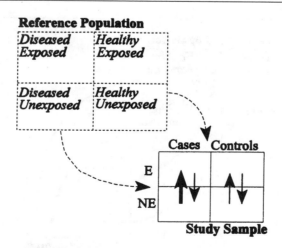

Figure 4–3 Misclassification (information) bias: some degree of misclassification of the exposure information exists in both cases and controls, but unexposed cases in this example tend to mistakenly report past exposure to a greater extent than do controls. E, exposed; NE, nonexposed.

ticularly when this bias occurs in case-control studies of hospitalized patients.[2,3]

A hypothetical depiction of selection bias in the context of a case-control study is seen in Tables 4–1 through 4–4. In these tables, for ease of understanding, it is assumed that confounding is absent and that there is neither random variability nor information bias (ie, that there is no misclassification of either exposure or case-control status, see Section 4.3).

In Table 4–1 all true cases and true noncases in a reference population of 10,000 subjects are included in a case-control study assessing the relationship of risk factor A with disease Y. Table 4–1 thus shows the "true" results that can be used as the "gold standard" for assessing the results shown in Tables 4–2 through 4–4.

In Table 4–2 a 50% sample of cases and a 10% sample of controls are chosen from the total population shown in Table 4–1. Unbiased sampling such as this yields unbiased exposure odds in cases and controls and thus an unbiased odds ratio. (The use of a larger sampling fraction for cases than for controls in Table 4–2 is typical of many case-control studies for which a limited pool of cases is available. See Chapter 3, Section 3.4.1.) However, as long as the sampling fraction *within* the group of cases and that *within* the group of controls are unaffected by exposure, selection bias does not occur.

Table 4–1 Hypothetical Case-Control Study Including All Cases and All Noncases of a Defined Population; Assume No Confunding Effects and No Information Bias

Risk Factor A	Total Population	
	Cases	Noncases (Controls)
Present	500	1800
Absent	500	7200
Total	1000	9000
Exposure odds	500:500 = 1.0:1.0	1800:7200 = 1.0:4.0
Odds ratio	$\dfrac{\left(\dfrac{500}{500}\right)}{\left(\dfrac{1800}{7200}\right)} = 4.0$	

Note: The results in this table represent the "gold standard" against which to compare results in Tables 4–2, 4–3, and 4–4.

Table 4–2 Hypothetical Case-Control Study Including a 50% Unbiased Sample of Cases and a 10% Unbiased Sample of Noncases of the Reference Population Shown in Table 4–1

	Sample of the Total Population	
Risk Factor A	50% of Cases	10% of Noncases (Controls)
Present	250	180
Absent	250	720
Total	1000 × 0.50 = 500	9000 × 0.10 = 900
Exposure odds	250:250 = 1.0:1.0	180:720 = 1.0:4.0
Odds ratio		$\dfrac{\left(\dfrac{250}{250}\right)}{\left(\dfrac{180}{720}\right)} = 4.0$
Consequences	Unbiased exposure odds in cases and controls	Unbiased odds ratio

Table 4–3 Example of Selection Bias in Choosing Cases in a Hypothetical Case-Control Study Including a 50% Sample of Cases and a 10% Sample of Noncases of the Reference Population Shown in Table 4–1

	Total Population	
Risk Factor A	Cases	Noncases (Controls)
Present	500 × 0.60* = 300	180
Absent	500 × 0.40* = 200	720
Total	1000 × 0.50 = 500	9000 × 0.10 = 900
Exposure odds	300:200 = 1.5:1.0	180:720 = 1.0:4.0
Odds ratio		$\dfrac{\left(\dfrac{300}{200}\right)}{\left(\dfrac{180}{720}\right)} = 6.0$
Consequences	Biased exposure odds in cases Unbiased exposure odds in controls Biased odds ratio	

*Differential sampling fractions unintended by and unknown to the investigator.

Table 4–4 Example of the Same Level of Selection Bias in Choosing Cases and Controls in a Hypothetical Case-Control Study Including a 50% Sample of Cases and a 10% Sample of Noncases of the Defined Population Shown in Table 4–1

	Total Population	
Risk Factor A	*Cases*	*Noncases (Controls)*
Present	$500 \times 0.60^* = 300$	$1800 \times 0.136^* = 245$
Absent	$500 \times 0.40^* = 200$	$7200 \times 0.091^* = 655$
Total	$1000 \times 0.50 = 500$	$9000 \times 0.10 = 900$
Exposure odds	$300:200 = 1.5:1.0$	$245:655 = 1.0:2.67$

Odds ratio
$$\frac{\left(\frac{300}{200}\right)}{\left(\frac{245}{655}\right)} = 4.0$$

Consequences   Exposure odds biased to the same extent in cases and controls
Unbiased odds ratio

*Differential sampling fractions unknown to the investigator.

In contrast to the unbiased approaches shown in Tables 4–1 and 4–2, Table 4–3 provides an example of selection bias, whereby, *unbeknownst to the investigator*, selection of cases, but not that of controls, is biased in that it varies according to exposure status. In the hypothetical example shown in Table 4–3, the investigator decides to select 50% of cases and 10% of controls, as done in Table 4–2. However, the selection of cases is not independent of exposure status. As a consequence, even though the overall sampling fraction for cases is the intended 50%, a greater sampling fraction is applied to exposed than to unexposed cases, biasing the exposure odds in cases but not in controls and thus yielding a biased odds ratio. It is important to emphasize that the difference in sampling fraction according to the exposure status in cases is unintended by the investigator, who is under the impression that both exposed and unexposed cases are subjected to the same preestablished sampling fraction of 50% applied to the total case pool. The examples shown in Tables 4–1 through 4–3 apply to a hypothetical situation in which there is a defined reference population list from which to sample cases and noncases. Often, population listings are unavailable, and thus epidemiologists use convenience samples of cases and controls, making the occurrence of selection bias even more likely.

A hypothetical example of selection bias is a study of aplastic anemia in which cases are identified in a major referral hospital and controls are patients with nonmalignant, nonhematologic disorders identified in the same hospital. Because aplastic anemia patients may be often referred to this hospital for a bone marrow transplantation, some of their characteristics will differ from those of other patients: for example, these patients may be more likely both to come from large families (as they often have a genetically matched sibling donor) and to have health insurance or a higher income in order to defray the considerable costs involved in this procedure. As a result, exposures related to having a large family and/or a higher socioeconomic status may be differentially distributed between cases and controls, leading to a distortion of the exposure-disease associations.

Because differential bias of the type exemplified in Table 4–3 distorts the nature or magnitude of an association, investigators often attempt to "equalize" bias between the groups under comparison. In retrospective studies, for example, attempts are often made to obtain samples of cases and controls undergoing the same selection processes. Thus, for cases identified only in hospitals H1 and H2 out of several hospitals serving a given population A, an appropriate control group would be a sample of the population subset that, if diseased, would have chosen or been referred to hospitals H1 and H2. (This strategy is occasionally called *case-based, clinic-based,* or *hospital-based control selection.*[4,5]) Choice of controls, ignoring the selection process that made study cases seek hospitals H1 and H2 (eg, selecting controls from total population A), may well produce selection bias if, for example, the two hospitals where cases are identified cater to patients having characteristics related to the exposure being evaluated.

Possibly the best example of successful equalization of selection processes is given by case-control studies in which both cases and controls are identified from among women attending a screening program.[6] Women participating in a screening program of breast cancer are more likely to have higher prevalence rates of known breast cancer risk factors, such as family history. Thus, if cases diagnosed by screening were compared with a sample of noncases drawn from the general population, overestimation of the magnitude of the association with certain risk factors might occur. Selecting both case and control groups from among screened women, however, makes both groups equally prone to the higher likelihood of exposure to known risk factors. This process is schematically illustrated in the hypothetical example shown in Table 4–4. In this table, bias of the same magnitude resulted in the inclusion of higher proportions of exposed subjects in both the case and the control groups. As a consequence, although exposure odds are biased in both cases and controls vis-à-vis the true exposure odds shown in Tables 4–1 and 4–2, the relative odds ratio is unbiased.

Note that the magnitude of bias in the selection of cases is the same as for controls in Table 4–4, leading to what Schlesselman[4(p128)] has defined as *compensating bias*:

$$\text{Bias} = \frac{\text{Observed odds}_{\text{cases}}}{\text{True odds}_{\text{cases}}} = \frac{\dfrac{1.5}{1.0}}{\dfrac{1.0}{1.0}} = \frac{\text{Observed odds}_{\text{controls}}}{\text{True odds}_{\text{controls}}} = \frac{\dfrac{1.0}{2.67}}{\dfrac{1.0}{4.0}} = 1.5$$

For compensating bias to occur, the same bias factor (in this example, "× 1.5") needs to be present in both the numerator (exposure odds of cases, $\text{Odds}_{\text{exp/cases}}$) and the denominator (exposure odds of controls, $\text{Odds}_{\text{exp/controls}}$) of the odds ratio, so as to be canceled out:

$$\frac{\text{Odds}_{\text{exp/cases}} \times [\text{bias}]}{\text{Odds}_{\text{exp/controls}} \times [\text{bias}]} = \frac{\text{Odds}_{\text{exp/cases}}}{\text{Odds}_{\text{exp/controls}}} = \text{True odds ratio (OR)}$$

In the example,

$$\text{OR} = \frac{\left(\dfrac{1.0}{1.0}\right) \times 1.5}{\left(\dfrac{1.0}{4.0}\right) \times 1.5} = \frac{\left(\dfrac{1.5}{1.0}\right)}{\left(\dfrac{1.0}{2.67}\right)} = 4.0$$

In practice, it is difficult to make sure that the same bias applies to the exposure odds of both cases and controls, and attempts to introduce a compensating bias may even backfire, as in the aplastic anemia example discussed previously. Another example is a study examining the association of coffee intake and pancreatic cancer by MacMahon et al,[7] in which controls were selected from a group of patients seen by the same physicians who had diagnosed the cases' disease. The likely goal of this design was to make the selection process (including attending biases) of cases and controls similar. However, as the exposure of interest was coffee intake, and as patients seen by physicians who diagnose pancreatic cancer often have gastrointestinal disorders and are thus advised not to drink coffee, the investigators' attempt to introduce a compensating bias led to the selection of controls with an unusually low odds of exposure. This resulted in a (spurious) positive association between coffee intake and cancer of the pancreas that could not be subsequently confirmed.[8]

Whenever possible, study subjects should be chosen from defined reference populations. In case-control studies, a sample of the defined population from which cases originated (as when doing a case-cohort study) constitutes the best type of control group. Efforts to introduce a compensating bias when the control group selection is driven by the case characteristics may or may not be successful, although they underscore the possibility of obtaining valid measures of association even when it is not possible to obtain valid absolute measures of disease frequency (odds).

All the preceding examples are from case-control studies, because these studies (along with cross-sectional studies) provide the most likely setting in which the sampling probabilities of the different disease-exposure groups may turn out to be differential (Figure 4–2). In a cohort study, because study participants (exposed or unexposed) are selected (at least theoretically) *before* the disease actually occurs, differential selection according to disease status is less likely to occur. For diseases with a long preclinical phase (eg, certain cancers, atherosclerotic disease), biases resulting from changes related to prodromic manifestations of the disease (before it becomes fully clinically apparent) will often affect both exposed and unexposed individuals, resulting in a situation analogous to that shown in Table 4–4 (compensating bias).

The more important analogue of selection bias in the context of cohort studies relates to the problem of *differential losses to follow-up,* that is, whether individuals who are lost to follow-up over the course of the study are different from those who remain under observation up to the event or termination of the study. This analogy was discussed in Section 1.4.2, and Figures 1–13 and 1–18 underscore the theoretical equivalence between issues of selection of cases and controls (from a defined or a hypothetical cohort) and those related to differential losses in a cohort study. The biases on the estimates of incidence that can occur as a consequence of losses were discussed in Section 2.2. Individuals who are lost to follow-up (particularly when losses are because of mortality from causes other than the outcome of interest, refusal, or migration—see Table 2–4) tend to have different probabilities of the outcome than those who remain in the cohort over the entire span of the study. Thus, incidence estimates tend to be biased. However, as in the case-control study (Table 4–4), relative measures of association (relative risk, rate ratio) will be unbiased if the bias on the incidence estimates is of similar magnitude in exposed and unexposed individuals (compensating bias). In other words, a biased relative risk or rate ratio estimate will only ensue if losses to follow-up are biased according to *both* outcome and exposure.

4.3 INFORMATION BIAS

Information bias in epidemiologic studies results from either imperfect definitions of study variables or flawed data collection procedures. These errors may result in misclassification of exposure and/or outcome status for a significant proportion of study participants. Throughout this section, the terms *validity, sensitivity, specificity,* and *reliability* are frequently used. These concepts are defined in basic epidemiology texts (Exhibit 4–1) and will also be frequently used in Chapter 8, which is closely related to this chapter.

A *valid study* is equivalent to an "unbiased" study—a study that, based on its design, methods, and procedures, will produce (on average) overall results that are close to the truth. *Sensitivity* and *specificity* are defined as the two main components of validity. Note that in basic textbooks or chapters discussing issues related to diagnosis and screening (eg, Gordis[9]), these terms typically refer to the correct classification of *disease* status (ie, diagnosis). However, in this chapter (as well as in Chapter 8), *sensitivity* and *specificity* also refer to the classification of *exposure* status. In addition to the main exposure variable (eg, the main risk factor of interest in the study), misclassification of other variables, such as confounders, may also occur (see Chapter 7, Section 7.5).

Exhibit 4–1 Definitions of Terms Related to the Classification of Individuals in Epidemiologic Studies

- Validity: The ability of a test to distinguish between who has a disease (or other characteristic) and who does not.
  - –Sensitivity: The ability of a test to identify correctly those who have the disease (or characteristic) of interest.
  - –Specificity: The ability of a test to identify correctly those who do not have the disease (or characteristic) of interest.
- Reliability (repeatability): The extent to which the results obtained by a test are replicated if the test is repeated.

Source: Data from L Gordis, *Epidemiology,* pp 59 and 70, © 1996, WB Saunders Company.

4.3.1   Exposure Identification Bias

Problems in the collection of exposure data or an imperfect definition of the level of exposure may lead to bias. Exposure identification bias is mainly, but not exclusively, of concern in case-control studies. Thus, most examples dealing with this type of information bias come from case-control studies. Two of the main subcategories of exposure identification bias are recall bias and interviewer bias.

Recall Bias

Recall bias resulting from inaccurate recall of past exposure is perhaps the most often cited type of exposure identification bias. It is a concern especially in the context of case-control studies, when cases and controls are asked about exposures in the past. Errors in recall of these past exposures result in misclassification of exposure status, thus biasing the results of the study. If the recall error differs between cases and controls, the misclassification is said to be differential; if the recall error is of similar magnitude, the error is said to be nondifferential, as will be discussed in Section 4.3.3. An empirical example of recall bias was documented by Weinstock et al,[10] who collected information on hair color and tanning ability both at baseline and after the occurrence of melanoma in cohort participants of the Nurses' Health Study. In this study, cases of melanoma tended to overreport "low tanning ability" in the postmelanoma diagnosis interview, as compared with the interview carried out before the occurrence of the disease, a difference that was not seen among controls (results from this study are discussed in detail in Section 4.3.3).

Methods used to prevent recall bias include verification of responses from study subjects, use of diseased controls in case-control studies, use of objective markers of exposure, and use of the cohort study design, including the conduct of case-control studies within the cohort.

Verification of exposure information obtained from participants by review of pharmacy or hospital charts, or other sources, is occasionally done in case-control studies. Examples include the studies examining the relationships of past use of estrogens on breast cancer,[11] in which responses from samples of cases and controls were verified by contacting physicians. In cohort studies, a similar strategy can be used to confirm participant information pertaining to event outcomes (eg, myocardial infarction) or to identify and exclude prevalent cases from the baseline cohort in order to estimate incidence on follow-up. As an example, in the ongoing Atherosclerosis Risk in Communities (ARIC) study, information provided by cohort members during the periodic interviews on admissions for the main outcomes (eg, myocardial infarction) is systematically verified by review of the relevant medical charts.[12]

Because in case-control studies recall bias may be caused by "rumination" by cases regarding the causes of their disease, on occasion *a control group formed by diseased subjects* is selected as an attempt to introduce a similar bias in the exposure odds of controls: an example is a study by Mele et al[13] in which cases of leukemia were compared with a control group formed by symptomatic patients who, after evaluation in the same hematology clinics as the cases, were found not to have hematologic disorders. The problem with using a diseased control group, however, is that it is often unclear whether the "rumination" process related to the controls' diseases is equivalent to that of cases with regard to the magnitude of recall bias.

Objective markers of exposure or susceptibility are less prone to recall bias than direct responses from study subjects. An example can be found in the study of melanoma risk factors cited above.[10] In contrast to the bias in reporting "tanning ability" after the disease diagnosis, the responses of cases and controls regarding hair color did not show any significant change comparing the responses to the questionnaires applied before and after the disease diagnosis (see Section 4.3.3). A likely reason for this is that hair color is more objectively assessed than tanning ability.

Certain genetic markers, for example, constitute "exposures" that are not time dependent and can be measured even after the disease has occurred, thus possibly being less prone to bias (assuming that the genetic marker is not related to survival, see Section 4.3.3). An example is the assessment of DNA repair capabilities (DRC) as a genetic marker for susceptibility to ultraviolet light–induced nonmelanoma skin cancer in young cases and controls.[14] Regrettably, however, most environmental exposures that can be assessed by means of objective biologic markers represent current, rather than past exposures, such as the levels of cotinine to indicate cigarette smoking, and are thus of limited usefulness.[15]

Nested case-control or case-cohort studies when prospective data are available (see Section 1.4.2) allow the evaluation of certain hypotheses free of recall bias (or temporal bias; see Section 4.4.2). Typically, in these case-control studies, information on exposure and confounders is collected at baseline, before the cases occur, thus reducing the likelihood of systematic recall differences between cases and controls. The study discussed above examining the relationship of tanning ability and melanoma[10] (see above and Section 4.3.3) is an example of a case-control study within a cohort (the Nurses Health Study cohort); the application of the premelanoma diagnosis questionnaire avoids the recall bias that is observed when the analysis is based on information obtained from the postmelanoma questionnaire.[10]

Although exposure recall bias is typically a problem of case-control studies, it may also occur in cohort studies. In the latter type of study, it may be present at the outset of the study when categorization of individuals by level of exposure relies on recalled information from the distant or recent past, as when attempts are made to classify cohort participants at baseline by duration of exposure.

Interviewer Bias

When data collection in a case-control study is not masked with regard to the disease status of study participants, observer bias in ascertaining exposure, such as interviewer bias, may occur. Interviewer bias may occur as a consequence of trying to "clarify" questions when such clarifications are not part of the study protocol, failing to follow the probing, or skipping rules of questionnaires. More subtle deviations from the protocol, which may include emphasizing certain words to cases but not to controls (or vice versa), are difficult to identify.

Although it is difficult to recognize interviewer bias, it is important to be aware of it and to implement procedures to minimize the likelihood of its occurrence. Attempts to prevent interviewer bias involve the careful design and conduct of quality assurance and control activities (see Chapter 8), including development of a detailed manual of operations, training of staff, standardization of data collection procedures, and monitoring of data collection activities. Additional measures to prevent this bias are the performance of reliability/validity substudies and the masking of interviewers with regard to case-control status.

Reliability and validity substudies in samples will be described in more detail in Chapter 8, Section 8.3. They constitute an important strategy that needs to be carried out systematically, with quick feedback to interviewers who do not follow the protocol or who have encountered problems. It should be noted, however, that in contrast to reliability studies of laboratory measurements, reliability substudies of interviews are not easy to conduct. Assessing the reliability of interview data is difficult because of intraparticipant variability when interviews are done at separate points in time and recall of the previous responses on the part of the interviewee, with the resultant tendency to provide the same, albeit mistaken responses.

As for recall bias, validity studies using independent sources (eg, medical charts) can be conducted to assess accuracy of data collection by interviewers.

Masking of interviewers with regard to case-control status of study participants is difficult, but when feasible, it may remove an important source of bias, particularly when the interviewer is familiar with the study hypothesis. On occasion, by including a health question for which a frequent affirmative response is expected from both cases and controls, it is possible to mask the interviewers with regard to the main study hypothesis and have them believe that the hypothesis pertains to the "misleading" question. Such a strategy was employed in a case-control study of psychosocial factors and myocardial infarction in women, in which questions about hysterectomy, which were often answered positively in view of the high frequency of this intervention in the United States, led the interviewers to believe that the study was testing a hormonal hypothesis.[16]

A mistake made in an early study of lung cancer and smoking conducted by Doll and Hill,[17] in which some controls were erroneously classified as cases, suggests an additional strategy for assessing the possibility of interviewer bias. In this study, the odds of exposure to smoking in the misclassified controls was very similar to that of the nonmisclassified controls and much lower than that of cases, thus confirming the absence of interviewer bias. This example suggests the possibility of using "phantom" cases and controls and/or purposely misleading interviewers to believe that some cases are controls and vice versa in order to assess interviewer bias.

4.3.2 Outcome Identification Bias

Outcome (eg, disease) identification bias may occur in both case-control and cohort studies. The resulting misclassification of disease may be due to an imperfect definition of the outcome or to errors at the data collection stage.

Observer Bias

In a cohort study, decision as to whether the outcome is present may be affected by knowledge of the exposure status of the study participant, particularly when the outcome is "soft," such as migraine episodes or psychiatric symptoms. There may be observer bias at different stages of the ascertainment of the outcome, including application of pathologic or clinical criteria. A fairly crude example of observer bias is the assignment of a histologic specimen to a diagnosis of "alcoholic cirrhosis" when the pathologist knows that the patient is an alcoholic. A documented example of observer bias is the effect of the patient's race on the diagnosis of hypertensive end-stage renal disease (ESRD). In a simulation study conducted by Perneger et al,[18] a sample of nephrologists were sent case histories for seven patients with ESRD. For each case history, the simulated race of each patient was randomly assigned to be "black" or "white." Case histories that identified the patient's race as "black" were twice as likely to result in a diagnosis of hypertensive ESRD as case histories in which the patient's race was said to be "white."

As mentioned above, observer bias occurs when the ascertainment of outcome is not independent from the knowledge of the exposure status. Thus, measures aimed at *masking observers in charge of deciding whether the outcome is present by exposure status* would theoretically prevent observer bias. When masking of observers by exposure status is not practical, observer bias can be assessed by stratifying on certainty of diagnosis. For example, exposure levels can be assessed in relation to incidence of "possible," "probable," and "definite" disease. Observer bias should be suspected if an association is seen only for the "softer" categories (eg, "possible" disease).

Another strategy to prevent observer bias is to perform diagnostic classification with *multiple observers*. For example, two observers could independently classify an event, and if disagreement occurred, a third observer would adjudicate: that is, decision on the presence or absence of the outcome would have to be agreed on by at least two of three observers. This strategy, however, increases the study's costs and is thus often not feasible.

Respondent Bias

Recall and other informant biases are usually associated with identification of exposure in case-control studies. However, outcome ascertainment bias may occur during follow-up of a cohort when information on the outcome is obtained by participant response: for example, when collecting information on events for which it is difficult to obtain objective confirmation, such as episodes of migraine headaches.

Whenever possible, information given by a participant on a possible occurrence of the outcome of interest should be confirmed by more objective means, such as hospital chart review. When objective confirmation is not possible—for example, for nonhospitalized events, or events for which laboratory verification is impossible, such as acute panic attacks—detailed information not only on presence versus absence of a given event but also on related symptoms that may be part of a diagnostic constellation may be of help in preventing respondent bias. For example, the questionnaire on the occurrence of an episode of migraine headaches in a study by Stewart et al[19] included questions not only on whether a severe headache had occurred but also on presence of aura, nausea, and fatigue accompanying the headache. This strategy allowed more objectivity in classifying migraines than the simple determination of the presence or absence of pain. For several outcomes, such as angina pectoris and chronic bronchitis, standardized questionnaires are available (see Chapter 8). The validity and limitations of some of these instruments have been assessed. An example is the Rose questionnaire for the diagnosis of angina pectoris.[20–23]

4.3.3   The Result of Information Bias: Misclassification

Information bias leads to misclassification of exposure and/or outcome status. For example, when there is recall bias in a case-control study, some exposed subjects are classified as unexposed, and vice versa. In a cohort study, a positive outcome may be missed. Alternatively, a pseudoevent may be mistakenly classified as a positive outcome. The examples of both differential and nondifferential misclassification in this section refer to exposure levels in case-control studies. Misclassification of case-control status in case-control studies and of exposure and outcome in cohort studies can be readily inferred, although they are not specifically discussed so as to avoid repetition.

There are two types of misclassification bias: nondifferential and differential.

Nondifferential Misclassification

Nondifferential misclassification occurs when the degree of misclassification of exposure is independent of case-control status (or vice versa).

Nondifferential Misclassification When There Are Two Categories. A simplistic hypothetical example of nondifferential misclassification of (dichotomous) exposure in a case-control study is shown in Exhibit 4–2. In this example, misclassification of exposed subjects as unexposed occurs in 30% of cases and 30% of controls. Nondifferential misclassification tends to bias the association toward the null hypothesis when there are two exposure categories (for instance, "yes" or "no"). (See the next section for a discussion of misclassification of exposure variables with more than two categories.)

In the hypothetical example shown in Exhibit 4–2, misclassification occurs in only one direction: exposed individuals are misclassified as unexposed. However, often misclassification occurs in both directions: that is, exposed subjects are classified as unexposed or "false negatives" (ie, the correct classification of the truly exposed, or sensitivity, is less than 100%), and unexposed subjects are classified as exposed or "false positives" (ie, the correct classification of the unexposed, or specificity, is less than 100%). In a case-control study, nondifferential misclassification occurs when the sensitivity and specificity of the classification of exposure are the same for cases and controls but are less than 100%. Estimation of the total numbers of

---

Exhibit 4–2 Hypothetical Example of the Effect of Nondifferential Misclassification of Two Categories of Exposure, with 30% of Both Exposed Cases and Exposed Controls Misclassified as Unexposed

No Misclassification

Exposure	Cases	Controls
Yes	50	20
No	50	80

$$OR = \frac{\left(\dfrac{50}{50}\right)}{\left(\dfrac{20}{80}\right)} = 4.0$$

30% Exposure Misclassification in Each Group

Exposure	Cases	Controls
Yes	50 − **15** = 35	20 − **6** = 14
No	50 + **15** = 65	80 + **6** = 86

$$OR = \frac{\left(\dfrac{35}{65}\right)}{\left(\dfrac{14}{86}\right)} = 3.3$$

Effect of nondifferential misclassification with two exposure categories: to bias the OR toward the null value of 1.0. (It "dilutes" the association.)

Note: Bold numbers represent misclassified individuals

individuals classified as "exposed" or "unexposed" by using a study's data collection procedures and exposure level definitions is akin to the estimation of "test-positive" and "test-negative" individuals when applying a screening test. Thus, the notions of sensitivity and specificity, schematically represented in Figure 4–4, can be used to explore the issue of misclassification in more depth.

A hypothetical example showing nondifferential misclassification of exposure in a case-control study in both directions—that is, exposed subjects are misclassified as unexposed, and unexposed as exposed—is presented in Exhibit 4–3. The exhibit shows the effects of nondifferential misclassification resulting from an exposure ascertainment with a sensitivity of 90% and a specificity of 80%. The fact that these sensitivity and specificity values are the same for cases and controls identifies this type of misclassification as nondifferential.

The net effect of misclassifying *cases* at a sensitivity of 90% and a specificity of 80% is shown on column (III) of Exhibit 4–3. The totals in column (III) indicate the numbers of cases classified as "exposed" or "unexposed" in the study and reflect the misclassification due to the less-than-perfect sensitivity and specificity values. Thus, cases classified as "exposed" include both the 45 persons truly exposed

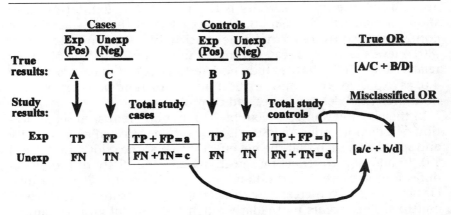

Pos = positives; Neg = negatives; TP = true positives; TN = true negatives; FP = false positives; FN = false negatives

Figure 4–4 Application of sensitivity/specificity concepts in misclassification of exposure: schematic representation of true and misclassified relative odds. Sensitivity of exposure ascertainment = TP ÷ (TP + FN); specificity of exposure ascertainment = TN ÷ (TN + FP).

Exhibit 4–3 Effects of Nondifferential Misclassification on the Odds Ratio
(Sensitivity = 0.90; Specificity = 0.80)

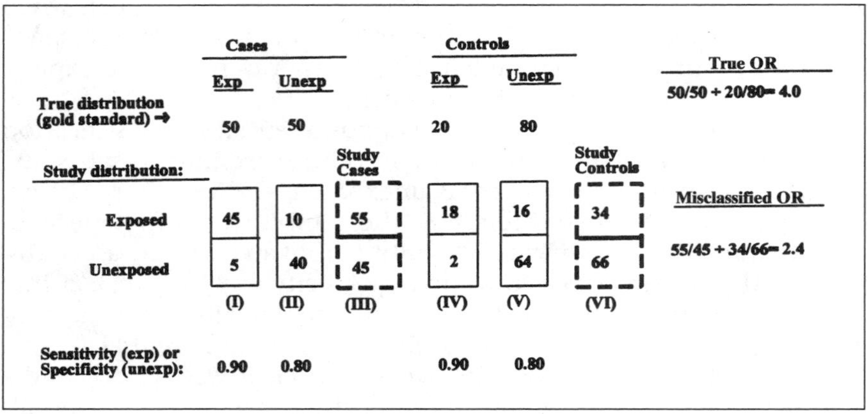

("true positives") and the 10 cases who, although unexposed, are misclassified as exposed ("false positives") due to a specificity less than 100% (see also Figure 4–4). Similarly, cases classified in the study as "unexposed" include both the 40 truly unexposed cases ("true negatives") and the 5 exposed cases misclassified as unexposed ("false negatives") because the sensitivity is less than 100%. Exhibit 4–3 also shows similar data for *controls*. The net effect of the classification of controls by exposure at the same sensitivity (90%) and specificity (80%) levels as those of cases is shown in column (VI). The observed relative odds of 2.4 in the study underestimates the true odds ratio of 4.0, as expected when misclassification of a dichotomous exposure is nondifferential between cases and controls.

In the example shown in Exhibit 4–3, nondifferential misclassification of a dichotomous exposure is shown to be affected by sensitivity and specificity, such that the net effect is to bias the odds ratio toward 1.0. In addition to reflecting sensitivity and specificity of the procedures for exposure definition and ascertainment, the degree of misclassification also increases with decreasing exposure prevalence in controls. This occurs particularly when the control group's sample size greatly outnumbers that of the case group: using the same sensitivity and specificity figures as in Exhibit 4–3, a hypothetical example is shown in Exhibit 4–4, in which a true odds ratio of 8.1 is severely biased toward 1.0 because of the large number of controls and their relatively low exposure prevalence. (This notion is akin to the effect of a low disease prevalence on positive predictive value when apply-

Exhibit 4–4 Effect of Nondifferential Misclassification on the Odds Ratio When the Exposure Prevalence in Controls Is Low and the Sample Size Is Much Greater in Controls than in Cases

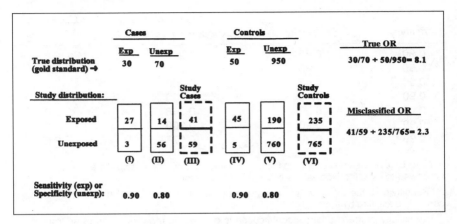

ing a test for early disease detection). Table 4–5 shows examples of the effects of sensitivity, specificity, and exposure prevalence in controls on the observed odds ratio when the true odds ratio is 4.0.

Nondifferential Misclassification When There Are More Than Two Categories. The rule that the direction of a nondifferential misclassification bias always dilutes the strength of the association may not hold in certain nondifferential misclassification situations involving more than two exposure categories. In a hypothetical example discussed by Dosemeci et al[24] involving three exposure levels in a case control study ("none," "low," and "high") (Table 4–6), 40% of both cases and controls in the "high" exposure category were misclassified as belonging to the adjacent category, "low"; the net effect was an increase in the odds ratio for the "low" category without a change for the "high." Misclassification for nonadjacent categories of exposure in the example—that is, between "high" and "none"—resulted in the disappearance of the truly graded relationship and, assuming no random error, the emergence of a J-shaped pattern. Additionally, as shown by Dosemeci et al, misclassification of nonadjacent exposure categories may invert the direction of the graded relationship.

Differential Misclassification

Differential misclassification occurs when the degree of misclassification differs between the groups being compared. Whereas the general tendency of nondifferential misclassification of a dichotomous

Table 4–5 Nondifferential Misclassification: Hypothetical Examples of the Effects of Sensitivity and Specificity of Exposure Identification and of Exposure Prevalence in Controls on a Study's Odds Ratio When the True Odds Ratio Is 4.0

Sensitivity*	Specificity†	Prevalence of Exposure in Controls	Observed Odds Ratio
0.90	0.85	0.200	2.6
0.60	0.85	0.200	1.9
0.90	**0.95**	0.200	3.2
0.90	**0.60**	0.200	1.9
0.90	0.90	**0.368**	3.0
0.90	0.90	**0.200**	2.8
0.90	0.90	0.077	2.2

Note: Bold figures represent the factor (sensitivity, specificity, or exposure prevalence) that is allowed to vary, for fixed values of the other two factors.

*Sensitivity of the exposure identification is defined as the proporton of all truly exposed correctly classified by the study.

†Specificity of the exposure identification is defined as the proportion of all truly unexposed correctly classified by the study.

exposure factor is to weaken a true association, differential misclassification may bias the association either toward or away from the null hypothesis. Furthermore, it is difficult to predict the direction of the bias when differential misclassification occurs, as it is the result of a complex interplay involving differences in sensitivity, specificity, and prevalence of exposure between cases and controls.

A hypothetical example of differential misclassification is given in Exhibit 4–5, in which the sensitivity of capturing the exposure in cases is 96% and that in controls is only 70%. Specificity in the example is 100% in both cases and controls. The better sensitivity among cases leads to a higher proportion of truly exposed subjects being identified in cases than in controls, yielding a biased odds ratio further away from 1.0 than the true odds ratio (true OR = 4.0, biased OR = 5.7). To underscore the difficulties in predicting results when there is differential misclassification, if the same calculations are done using a higher specificity in cases (100%) than in controls (80%), the odds ratio is biased toward the null hypothesis (Exhibit 4–6), as a poorer specificity in controls offsets the higher sensitivity in cases.

Examples of the isolated effects of sensitivity (for a specificity of 100%) or specificity (for a sensitivity of 100%) on the odds ratio in a hypothetical case-control study with differential misclassification of

Table 4–6 Examples of the Effects of Nondifferential Misclassification Involving Three Exposure Categories; Misclassification of 40% Between "High" and "Low" **(A)** and Between "High" and "None" **(B)**

Case-Control Status	Exposure Status		
	None	Low	High
True distribution			
Cases	100	200	600
Controls	100	100	100
Odds ratio	1.00	2.00	6.00
A. Adjacent categories: 40% of cases and controls in "high" misclassified as "low"			
Cases	100	200 CC + 240 MC = 440	600 CC − 240 MC = 360
Controls	100	100 CC + 40 MC = 140	100 CC − 40 MC = 60
Odds ratio	1.00	3.14	6.00
B. Nonadjacent categories: 40% of cases and controls in "high" misclassified as "none"			
Cases	100 CC + 240 MC = 340	200	600 CC − 240 MC = 360
Controls	100 CC + 40 MC = 140	100	100 CC − 40 MC = 60
Odds ratio	1.00	0.82	2.47

Note: CC, correctly classified; MC, misclassified.
Source: Data from M Dosemeci,S Wacholder, and JH Lubin, Does Nondifferential Misclassification of Exposure Always Bias a True Effect Toward the Null Value? *American Journal of Epidemiology,* Vol 132, pp 746–748, © 1990, The Johns Hopkins University School of Hygiene & Public Health.

Exhibit 4–5 Hypothetical example of the Effect of Differential Misclassification on the Odds Ratio, in Which, for Sensitivity, Cases > Controls, and, for Specificity, Cases = Controls

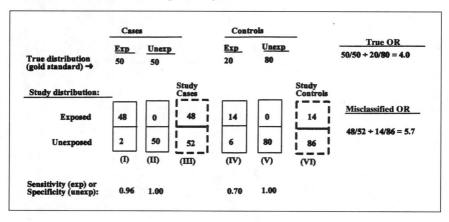

Exhibit 4–6 Hypothetical Example of the Effect of Differential Misclassification on the Odds Ratio, in Which for Both Sensitivity and Specificity, Cases > Controls

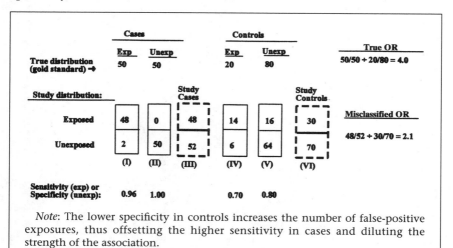

Note: The lower specificity in controls increases the number of false-positive exposures, thus offsetting the higher sensitivity in cases and diluting the strength of the association.

exposure and a control exposure prevalence of 10% are shown in Table 4–7.

An example of differential misclassification of exposure was documented by Weinstock et al.[10] This example was used above to illustrate the concept of recall bias (see Section 4.3.1). In this study, melanoma cases and controls selected from participants of the Nurses Health Study cohort were compared with regard to their report of "hair color" and "tanning ability" both at baseline and after the case was diagnosed. In this example, the differential misclassification probably occurred because the disease status was known to the participant and had the potential to affect recall of exposure. Therefore, the premelanoma diagnosis interview is assumed to accurately reflect the true association. The main results of the study are summarized in Table 4–8. For the discussion that follows, the categories associated with an increase in odds using the case-control data obtained after the occurrence of melanoma were regarded as "exposed" ("red or blond" and "no tan or light tan" for hair color and tanning ability, respectively).

Compared with the pre–disease development data, the odds for hair color increased slightly only for controls when the postmelanoma interview data were used (from 37:197 to 41:193); as a result, the odds ratio changed relatively little (prediagnosis OR = 2.5, postdiagnosis OR = 2.3). The effect of differential misclassification of tanning ability, however, was severe, leading to a reversal of the direction of the

---

Table 4–7 Examples of the Effects of Differential Sensitivity and Specificity of Exposure Ascertainment on the Odds Ratio (OR) for a True OR of 3.86 and a Control Exposure Prevalence of 0.10

Exposure Ascertainment				
Sensitivity*		Specificity†		
Cases	Controls	Cases	Controls	Odds Ratio
0.90	0.60	1.00	1.00	5.79
0.60	0.90	1.00	1.00	2.22
1.00	1.00	0.90	0.70	1.00
1.00	1.00	0.70	0.90	4.43

*Sensitivity of the exposure identification is defined as the proportion of all truly exposed correctly classified by the study.

†Specificity of the exposure identification is defined as the proportion of all truly unexposed correctly classified by the study.

Table 4–8 Reported Hair Color and Tanning Ability among Incident Cases and Controls in a Case-Control Study of Melanoma Within the Nurses Health Study Cohort

	Premelanoma Diagnosis Information ("Gold Standard")		Postmelanoma Diagnosis Information	
	Cases	Controls	Cases	Controls
Hair Color				
Red or blond (exposed)	11	37	11	41
Brown or black (unexposed)	23	197	23	193
Odds ratio	2.5		2.3	
Tanning Ability				
No tan, practically no tan, or light tan (exposed)	9	79	15	77
Medium, average, deep, or dark tan (unexposed)	25	155	19	157
Odds ratio	0.7		1.6	

Source: Data from MA Weinstock et al, Recall (Report) Bias and Reliability in the Retrospective Assessment of Melanoma Risk, *American Journal of Epidemiology*, Vol 133, pp 240–245, © 1991, The Johns Hopkins University School of Hygiene & Public Health.

association: assuming no random variability, the true association (ie, that detected using the premelanoma diagnosis information) denotes a protective effect (OR = 0.7), whereas the observed postdiagnosis association (OR = 1.6) suggests a greater melanoma odds associated with a low tanning ability. It is of interest that the misclassification of exposure as measured by tanning ability seems to have been slight in controls (the odds of exposure changed from 79/155 to 77/157). In cases, however, the misclassification effect was substantial, with the number of individuals classified as "exposed" increasing from 9 to 15 between the first and the second interviews.

The cross-tabulation of the pre- and postmelanoma diagnosis data enables the calculation of sensitivity and specificity of tanning ability ascertainment in cases. As shown in Table 4–9, the sensitivity of 89% of the postmelanoma diagnosis interviews resulted in the correct classification of eight of the nine truly exposed cases. However, a specificity of only 72% led to a relatively large number of unexposed persons in the "false-positive" cell and thus to a marked increase in the postdiagnosis exposure odds (true exposure odds in cases, 9:25 or

Table 4–9 Distribution of Incident Cases in the Nurses' Health Study Cohort, 1976 to 1984, According to Responses Given with Regard to Tanning Ability Prior to the Development of Melanoma and after Diagnosis Was Made

| Postmelanoma Diagnosis Information | *Premelanoma Diagnosis Information ("Gold Standard")* | | |
	No Tan, Practically No Tan, or Light Tan ("Exposed")	*Medium, Average,Deep, or Dark Tan ("Unexposed")*	*Total (Case-Control Classification)*
No tan, practically no tan, or light tan ("exposed")	8 (TP)	7 (FP)	15
Medium, average, deep, or dark tan ("unexposed")	1 (FN)	18 (TN)	19
Total ("true" classification)	9	25	34
	Sensitivity: 8/9 = 89%	Specificity: 18/25 = 72%	

Note: TP, true positives; FP, false positives; FN, false negatives; TN, true negatives.

Source: Data from MA Weinstock et al, Recall (Report) Bias and Reliability in the Retrospective Assessment of Melanoma Risk, *American Journal of Epidemiology*, Vol 133, pp 240–245, © 1991, The Johns Hopkins University School of Hygiene & Public Health.

0.36:1.0; biased exposure odds, 15:19 or 0.79:1.0) such that the odds ratio in the postdiagnosis study is in a direction opposite to that of the true value. As mentioned previously (Section 4.3.1), differential misclassification in the study by Weinstock et al[10] probably occurred because of recall bias. Additional misclassification may have occurred because the questions on hair color and tanning ability were not exactly the same in the interviews conducted before and after diagnosis.

Effect of Misclassification of a Confounding Variable

Misclassification also affects the efficiency of adjustment for confounding effects. Whereas a nondifferential misclassification of a potential risk factor tends to bias the measure of association toward the null hypothesis, nondifferential misclassification of a confounding variable results in an imperfect adjustment due to residual confounding (see Section 7.5).[25]

Prevention of Misclassification

Misclassification has been extensively discussed in the epidemiological literature,[26-29] reflecting its importance in epidemiologic studies. As seen in the examples described in this section, misclassification may severely distort the magnitude of an association between a risk factor and a disease. If the true relative risk or odds ratio is close to 1.0, a nondifferential misclassification may completely mask the association: for example, for an exposure with a prevalence as high as 16% (not unlike that of many risk factors), if the true odds ratio is approximately 1.3, the observed odds ratio may be virtually 1.0 if a nondifferential misclassification resulted from a measurement procedure with both sensitivity and specificity levels of about 70%. Differential misclassification, on the other hand, may either dilute or strengthen an association or even produce a spurious one. When the exposure is common, failing to demonstrate a real relationship or inferring that a real association exists when it is spurious may have serious public health consequences.

Data are usually not available to allow a comparison between correctly classified and misclassified individuals in terms of available characteristics (eg, educational level), but when they are, they may be informative. As seen in Table 4-9, of the 34 incident cases included in the case-control study nested in the Nurses' Health Study cohort, 26 were correctly classified (8 true positives and 18 true negatives),[10] and 8 were misclassified (7 false positives and 1 false negative). A comparison could be made, for example, between the false positives and true negatives on the one hand (addressing the issue of specificity) and between the false negatives and true positives on the other (addressing the issue of sensitivity). In the Nurses' Health Study, the authors reported no important differences between the correctly and the incorrectly classified cases. (When studying tanning ability, it would not be unreasonable to postulate that recall of tanning ability could be influenced by factors such as family history of skin diseases or involvement in outdoor activities.) Similarity in pertinent characteristics of correctly classified and misclassified persons may perhaps indicate that recall bias is not a probable explanation for the misclassification and raises the possibility that the information bias originated from problems related to the instrument or the observer. Thus, the comparison between misclassified and nonmisclassified subjects need not be limited to respondent characteristics and should also include potential problems in the data collection procedures. When interviews are taped, adherence to the protocol by interviewers can be compared. Additionally, information should be obtained on the reliability and validity of the instrument (eg, a questionnaire), as discussed in Chapter 8.

Prevention of misclassification of exposure and outcome is a function of the "state-of-the-art" measurement techniques that can be safely applied to the large number of subjects participating in epidemiologic studies. Use of objective (eg, biologic) markers of exposure and more accurate diagnostic techniques for ascertainment of outcomes, such as the use of ultrasound to diagnose asymptomatic atherosclerosis,[12] constitutes the most efficient approach for ameliorating the problems related to misclassification bias. In the meantime, if sensitivity and specificity of outcome or exposure measurements are known, it is possible to correct for misclassification using available formulas that estimate a "corrected RR," for example, as a function of the "observed RR" and the estimated sensitivity and specificity of exposure classification in the study.[27–30] Furthermore, correction methods that can be applied to situations in which measurement errors affect both exposure variables and covariates (either categorical or continuous variables) have been described.[31]

4.4 COMBINED SELECTION/INFORMATION BIASES

This section discusses biases that have both selection and information components. These include biases related to medical surveillance, cross-sectional studies, and screening evaluation. The sections on cross-sectional and screening evaluation biases may seem somewhat repetitious vis-à-vis previous discussions on selection and information biases in this chapter. They have, however, been included here because they include examples specific to these areas and thus may be of special value to those especially interested in cross-sectional and screening intervention studies.

4.4.1 Medical Surveillance (or Detection) Bias

In this type of bias, the occurrence of a presumably medically relevant exposure leads to a closer surveillance for study outcomes that, particularly if subclinical, may result in a higher probability of detection in exposed individuals. Thus, medical surveillance bias occurs when the identification of the outcome is not independent of the knowledge of the exposure. For example, certain exposures may lead to a closer medical surveillance, expressed by more frequent medical encounters or more thorough questioning and examination of patients during an encounter.

Medical surveillance bias is particularly likely when the exposure is a medical condition or therapy that leads to frequent and detailed checkups—such as diabetes or use of oral contraceptives—and the outcome is a disease characterized by a high proportion of subclinical cases and thus more likely to be diagnosed during the frequent medical encounters resulting from the need to monitor the "exposure." For example, although there may be no basis to believe that oral contraceptive use can lead to renal failure, a spurious association would be observed if women taking oral contraceptives were more likely to have medical checkups, including repeated measurements of serum creatinine concentration.

Medical surveillance bias can be regarded as a type of either selection bias, because the identification of the outcome is influenced by the presence of the exposure, or information bias, because the exposed undergo a more thorough examination than the unexposed individuals.

Medical surveillance bias is more likely to occur when the outcome is ascertained through regular medical channels. Alternatively, *when the outcome is assessed systematically, regardless of exposure, using a concurrent prospective design,* medical surveillance bias is less likely to occur.[3] Thus, meticulously standardized methods of outcome ascertainment are routinely used in most major cohort studies, such as the classical Framingham study[32] or the ARIC study.[12]

Another strategy to prevent medical surveillance bias that can be used when conducting cohort studies is to *mask exposure status when ascertaining the presence of the outcome.* If these strategies are not feasible, as when carrying out a case-control study in which the disease diagnosis may have already been affected by the presence of the exposure, *information should be obtained on the frequency, intensity, and quality of medical care received by study participants for analytic purposes.* For example, to assess the relationship between use of hormone replacement therapy and a given disease with a subclinical component (eg, non–insulin-dependent diabetes) using a traditional case-control design, it is important to take into account medical care indicators, such as the frequency of medical visits in the past and whether the individual has medical insurance. Because education and socioeconomic status are usually related to availability and use of medical care, they too should be taken into consideration when trying to prevent surveillance bias.

It also is possible to *obtain information on variables that indicate awareness of health problems,* such as compliance with screening exams and knowledge of subclinical disease or of results of blood measurements. For example, in a prospective study of the relationship of vasectomy to the risk of prostatic cancer, the possibility of surveillance bias was assessed by examining variables that might reflect greater utilization of medical care.[33] No differences were found between subjects who had and those who had not had vasectomy with regard to their knowledge of their blood pressure or serum cholesterol levels. The percentages who had had screening sigmoidoscopy were also similar, leading the authors to conclude that men with vasectomy were not under a greater degree of medical surveillance. In addition, the frequency of digital rectal examinations was similar between the vasectomized (exposed) and the nonvasectomized (unexposed) groups, implying equal access to a procedure that may lead to the diagnosis of the study outcome.

Finally, when medical surveillance bias occurs, the disease tends to be diagnosed earlier in exposed than in unexposed individuals; as a result, the proportion of less advanced disease in a cohort study is higher in the exposed group. In a case-control study, the bias is denoted by the fact that the association is found to be stronger or present only for the less advanced cases. In the cohort study discussed above, Giovannucci et al[33] found that the histological severity staging of prostate cancer was similar for vasectomized and nonvasectomized persons, a finding inconsistent with what would be expected if medical surveillance had been more intensive in the vasectomized group. *Stratification by disease severity at diagnosis* is thus an additional strategy to examine and take into consideration the possibility of surveillance bias.

4.4.2 Cross-Sectional Biases

Cross-sectional biases can be classified as incidence-prevalence bias and temporal bias. The former is a type of selection bias, whereas the latter can be regarded as an information bias.

Incidence-Prevalence Bias

Incidence-prevalence bias results from the inclusion of prevalent cases into the study. As discussed in Chapter 3 (Section 3.3), the strength of an association is sometimes estimated using the prevalence rate ratio rather than the relative risk, as when analyzing data from a cross-sectional survey or when assessing cross-sectional associations at baseline in a cohort study. If the investigator is interested in assessing potentially causal associations, the use of the prevalence rate ratio as an estimate of the incidence rate ratio is subject to bias.

Equation 2.3, described in Chapter 2 (Section 2.3), shows the dependence of the point prevalence odds [Prev/(1 − Prev)] on incidence (Inc) and disease duration (Dur), assuming that incidence and duration are approximately constant:

$$\frac{\text{Prev}}{1.0 - \text{Prev}} = \text{Inc} \times \text{Dur}$$

Equation 2.3 can be rewritten as Equation 2.4:

$$\text{Prev} = \text{Inc} \times \text{Dur} \times (1.0 - \text{Prev})$$

thus demonstrating that, in addition to incidence and duration, prevalence is a function of the term (1.0 − Prev) (which, in turn, obviously depends on the magnitude of the point prevalence rate).

Equation 2.4 shows that a point prevalence rate ratio (PRR) comparing exposed (denoted by subscript "+") and unexposed (denoted by subscript "−") individuals, obtained in cross-sectional studies, is a function of (1) the incidence rate ratio (IRR), (2) the ratio of the disease duration in exposed individuals to that in unexposed individuals, and (3) the ratio of the term (1.0 − Prev) in exposed individuals to the same term in unexposed individuals. Ratios 2 and 3 represent two types of incidence-prevalence bias, ie, the *duration ratio bias* and the *point prevalence complement ratio bias*, respectively, when the PRR is used to estimate the IRR (see Section 3.3):

$$\text{PRR} = \left(\frac{\text{Inc}_+}{\text{Inc}_-}\right) \times \left(\frac{\text{Dur}_+}{\text{Dur}_-}\right) \times \left(\frac{1.0 - \text{Prev}_+}{1.0 - \text{Prev}_-}\right)$$

Duration Ratio Bias. This type of bias (which can be thought of as a type of selection bias) occurs when one is using the PRR as a measure of association and the duration of the disease after its onset is different between exposed and unexposed persons. (Since duration of a chronic disease is so often related to survival, this type of bias may be also designated as *survival bias*.) For diseases of low prevalence, when the duration (or prognosis) of the disease is independent of the exposure (ie, duration is the same in exposed and unexposed), the PRR is a virtually unbiased estimate of the IRR. On the other hand, when exposure not only increases disease risk but also affects its prognosis, bias will be present, as shown in the examples below.

Point Prevalence Complement Ratio Bias. If duration is independent of exposure, regardless of the direction of the effect of the factor on the outcome, the PRR tends to underestimate the *strength* of the association between the exposure and the outcome (ie, it biases the IRR toward 1.0). The magnitude of this bias depends on both the PRR and the absolute magnitude of the point prevalence rates. When the point prevalence rate is higher in exposed than in unexposed individuals (PRR > 1.0), the point prevalence complement ratio, $(1.0 - \text{Prev}_+)/(1.0 - \text{Prev}_-)$, is less than 1.0. It is close to 1.0 when the point prevalence rates are low in both exposed and unexposed, even if the PRR is relatively high. For example, if the prevalence of the disease in exposed subjects is 0.04 and that in unexposed subjects is 0.01, the PRR is high ($0.04/0.01 = 4.0$), but the bias resulting from the point prevalence complement ratio is merely $0.96/0.99 = 0.97 \approx 1.0$. On the other hand, when the prevalence is relatively high in exposed individuals, the point prevalence complement ratio can be markedly less than 1.0, thus resulting in important bias. For example, if the prevalence of the disease in exposed subjects is 0.40 and that in unexposed subjects is 0.10, the PRR is the same as in the previous example (4.0); however, the point prevalence complement ratio is $0.6/0.90 = 0.67$: that is, the PRR underestimates the IRR by 33%. The influence of the magnitude of prevalence is sometimes felt even for a low PRR. For example, if the point prevalence rates are 0.40 in exposed and 0.25 in unexposed subjects, the PRR is fairly small (1.6), but the bias factor is 0.80: that is, the PRR underestimates the IRR by 20%. Obviously, the bias will be greatest when both the PRR and the prevalence rate in one of the groups (exposed or unexposed) are high. For studies of factors that decrease the prevalence of the disease (ie, PRR < 1.0), the reciprocal reasoning applies: that is, $(1.0 - \text{Prev}_+)/(1.0 - \text{Prev}_-)$ will be greater than 1.0, and the magnitude of the bias will also be affected by the absolute rates.

Examples of Incidence-Prevalence Biases. In the examples that follow, it is assumed that incidence and duration according to exposure have remained stable over time.

- *Gender and acute myocardial infarction in US whites*: White US males have a much higher risk of myocardial infarction than females. However, some studies have shown that, even after careful age adjustment, females have a shorter average survival than males.[34] Thus, the ratio ($\text{Dur}_{males}/\text{Dur}_{females}$) tends to be greater than 1.0, and as a consequence, the PRR expressing the relationship of sex to myocardial infarction overestimates the IRR.
- *Current smoking and emphysema*: Smoking substantially increases the risk of emphysema. In addition, survival (and thus duration of the disease) in emphysema patients who continue to smoke after diagnosis is shorter than in those who quit smoking. As a result, PRRs estimated in cross-sectional studies evaluating the asso-

ciation between current smoking and emphysema tend to underestimate the IRR.

- *PPD reaction and clinical tuberculosis*: In assessments of the relationship between the size of the PPD skin test reaction and clinical tuberculosis, PRRs were shown to underestimate IRRs in a
population-based study carried out by George Comstock and colleagues (unpublished observations) a few decades ago (Figure
4–5). This underestimation was likely due to the relatively high
prevalence of clinical tuberculosis in this population at the time
the study was carried out and thus to the occurrence of prevalence complement ratio bias.

Prevention of Incidence-Prevalence Bias. If the goal is to evaluate potential disease determinants, whenever possible, incident cases
should be used in order to avoid incidence-prevalence bias. Inci-

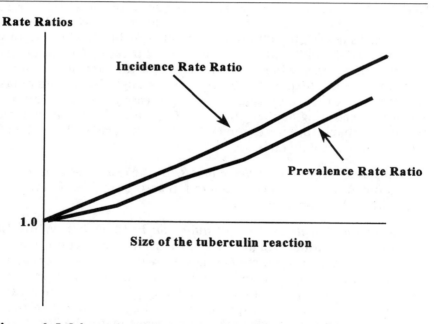

Figure 4–5 Schematic representation of the results of the study by Comstock et al (unpublished) evaluating the relationship of size of PPD reaction
to clinical tuberculosis. After an initial cross-sectional survey conducted in
1946, the cohort was followed over time for determinaton of incidence rates.
Source: Data from GW Comstock et al, personal communication.

dence-prevalence bias, although more easily conceptualized by comparing incidence with prevalence (cross-sectional) rate ratio data, may also occur in case-control studies when prevalent rather than only newly developed (incident) cases are used. For example, if smoking decreases survival after diagnosis, thereby decreasing the disease's duration (as in myocardial infarction), a case-control study based on prevalent cases may include a higher proportion of nonsmoking cases (as smokers would have been selected out by death) than would a study based on incident cases, thus diluting the strength of the association (see Chapter 1, Figure 1–19).

Another problem in case-control studies is that newly *diagnosed* cases are used as proxies for newly *developed* cases. Thus, for diseases that may evolve subclinically for many years prior to diagnosis, such as chronic lymphocytic leukemia, diabetes, or renal failure, presumed incident cases are in fact a mix of incident and prevalent cases, and incidence-prevalence bias may occur unbeknownst to the investigator. A cohort study efficiently prevents incidence-prevalence bias if its procedures include the careful ascertainment and exclusion of prevalent cases at baseline and a systematic and periodic search of newly developed clinical and subclinical outcomes.

Temporal Bias

Temporal bias occurs when the proper temporal sequence needed to establish causality, risk factor $\rightarrow$ disease, cannot be firmly established. In other words, it is difficult to know which came first, the exposure to the potential risk factor or the disease.

Temporal bias typically occurs in cross-sectional surveys when information is lacking on the time sequence with regard to the presumed risk factor and the outcome. For example, because exposure and outcome data are collected at the same point in time, results from a prevalence survey may establish a statistical association between high serum creatinine levels and the occurrence of high blood pressure. Because the time sequence cannot be established, a cross-sectional association between these variables may mean either that high serum creatinine (a marker of kidney failure) leads to hypertension or vice versa. A prospective study in which blood pressure levels are measured in persons with normal serum creatinine levels who are then followed over time for ascertainment of hypercreatininemia can obviously identify the proper temporal sequence and thus lend support to the conclusion that HBP predicts incipient renal insufficiency.[35]

Temporal bias may also occur in case-control studies—even those including only newly developed (incident) cases—when the suspected exposure is measured after disease diagnosis in cases. For example, because clinically detected viral hepatitis is myelotoxic, it has been suggested that exposure to hepatitis B virus (HBV) may be an etiologic factor for the so-called idiopathic aplastic anemia (AA).[36] However, temporal bias could explain the relationship between HBV and AA in a case-control study if serum samples for determination of HBV antibody and antigen levels had been collected after AA onset, as individuals with undiagnosed aplastic anemia may receive transfusions of blood contaminated with HBV even before a diagnosis is made. Thus, the inferred sequence is HBV → AA, but the true sequence is undiagnosed AA → blood transfusion → diagnosed AA.

An example of the reasoning underlying the possibility of temporal bias is given by the association between estrogen replacement therapy (ERT) in postmenopausal women and endometrial cancer.[37] Although the causal nature of this association is currently well established, it was initially disputed on the grounds that a higher likelihood of using ERT resulted from symptoms occurring as a consequence of incipient, undiagnosed endometrial cancer.[38] Thus, instead of the sequence ERT → endometrial cancer, the true sequence would be undiagnosed endometrial cancer → symptoms → ERT → diagnosed endometrial cancer.

Another example of temporal bias is given by a cross-sectional study of Dutch children, in which negative associations were found of pet ownership with allergy, respiratory symptoms, and asthma.[39] As aptly postulated by the study's investigators, these results may well have resulted from the fact that families are likely to remove from the home (or not acquire) pets after such manifestations occur. This study also underscores why the term *reverse causality* is occasionally used in connection with a temporal bias of this sort.

Another example of this type of bias was suggested by Nieto et al,[40] who found that the relationship of current smoking to clinical atherosclerosis (defined by self-reported physician-diagnosed heart attack or cardiac surgery) was much stronger when using longitudinal than when using cross-sectional data (in contrast to the association between smoking and subclinical atherosclerosis, which was about equally strong for the longitudinal and the cross-sectional data). Among the possible explanations offered by these authors for these findings was that occurrence of a heart attack (but not the presence of subclinical atherosclerosis) may lead to smoking cessation and thus to a dilution of the association when using prevalent cases (cross-sectionally). This type of bias may occur even in prospective analyses when the outcome of interest is mortality. For example, the short-term mortality from lung cancer can be higher in former than in current smokers due to the tendency of symptomatic individuals or those for whom a diagnosis has been made to quit smoking. Epidemiologists usually handle this bias by excluding from the analysis the deaths that occur within a specified period after the beginning of the study.

To prevent temporal bias, in a cross-sectional survey, it is occasionally possible to improve the information on temporality when obtaining data through questionnaires. Temporality pertaining to potential risk factors such as smoking, physical activity, and occupational exposures can be ascertained in cross-sectional samples by means of questions such as "When were you first exposed to. . . ?" For some chronic diseases, such as angina pectoris, it is also possible to obtain information on the date of onset. The investigators can then establish the temporal sequence between risk factor and disease—assuming, of course, that the information from surveyed individuals is accurate. (Obviously, even if temporality can be established in a cross-sectional study, the investigator will still have the incidence-prevalence bias to contend with.) When the date of the beginning of the exposure is unknown, as in the example of viral hepatitis and aplastic anemia, the only solution is to use prospective data on exposure and outcome (a formidable challenge in this example, given the rarity of aplastic anemia).

Finally, it may be possible to assess temporal bias occurring because the presumed exposure is a consequence of undiagnosed disease—as in the example of ERT and endometrial cancer above—by considering why the exposure occurred. In the study of Antunes et al,[37] for instance, data can be stratified according to indication for ERT use, such as bleeding; if temporal bias is not a likely explanation for the relationship of estrogen to endometrial cancer, the association will be observed both for individuals who were prescribed estrogens because they were bleeding and for those who were given estrogens for other reasons (eg, prevention of osteoporosis).

4.4.3 Biases Related to the Evaluation of Screening Interventions

Like any other epidemiologic study, studies of the evaluation of screening interventions are also prone to biases, of which four types are particularly relevant: selection bias, incidence-prevalence bias, length bias, and lead time bias. (For a better understanding of these types of bias, the reader should review the concepts underlying the natural history of disease; see, eg, Gordis.)[9]

Selection Bias

Selection bias stems from the fact that when the evaluation of screening relies on an observational design, the groups under comparison may differ substantially with regard to the reasons for screening. Thus, for example, persons who attend a screening program may be of a higher socioeconomic status than those who do not and may therefore have a better prognosis regardless of the effectiveness of the screening program. *Prevention* of this type of selection bias is best carried by using an experimental design. Whereas this type of bias affects the internal validity of the study, a bias affecting its external validity occurs when the effectiveness of screening (or of any other intervention) varies according to the characteristics of the study population, making it difficult to generalize its results to other populations.

Incidence-Prevalence Bias

Survival bias results from comparing prognosis in prevalent cases detected in the first screen, which is akin to a cross-sectional survey, with that in incident cases detected in subsequent screenings. This bias occurs because prevalent cases include long-term survivors, who have a better average survival than that of incident cases, in whom the full spectrum of severity is represented. This type of bias may occur in "pre-post" studies, as when comparing a screening strategy used in the first screening exam ("pre") that identifies prevalent cases with a different strategy used in subsequent screens identifying incident cases ("post").

A related bias is the so-called *length bias*, which occurs when a better prognosis for cases detected directly by the screening procedure (eg, occult blood test for colorectal cancer) than for cases diagnosed between screening exams is used as evidence that the screening program is effective. To understand this type of bias, it is important to briefly review some key concepts related to the natural history of a disease and screening.

The effectiveness of screening is positively related to the length of the detectable preclinical phase (DPCP; see Figure 4–6 and, for definitions, Table 4–10), which in turn reflects the rate at which the disease progresses. This means that for diseases with a rapid progression, it is difficult, if not outright impossible, to improve prognosis by means of early detection. For example, a short average DPCP and its attending

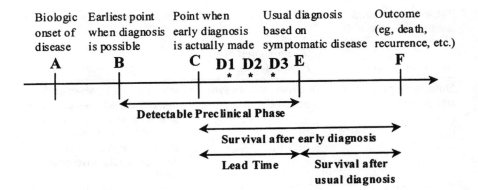

* Critical points

Figure 4–6 Natural history of a disease. *Source*: Reprinted with permission from L Gordis, *Epidemiology*, p 231, © 1996, WB Saunders Company.

poor survival characterizes most cases of lung cancer, for which screening generally is not effective. On the other hand, the long DPCP of in situ cervical cancer explains why treatment following a positive Pap smear denoting carcinoma in situ is related to a cure rate of virtually 100%.

Even for the same disease, regardless of screening, it can be shown that patients whose disease has a longer DPCP have a better prognosis than those whose disease has a shorter DPCP (eg, post- vs premenopausal breast cancer, respectively). For example, in the Health Insurance Plan (HIP) study of the efficacy of screening for breast cancer, the so-called "interval" cases—that is, cases who were clinically diagnosed during the interval between the screening exams—had, on average, a higher case fatality rate than subclinical cases diagnosed as a result of the screening exam.[41] Although some of these cases may have been false negatives missed by the screening exam and therefore not true interval cases, many were probably characterized by rapidly growing tumors—that is, by a short DPCP (Figure 4–7). It follows that when evaluating a screening program, one must take into careful consideration the fact that cases detected by the screening procedure (eg, mammography), who thus tend to have a longer DPCP, have an inherently better prognosis than the "interval" cases, *regardless of the effectiveness of screening*. Failure to do so results in length bias, which occurs when a better prognosis for screening-detected cases is used as evidence that the screening program is effective, when in reality it

Table 4–10 Natural History of a Disease: Definitions of Components Represented in Figure 4–6

Component	Represented in Figure 4–6 as. . .	Definition
Detectable preclinical phase	The interval between points B and E	Phase that starts when early diagnosis becomes possible and ends with the point in time when usual diagnosis based on symptomatic disease would have been made.
Critical points	D1, D2, and D3	Points beyond which early detection and treatment are less and less effective vis-à-vis treatment following usual diagnosis. Treatment is totally ineffective after the last critical point (point D3 in the figure).
Lead time	The interval between points C and E	Period between the point in time when early diagnosis was made and the point in time when the usual diagnosis (based on symptoms) would have been made.

Source: Data from L Gordis, *Epidemiology,* © 1996, WB Saunders Company.

may be due to the longer DPCP of these cases, reflecting a slower growing disease than that of interval cases.

Prevention of length bias can be accomplished by using an experimental approach and comparing the prognosis of *all* cases—which include cases with both short and long DPCPs—occurring in individuals randomly assigned to a screening program with that of all cases occurring in randomly assigned controls who do not undergo the screening exams.

Lead Time Bias

Lead time is the time by which diagnosis can be advanced by screening. It is the time between early diagnosis (Figure 4–6, point C) and the usual time when diagnosis would have been made if an early diagnosis test(s) had not been applied to the patient (Figure 4–6, point

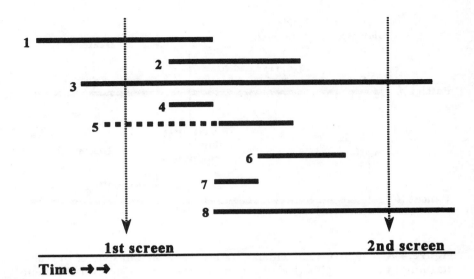

Figure 4–7 Schematic representation of the length of the detectable preclinical phase (DPCP) in cases occurring during a screening program. Cases with a longer DPCP (cases no. 1, 3, and 8) have a higher probability of identification at each screening exam. Cases with a shorter DPCP occurring between screening exams are the "interval" cases (cases no. 2, 4, 6, and 7). Case no. 5 is a false negative (missed by the first exam).

E; see also Table 4–10). The lead time, therefore, is contained within the DPCP.

When evaluating effectiveness of screening, lead time bias occurs when survival (or recurrence-free time) is counted from the point in time when early diagnosis was made. Thus, even if screening is ineffective, the early diagnosis adds lead time to the survival counted from the time of usual diagnosis. Survival may then be increased from time of early diagnosis but not from the biologic onset of the disease (Figure 4–8).[42]

Lead time bias occurs only when estimating survival (or time-to-event) from time of diagnosis. Thus, lead time bias can be avoided by calculating the mortality risk or rate among all screened and control subjects rather than the cumulative probability of survival (or its complement, the cumulative case fatality probability) from diagnosis among cases.[9] If survival from diagnosis is chosen as the strategy to describe the results of the evaluation of a screening approach, the average duration of lead time must be estimated and taken into account when comparing survival after diagnosis between screened and non-

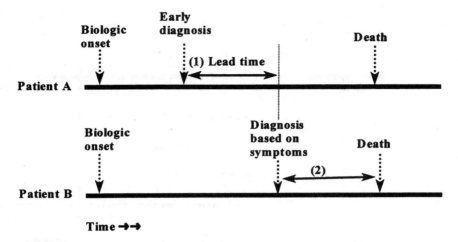

Figure 4–8 Schematic representation of lead time bias: in spite of the early diagnosis by screening, survival of patient A is the same as survival of patient B, whose disease was diagnosed because of clinical symptoms, because Survival(A) = (1) lead time + (2) Survival(B). *Source:* Reprinted with permission from L Gordis, *Epidemiology,* p 235, © 1996, WB Saunders Company.

screened groups. For survival to be regarded as increased from the biologic onset, it has to be corrected for lead time: that is, it should be greater than the survival after usual diagnosis plus lead time (Figure 4–9). It is thus important to estimate average lead time.

If the disease for a given individual is identified through screening, it is impossible to know when "usual" diagnosis would have been made if screening had not been carried out. Thus, it is not possible to estimate the lead time for individual patients, only an *average* lead time. What follows is a simplified description of the basic approach used to estimate average lead time. A more detailed account of lead time estimation is beyond the scope of this intermediate methods text and can be found elsewhere.[42]

The first step in the estimation of the average lead time is the estimation of the average duration of the DPCP. As mentioned previously, the lead time is a component of the DPCP. Thus, to estimate the average lead time, it is first necessary to estimate the average duration of the DPCP (Dur_{DPCP}), using the known relationship between prevalence ($Prev_{DPCP}$) and incidence (Inc_{DPCP}) of preclinical cases: that is, cases in the DPCP (see also Chapter 2, Section 2.3, Equation 2.4):

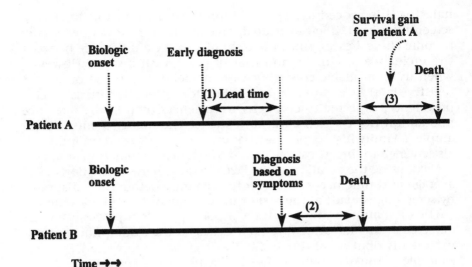

Figure 4–9 Schematic representation of lead time bias: survival of patient A from early diagnosis is better than survival of patient B, because Survival(A) > (1) lead time + (2) Survival(B). *Source:* Reprinted with permission from L Gordis, *Epidemiology*, p 235, © 1996, WB Saunders Company.

$$\text{Prev}_{\text{DPCP}} = \text{Inc}_{\text{DPCP}} \times \text{Dur}_{\text{DPCP}} \times (1.0 - \text{Prev}_{\text{DPCP}})$$

The duration of the DPCP can then be easily derived as

$$\text{Dur}_{\text{DPCP}} = \frac{\text{Prev}_{\text{DPCP}}}{\text{Inc}_{\text{DPCP}} \times (1.0 - \text{Prev}_{\text{DPCP}})}$$

If the prevalence of the disease is not too high (eg, no greater than about 5%), $1.0 - \text{Prev}_{\text{DPCP}}$ will be close to 1.0, and thus the equation above can be simplified:

$$\text{Dur}_{\text{DPCP}} \approx \frac{\text{Prev}_{\text{DPCP}}}{\text{Inc}_{\text{DPCP}}}$$

To apply this formula, the $\text{Prev}_{\text{DPCP}}$ is estimated using data from the first screening exam of the target population, which is equivalent to a cross-sectional survey. The Inc_{DPCP} can be estimated in successive screening exams among screenees found to be disease-free at the time of the first screening. An alternative way to estimate Inc_{DPCP}, and one that does not require following-up screenees, is to use the incidence of clinical disease in the reference population, if available. The rationale for this procedure, and an important assumption justifying screening, is that, if left untreated, preclinical cases would necessarily become clinical cases; thus, there should not be a difference between the incidence of clinical and that of preclinical disease. However, when using available clinical disease incidence (eg, based on cancer registry data), it is important to adjust for differences in risk factor prevalence, expected to be higher in screenees than in the reference population from which clinical incidence is obtained. Thus, for example, a family history of breast cancer is more prevalent in individuals screened for breast cancer than in the female population at large.

Next, using the duration of the DPCP estimate, the estimation of the average lead time needs to take into account whether early diagnosis by screening is made at the first or in subsequent screening exams.

The estimation of the lead time of point prevalent preclinical cases detected at the first screening exam relies on the assumptions regarding the distribution of times of early diagnosis during the DPCP. For example, if the distribution of early diagnosis by screening can be assumed to be homogeneous throughout the DPCP—that is, if the sensitivity of the screening test is independent of time within the DPCP (Figure 4–10A)—the lead time of point prevalent preclinical cases can be simply estimated as

$$\text{Lead time} = \frac{\text{DPCP}}{2}$$

The latter assumption, however, may not be justified in many situations. For most diseases amenable to screening (eg, breast cancer), the sensitivity of the screening test, and thus the probability of early diagnosis, is likely to increase during the DPCP (Figure 4–10B) as a result of the progression of the disease as it gets closer to its symptomatic (clinical) phase. If this is the case, a more reasonable assumption would be that the average lead time is less than one half of the DPCP. Obviously, the longer the DPCP, the longer the lead time under any distributional assumption. Also, because the average lead time is a function of the validity of the screening exam, it becomes longer as more sensitive screening tests are developed.

The duration of the lead time for *incident* preclinical cases identified in a program where repeated screening exams are carried out is a function of how often the screenings are done—that is, the length of the interval between successive screenings. The closer in time the screening exams are, the greater the probability that early diagnosis will occur closer to the onset of the DPCP—and thus, the more the lead time will approximate the DPCP.

**A. Sensitivity of screening exam
is same throughout the detectable
preclinical phase (DPCP):
Average lead time ≈ ½ DPCP**

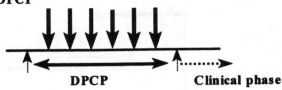

**B. Sensitivity of screening exam
increases during the detectable preclinical phase (DPCP) as a result of
the progression of the disease:
Average lead time < ½ DPCP**

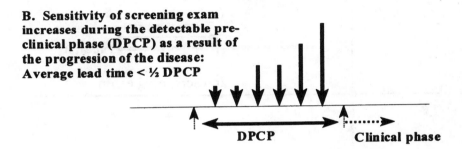

Figure 4–10 Estimation of lead time as a function of the variability of the sensitivity of the screening exam during the detectable preclinical phase.

Figure 4–11 illustrates schematically short and long between-screening intervals and their effect on the lead time. Assuming two persons with similar DPCPs whose disease starts soon after the previous screening, the person with the shorter between-screening interval (a to b, patient A) has his or her newly developed preclinical disease diagnosed nearer the beginning of the DPCP than the person with the longer between-screening interval (a to c, patient B). Thus, the duration of the lead time is closer to the duration of the DPCP for patient A than for patient B. The maximum lead time obviously cannot be longer than the DPCP.[43]

4.5 BIASES IN REPORTING STUDY RESULTS: PUBLICATION BIAS

Some common problems that may influence the quality of reporting of epidemiologic studies and that could potentially create report-

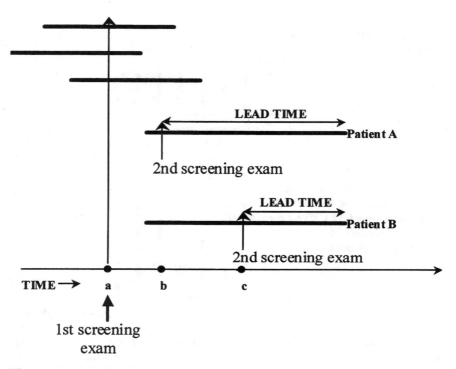

Figure 4–11 Relationship between frequency of screening and duration of lead time. Horizontal lines represent duration of detectable preclinical phase (DPCP). In patient A, the second screening exam is carried out soon after the first screening exam: lead time ≈ DPCP. In patient B, the between-screening interval is longer: lead time ≈ (.05) × DPCP.

ing biases are discussed in detailed in Chapter 9. In this section, we focus on a special type of reporting bias: *publication bias*.

Acceptance of the validity of published findings as applied to a given reference population is conditional on two important assumptions: (1) that each published study is unbiased and (2) that published studies constitute an unbiased sample of a theoretical "population" of unbiased studies (Figures 4–12 and 4–13). When these assumptions are not met, a literature review based on either meta-analytic or conventional narrative approaches will give a distorted view of the exposure-outcome association of interest. Whether assumption 1 above is met depends on several factors, including the soundness of the study designs and the quality of peer review. Publication bias, as conventionally defined, occurs when assumption 2 cannot be met because,

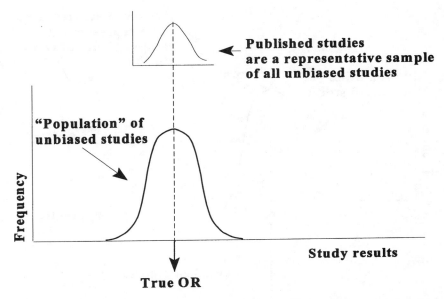

Figure 4-12 Published studies constitute a representative sample of a theoretical reference "population" of unbiased studies (no publication bias).

besides the quality of the report, other factors dictate acceptability for publication. Direction of findings is one such factor. For example, in a study carried out a few decades ago, Sterling[44] demonstrated that 97% of papers published in four psychology journals showed statistically significant results at the alpha level of 5%, thus strongly suggesting that results were more likely to be published if they had reached this conventional significance level.

Subsequent research[45-49] has confirmed the tendency to publish "positive" results. In a study by Dickersin[47] comparing published randomized clinical trials with completed yet unpublished randomized trials by the same investigators, 55% of the published, but only 15% of the unpublished studies favored the new therapy being assessed.

A possible reason for publication bias is the reluctance of journal editors and reviewers to accept negative ("uninteresting"?) results. For example, in a study by Mahoney,[50] a group of 75 reviewers were asked to review different versions (randomly assigned) of a fictitious manuscript. The "Introduction" and "Methods" sections in all versions were identical, whereas the "Results" and "Discussion" sections were different, ranging from "positive" to "ambiguous" to "negative" results. Reviewers were asked to evaluate the methods, the data presen-

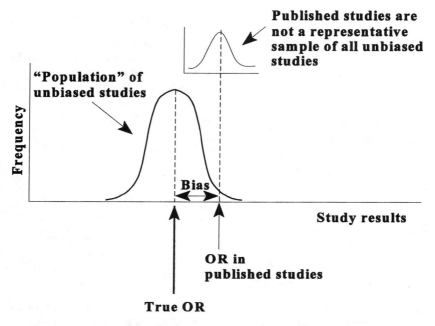

Figure 4–13 Publication bias: published studies constitute a biased sample of a theoretical reference "population" of unbiased studies (publication bias).

tation, the scientific contribution, and the publication merit. Compared with negative or ambiguous studies, the manuscripts with "positive" results systematically received higher average scores for all categories, including the category for evaluation of methods, even though the "Methods" section was identical in all sets.

Interestingly, however, editors and reviewers may not be the only source of publication bias. For example, in Dickersin et al's study,[47] for only 12% of unpublished yet completed studies, publication was intended by the authors. Reasons given by the authors why publication was not intended for the remaining 88% included "negative results" (28%), "lack of interest" (12%), and "sample size problems" (11%).

Even source of support seems to interfere with the likelihood of publication. Davidson,[51] for example, found that clinical trials favoring a new over a traditional therapy funded by the pharmaceutical industry had a publication odds 5.2 greater than that of trials supported by other sources, such as the National Institutes of Health.

Some forms of publication bias are rather subtle, such as "language bias" (ie, publication in an English language-journal vs publication in a journal in another language). For example, Egger et al[52] compared randomized clinical trials published by German investigators in either German journals or English journals from 1985 through 1994. When pairs of articles with the same first author were compared, no evidence of differences in quality between the papers written in German or English was found. In contrast, a strong, statistically significant difference with regard to the *significance* of findings was present: 63% of the articles published in English reported a statistically significant result, compared to only 35% of articles published in German (OR = 3.8; 95% confidence limits 1.3–11.3). These results strongly suggest that using language as one of the criteria to select studies to be included in a meta-analysis (a criterion that is frequently adopted because of practical reasons or reasons related to access) can seriously undermine the representativeness of published reviews, including those using meta-analysis methods.

The two most often cited systematic approaches to avoid publication bias are the creation of study registers[49] and advance publication of research designs.[53] Prevention of publication bias obviously requires efforts on the part of the scientific community as a whole, including researchers, peer reviewers, and journal editors. The latter should be aware that direction of findings and absence of "significant" results should not be used as criteria for rejection or acceptance of a paper.

REFERENCES

1. Sackett DL. Bias in analytical research. *J Chron Dis.* 1979;32:51–63.
2. Last JM. *A Dictionary of Epidemiology.* 3rd ed. New York, NY: Oxford University Press; 1995:15.
3. Lilienfeld DE, Stolley PD. *Foundations of Epidemiology.* New York, NY: Oxford University Press; 1994.
4. Schlesselman JJ. *Case-Control Studies: Design, Conduct, Analysis.* New York, NY: Oxford University Press; 1982.
5. Rothman KJ, Greenland S. *Modern Epidemiology.* 2nd ed. Philadelphia, Pa: Lippincott-Raven Publishers; 1998.
6. Byrne C, Brinton LA, Haile RW, et al. Heterogeneity of the effect of family history on breast cancer risk. *Epidemiology.* 1991;2:276–284.
7. MacMahon B, Yen S, Trichopoulus D, et al. Coffee and cancer of the pancreas. *N Engl J Med.* 1981;304:630–633.
8. Hsieh CC, MacMahon B, Yen S, et al. Coffee and pancreatic cancer. *N Engl J Med.* 1986;315:587–588. Letter.

9. Gordis L. *Epidemiology*. Philadelphia, Pa: WB Saunders; 1996.

10. Weinstock MA, Colditz GA, Willett WC, et al. Recall (report) bias and reliability in the retrospective assessment of melanoma risk. *Am J Epidemiol*. 1991;133:240–245.

11. Brinton LA, Hoover RN, Szklo M, et al. Menopausal estrogen use and risk of breast cancer. *Cancer*. 1981;47:2517–2522.

12. Chambless LE, Heiss G, Folsom AR, et al. Association of coronary heart disease incidence with carotid arterial wall thickness and major risk factors: the Atherosclerosis Risk in Communities (ARIC) study, 1987-1993. *Am J Epidemiol*. 1997;146:483–494.

13. Mele A, Szklo M, Visani G, et al. Hair dye use and other risk factors for leukemia and pre-leukemia: a case-control study. Italian Leukemia Study Group. *Am J Epidemiol*. 1994;139:609–619.

14. Wei Q, Matanoski GM, Farmer ER, et al. DNA repair and susceptibility to basal cell carcinoma: a case-control study. *Am J Epidemiol*. 1994;140:598–607.

15. Commonwealth of Australia, National Health and Medical Research Council. *The Health Effects of Passive Smoking*. November 1997. Canberra: Australian Government Publishing Service.

16. Szklo M, Tonascia J, Gordis L. Psychosocial factors and the risk of myocardial infarctions in white women. *Am J Epidemiol*. 1976;103:312–320.

17. Doll R, Hill AB. Smoking and carcinoma of the lung: preliminary report. *B Med J*. 1950;2:739–748.

18. Perneger TV, Whelton PK, Klag MJ, Rossiter KA. Diagnosis of hypertensive end-stage renal disease: effect of patient's race. *Am J Epidemiol*. 1995;141:10–15.

19. Stewart WF, Linet MS, Celentano DD, et al. Age- and sex-specific incidence rates of migraine with and without visual aura. *Am J Epidemiol*. 1991;134:1111–1120.

20. Rose GA. Chest pain questionnaire. *Milbank Mem Fund Q*. 1965;43:32–39.

21. Bass EB, Follansbee WP, Orchard TJ. Comparison of a supplemented Rose questionnaire to exercise thalium testing in men and women. *J Clin Epidemiol*. 1989;42:385–393.

22. Garber CE, Carleton RA, Heller GV. Comparison of "Rose questionnaire angina" to exercise thalium scintigraphy: different findings in males and females. *J Clin Epidemiol*. 1992;45:715–720.

23. Sorlie PD, Cooper L, Schreiner PJ, et al. Repeatability and validity of the Rose questionnaire for angina pectoris in the Atherosclerosis Risk in Communities study. *J Clin Epidemiol*. 1996;49:719–725.

24. Dosemeci M, Wacholder S, Lubin JH. Does nondifferential misclassification of exposure always bias a true effect toward the null value? *Am J Epidemiol*. 1990;132:746–748.

25. Greenland S. The effect of misclassification in the presence of covariates. *Am J Epidemiol*. 1980;112:564–569.

26. Wacholder S. When measurement errors correlate with truth: surprising effects of nondifferential misclassification. *Epidemiology*. 1995;6:157–161.

27. Flegal KM, Brownie C, Haas JD. The effects of misclassification on estimates of relative risk. *Am J Epidemiol*. 1986;123:736–751.

28. Flegal KM, Keyl PM, Nieto FJ. Differential misclassification arising from nondifferential errors in exposure measurement. *Am J Epidemiol*. 1991;134:1233–1244.

29. Willet W. An overview of issues related to the correction of non-differential exposure measurement error in epidemiologic studies. *Stat Med*. 1989;8:1031–1040.

30. Thomas D, Stram D, Dwyer J. Exposure measurement error: influence on exposure-disease. Relationships and methods of correction. *Annu Rev Public Health*. 1993;14:69–93.

31. Armstrong BG. The effects of measurement errors on relative risk regressions. *Am J Epidemiol*. 1990;132:1176–1184.

32. Kannel WB. CHD risk factors: a Framingham study update. *Hosp Prac*. 1990;25: 93–104.

33. Giovannucci E, Ascherio A, Rimm EB, et al. A prospective cohort study of vasectomy and prostate cancer in US men. *JAMA*. 1993;269:873–877.

34. Goldberg RJ, Gorak EJ, Yarzebski J. A communitywide perspective of sex differences and temporal trends in the incidence and survival rates after acute myocardial infarction and out-of-hospital deaths caused by coronary heart disease. *Circulation*. 1993;87:1947–1953.

35. Perneger TV, Nieto FJ, Whelton PK. A prospective study of blood pressure and serum creatinine: results from the "CLUE" study and the ARIC study. *JAMA*. 1993; 269:488–493.

36. Szklo M. Aplastic anemia. In: Lilienfeld AM, ed. *Reviews in Cancer Epidemiology*, vol 1. New York, NY: Elsevier North-Holland; 1980:115–119.

37. Antunes CM, Stolley PD, Rosenshein NB. Endometrial cancer and estrogen use: report of a large case-control study. *N Engl J Med*. 1979;300:9–13.

38. Horwitz RI, Feinstein AR. Estrogens and endometrial cancer: responses to arguments and current status of an epidemiologic controversy. *Am J Med*. 1986; 81:503–507.

39. Brunekreef B, Groot B, Hoek G. Pets, allergy and respiratory symptoms in children. *Int J Epidemiol*. 1992;21:338–342.

40. Nieto FJ, Diez-Roux A, Szklo M, Comstock GW, Sharret AR. Short and long term prediction of clinical and subclinical atherosclerosis by traditional risk factors. *J Clin Epidemiol*. 1999;52:559–567.

41. Shapiro S, Venet W, Strax P. Selection, follow-up, and analysis in the Health Insurance Plan study: a randomized trial with breast cancer screening. *Natl Cancer Inst Monogr*. 1985;67:65–74.

42. Hutchison GB, Shapiro S. Lead time gained by diagnostic time screening for breast cancer. *J Natl Cancer Inst*. 1968;41:665.

43. Morrison AS. *Screening in Chronic Disease*. New York, NY: Oxford University Press; 1985. Monographs in Epidemiology and Biostatistics, vol. 7.

44. Sterling TD. Publication decisions and their possible effects on inferences drawn from tests of significance or vice versa. *J Am Stat Assoc*. 1959;54:30–34.

45. Dickersin K, Hewitt P, Mutch L, et al. Perusing the literature: comparison of MEDLINE searching with a Perinatal Trials database. *Control Clin Trials*. 1985;6:306–317.

46. Dickersin K, Chan S, Chalmers TC, et al. Publication bias and clinical trials. *Control Clin Trials*. 1987;8:343–353.

47. Dickersin K, Min Y-I, Meinert CL. Factors influencing publication of research results. *JAMA*. 1992;267:374–378.

48. Easterbrook PJ, Berlin JA, Gopalan R, et al. Publication bias in clinical research. *Lancet.* 1991;337:867–872.

49. Dickersin K. Report from the Panel on the Case for Registers of Clinical Trials at the eighth annual meeting of the Society for Clinical Trials. *Control Clin Trials.* 1988;9:76–81.

50. Mahoney MJ. Publication prejudices: an experimental study of confirmatory bias in the peer review system. *Cog Ther Res.* 1977;1:161–175.

51. Davidson RA. Source of funding and outcome of clinical trials. *J Gen Intern Med.* 1986;1:155–158.

52. Egger M, Zellweger-Zahner T, Schneider M, et al. Language bias in randomised controlled trials publishd in English and German. *Lancet.* 1997;350:326–329.

53. Piantadosi S, Byar DP. A proposal for registering clinical trials. *Control Clin Trials.* 1988;9:82–84.

CHAPTER 5

Identifying Noncausal Associations: Confounding

5.1 INTRODUCTION

The term *confounding* refers to a situation in which a noncausal association between a given exposure and an outcome is observed as a result of the influence of a third variable (or group of variables), usually designated as a *confounding variable*, or merely a *confounder*. As discussed below, the confounding variable must be related to both the putative risk factor and the outcome under study. In an observational cohort study, for example, a confounding variable would differ between exposed and unexposed subjects and would also be associated with the outcome of interest. As shown in the examples that follow, this may result either in the appearance or strengthening of an association not due to a direct causal effect or in the apparent absence or weakening of a true causal association.

From the epidemiological standpoint, it is useful to conceptualize confounding as distinct from bias in that a confounded association, though not causal, is real (for further discussion of this concept, see Section 5.4.7). This distinction has obvious practical implications with respect to the relevance of exposures as *markers* of the presence or risk of disease for screening purposes (secondary prevention). If, on the other hand, the goal of the researcher is to carry out primary prevention, it becomes crucial to distinguish a causal from a noncausal association, the latter resulting from either bias or confounding. A number of statistical techniques are available to control for confounding; as described in detail in Chapter 7, the basic idea underlying adjustment is to use some *statistical model* to estimate what the association between the exposure and the outcome would be, given a constant value or level of the suspected confounding variable(s).

Confounding is more likely to occur in observational than in experimental epidemiology studies because the likelihood that groups under comparison (eg, exposed and unexposed) differ with regard to confounding variables is minimized in experimental studies as a result of random allocation. In these studies, random subsamples of the reference population are selected that are expected to be comparable regarding the distribution of both known and unknown confounders, particularly when large sample sizes are involved. However, even if the randomization approach is unbiased and the samples are large, there may be random differences between the experimental (eg, vaccinated) and the control (eg, those receiving placebo) groups, possibly leading to confounding (Exhibit 5–1). In an observational study, in addition to random differences between the comparison groups, factors related to the exposure may confound the association under study, as illustrated in the examples that follow and as further discussed in the next section.

- *Example 1.* The overall crude mortality rates in 1986 for six countries in the Americas[1] were as follows:
  - –Costa Rica: 3.8 per 1000
  - –Venezuela: 4.4 per 1000
  - –Mexico: 4.9 per 1000
  - –Cuba: 6.7 per 1000
  - –Canada: 7.3 per 1000
  - –US: 8.7 per 1000

  Assuming that this mortality ranking is accurate, the literal (and correct) interpretation of these crude data is that the United States and Canada had the highest rates of death during 1986. Although this interpretation of crude data is useful for public health planning purposes, it may be misleading when using mortality rates as indicators of health status, as it fails to take into consideration interpopulation age differences. In this example, the higher mortality rates in Canada and the United States reflect the fact that there is a much higher proportion of older individuals in these populations; because age is a very strong "risk factor" for mortality, these age differences result in these countries having the highest mortality rates. Inspection of age-specific mortality rates (see Chapter 7, Section 7.2) results in a very different picture, with the lowest mortality rates observed in Canada, the United States, and Costa Rica for every age group. With adjustment for age (using the direct method and the 1960

Exhibit 5–1 Confounding in Experimental and Nonexperimental Epidemiologic Studies

Study Design	Experimental: Randomized Clinical Trial	Observational: Prospective Study
Approach	Random allocation $\swarrow \quad \searrow$ A B	Nonrandom allocation $\swarrow \quad \searrow$ A B
Example	A = vaccine B = placebo	A = smokers B = nonsmokers
Source of confounding (difference(s) between groups)	Random difference(s)	Random difference(s) *and* factors associated with the exposure of interest

population of Latin America as the standard, see Chapter 7, Section 7.3.1), the relative rankings of the United States and Canada are reversed (mortality per 1000: Costa Rica: 3.7; Venezuela: 4.6; Mexico: 5.0; Cuba: 4.0; Canada: 3.2; United States: 3.6). Age is therefore a confounder of the observed association between country and mortality.

- *Example 2.* In a cohort study conducted in England,[2] participants who reported a higher frequency of sexual activity at baseline (as indicated by their reported frequency of orgasm) were found to have a decreased risk of 10-year mortality compared with those who reported lower sexual activity. Does sexual activity *cause* lower mortality? Or are people with higher levels of sexual activity (or capacity to have orgasms) healthier in general and thus, by definition, at lower risk of mortality? Although the authors of this study, aware of this problem, attempted to control for it by adjusting for a number of health-related surrogate variables (see Chapter 7), the possibility of a "residual confounding" effect remains open to question (see Section 5.4.3 and Chapter 7, Section 7.5).

- *Example 3.* A reported side effect of calcium channel blockers, used for the treatment of hypertension, is gastrointestinal bleeding. However, it has been suggested that this complication results from the concurrent use of other drugs often used by patients on calcium channel blockers, or from comorbidities found in these patients.[3] Acting as confounders, these comorbidities and/or the use of additional medications may therefore be partially or entirely responsible for the observed association between calcium channel blockers and digestive hemorrhage.

- *Example 4.* In a nested case-control study among American Japanese men, low dietary vitamin C has been found to be related to colon cancer risk.[4] Although it is possible that this relationship is causal, an alternative explanation is that individuals who consume more vitamin C tend to have a healthier lifestyle in general and thus to be exposed to true protective factors (eg, other dietary items, physical exercise) acting as confounders.

5.2   THE NATURE OF THE ASSOCIATION BETWEEN THE CONFOUNDER, THE EXPOSURE, AND THE OUTCOME

5.2.1   General Rule

The common theme with regard to confounding is that the association between an exposure and a given outcome is induced, strengthened, weakened, or eliminated by a third variable or group of variables (confounders). The essential nature of this phenomenon can be stated as follows:

The confounding variable is causally associated with the outcome

and

noncausally or causally associated with the exposure

but

is not an intermediate variable in the causal pathway between exposure and outcome.

This general rule is schematically represented in Figure 5–1. The association of interest (ie, whether a given exposure is causally related to the outcome) is represented by a dotted line and a question mark; note that this line has an arrow pointing to the outcome, since the question of interest here is whether the exposure *causes* the outcome. (An association between exposure and outcome can also occur because the "outcome" causes changes in "exposure": ie, *reverse causality*, a situation that is discussed in Chapter 4, Section 4.4.2.)

Some exceptions to the above general rule for the presence of confounding are discussed in Section 5.2.3; its components are dissected in the next section (5.2.2), using the previously discussed examples as illustrations (Figure 5–2). Note that the confounding variables in Fig-

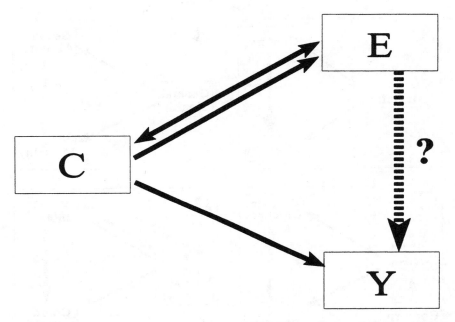

Figure 5–1 General definition of confounding. The confounder (C) is causally associated with the outcome of interest (Y) and either causally or noncausally associated with the exposure (E); these associations may distort the association of interest: whether E causes Y. A unidirectional arrow indicates that the association is causal; a bidirectional arrow indicates a noncausal association.

ure 5–2A and 5–2B are denoted as simple, and possibly oversimplified, characteristics ("age distribution" and "general health," respectively). In Figure 5–2C and D, the postulated "confounding variables" are represented by more or less complex sets of variables. In Figure 5–2C, "other medications" are related to the presence of comorbidities (other disease manifestations that are associated with hypertension, the indication for the prescription of calcium channel blockers). In Figure 5–2D, the "confounder" is a constellation of variables related to general socioeconomic status (SES) and lifestyle characteristics that have their own interrelations. There is usually a trade-off in choosing simplicity over complexity in the characterization of these variables and in the conceptualization of their interrelations; this trade-off is directly relevant to the art of statistical "modeling" and is the core of

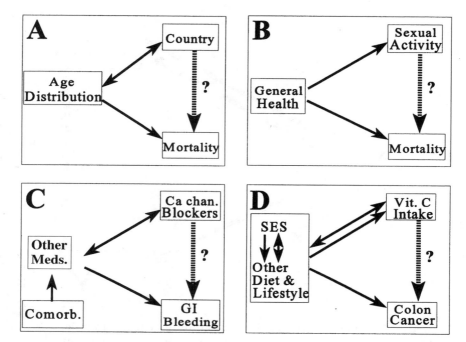

Figure 5–2 Schematic representation of the hypothetical relations of confounders, exposures of interest, and outcomes, based on the examples in the text. A unidirectional arrow indicates that the association is causal; a bidirectional arrow indicates a noncausal association. A dotted arrow with a question mark indicates the research question of interest. GI, gastrointestinal; SES, socioeconomic status.

the science of multivariate analysis, a key tool in analytical epidemiology (see Chapter 7, Section 7.4).

5.2.2   Elements of the General Rule for Defining the Presence of Confounding

"The Confounding Variable Is Causally Associated with the Outcome"

In all the examples illustrated in Figure 5–2, the confounding variables (age distribution, general health, other medications, and SES/other lifestyle characteristics) determine the likelihood of the outcome (mortality rate, risk of death, gastrointestinal bleeding, and risk of colon cancer, respectively) to a certain degree.

"And Noncausally or Causally Associated with the Exposure"

The examples in Figure 5–2 illustrate the different forms assumed by the relationships between the postulated confounders and the respective exposures of interest (country, sexual activity, calcium channel blockers, and vitamin C intake). In Figures 5–2A and C, in addition to causal relationships with the outcomes, the confounders are related to the exposures in a noncausal fashion, a situation that is consistent with the traditional definition of confounding. For example, in Figure 5–2A, the relationship of age (the confounder) to country (the variable of interest) is postulated as being contextual rather than causal—that is, determined by a set of historical and social circumstances that are not unique to any given country. Similarly, in Figure 5–2C, the association between calcium channel blockers and concurrent medications is conceptualized as noncausal, so that, for example, hypertensives who have been prescribed calcium channel blockers are also likely to use aspirin (the "true" cause of gastrointestinal bleeding) because of hypertension-induced headaches, but *not* because aspirin *causes* physicians to prescribe calcium channel blockers. Aspirin, however, is causally related to gastrointestinal bleeding.

The confounding variables may be also related to the exposure in a causal fashion, as in the case of the postulated relationship between "good health" and sexual activity exemplified in Figure 5–2B. Finally, the example in Figure 5–2D shows the different types of relationship of the exposure of interest to the constellation of factors included in the "confounding complex": for example, lower SES may be causally related to vitamin C intake to the extent that it determines degree of access to food products that are rich in vitamin C (causal association). On the other hand, some other lifestyle characteristics related to SES (eg, physical exercise) may be related to vitamin intake in a noncausal fashion.

An additional illustration of the rule that confounding may result when the confounding variable is causally related to the exposure of interest is given by smoking and high-density lipoprotein (HDL) cholesterol (not shown in Figure 5–2). Smoking, for example, is known to cause a decrease in HDL levels,[5] thus explaining the possible relationship of low HDL and lung cancer.

"But Is Not an Intermediate Variable in the Causal Pathway Between Exposure and Outcome"

The general rule defining a confounding variable excludes the situation where the exposure determines the presence or level of the presumed confounder. In the above examples, the assumption that this type of situation does not exist may not be entirely justified. For example, in the example illustrated in Figure 5–2B, a reverse association between the exposure and the confounder may exist: that is, increased sexual activity may *cause* an improvement in general health, which in turn results in a decrease in mortality (Figure 5–3). If this type of relationship occurs, and particularly if it constitutes the only mechanism whereby sexual activity is related to mortality (see Section 5.2.3), "general health" should not be considered a true confounder, as it is the link between sexual activity and mortality.

Another example relates to the hypothesized causal relation between obesity and increased risk of mortality. Although it could be argued that this association is due to the "confounding" effect of hypertension, an alternative explanation is that hypertension is a *mediator* of the association between obesity and mortality rather than a confounder.[6]

5.2.3 Exceptions to the General Rule for the Presence of Confounding

"Confounding" Due to Random Associations

Although the general rule is that the confounding variable must be causally associated with the outcome (Figure 5–1), in practice it is possible to encounter situations where a noncausal (statistical) association leads to confounding. Thus, for example, in a case-control study, sampling (random) variability may create an imbalance between cases and controls with regard to a given variable, even though there is no such imbalance in the total reference population. Even in randomized clinical trials, particularly if the sample size is small, imbalances pertaining to variables related to the outcome(s) may happen by chance. In these trials, too, investigators take into account a (randomly produced) confounding effect using one of the available adjustment techniques (see Chapter 7).

The "Confounder" as an Intermediate Variable in the Causal Pathway of the Relation Between Exposure and Outcome

As discussed above, the potential confounder should not be an intermediate variable in the causal pathway between the suspected risk factor and the outcome. It follows that it is inappropriate to adjust for such a variable. Although this rule is generally sound, exceptions to it occur when the investigator deliberately explores alternative mecha-

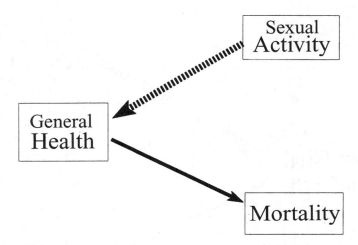

Figure 5–3 Alternative hypothesized model for the relationships in Figure 5–2B: "general health" is in the causal pathway of the relation between sexual activity and mortality.

nisms explaining the association between the exposure and the outcome of interest.

The association of maternal smoking during the index pregnancy with an increased risk of perinatal death provides an example of a situation in which it may be appropriate to adjust for an intermediate variable. Low birth weight is known to be an important link in the causal chain between smoking and perinatal death (Figure 5–4). Thus, if the study question is "Does smoking cause perinatal death?" (which does not address a specific mechanism, as may be the case when first examining a hypothesis), it is clearly inappropriate to adjust for a possible mechanism, particularly a key mechanism such as low birth weight. However, once the principal link in the causality chain (low birth weight) is established, a different question may be asked: "Does smoking cause perinatal death through mechanism(s) *other than low birth weight*?" (Figure 5–5). In this situation, to treat birth weight as a "confounder" (at least in the sense that to control for it is warranted) is appropriate; the presence of a residual (birth weight–adjusted) effect of smoking on perinatal mortality would indicate that in addition to lowering birth weight, smoking may have a direct toxic effect.[7]

In the above-mentioned obesity-hypertension example, even if the main mechanism whereby obesity increases mortality is an increase

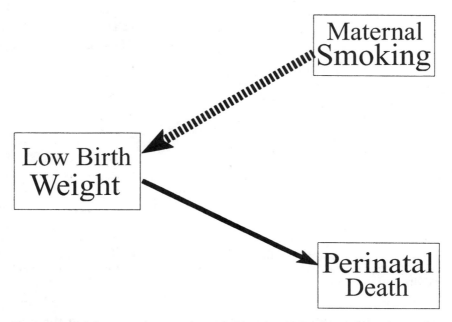

Figure 5–4 Schematic representation of low birth weight as the only mechanism for the relationship between maternal smoking and perinatal death.

---

in blood pressure levels,[6] it may be of interest to examine the hypertension-adjusted association between obesity and mortality with the purpose of exploring the possibility that other mechanisms could explain the hypothesized relationship.

The degree to which a given mechanism (or positive confounding) explains the relationship of interest is given by the comparison of adjusted (A) and unadjusted (U) measures of association (eg, a relative risk, RR). This comparison can be made using the ratio of the unadjusted RRs, RR_U/RR_A,[8] or the percent excess risk explained by the variable(s) adjusted for:

$$\% \text{ Excess Risk Explained} = \frac{RR_U - RR_A}{RR_U - 1.0} \times 100$$

As an example of the application of the percent excess risk formula, if the adjusted relative risk is 2.0, and the unadjusted relative risk is 3.0, the mechanism represented by the variable adjusted for (eg, low birth weight) can be regarded as responsible for 50% of the association. It is important to keep in mind, however, that if a residual association persists after a potentially intermediate variable is controlled for, it does

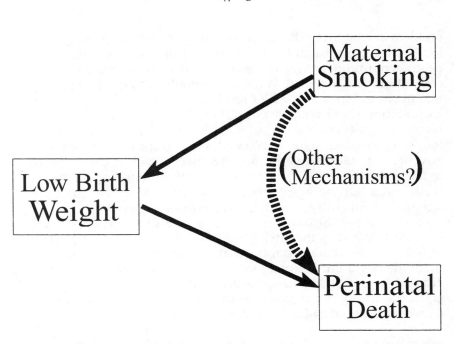

Figure 5-5 Schematic representation of mechanism(s) other than low birth weight to explain the relationship between maternal smoking and perinatal death.

not necessarily follow that there must be other causal pathways or mechanisms; the residual association may be due to *residual confounding* (see Section 5.4.3 and Chapter 7, Section 7.5). For example, even if hypertension were an important mechanism, a residual association between obesity and mortality could still be observed after controlling (adjusting) for blood pressure levels because of measurement error and thus incomplete adjustment for blood pressure, leading to residual confounding.

In summary, the approach to confounding when exposure and confounder are part of the same causal pathway is a function of the hypothesis being evaluated: in other words, it depends on the conceptual model that is translated into the study questions and goals.

Excessive Correlation Between the Confounder and the Exposure of Interest

Although, by definition, a confounding variable is correlated with the exposure of interest (Figure 5-1), on occasion the correlation is so strong that adjustment becomes difficult, if not impossible. This is a problem analogous to the situation known in biostatistics as *collinearity*. Consider, for example, the exposure "air pollution" and the suspected confounder "area of residence." Given the virtually perfect correlation between these variables, it would be difficult (or impossible) to control for the effect of residence when assessing the effect of air pollution on respiratory symptoms. Figure 5–6 schematically represents a perfect correlation between dichotomous exposure and confounding variables, which makes adjustment for the confounder impossible. The ideal situation for effective control of confounding is that in which there is a clear-cut correlation between exposure and confounder but the variability is sufficient to allow adequate representation of all cross-tabulated cells shown in Figure 5–7.

An example of the difficulty posed by excessive correlations among variables is given by the assessment of the role of dietary components as risk factors. When examining the observational association between dietary animal protein intake and a given outcome, it may be difficult to control for the possible confounding role of dietary fat, given the strong correlation between animal protein and fat intake.[9] Other examples of collinearity include education/income, serum HDL

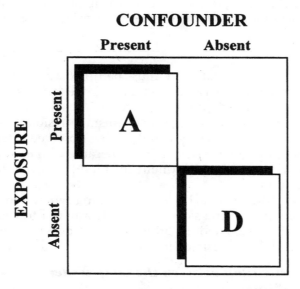

Figure 5–6 Perfect correlation between dichotomous exposure of interest and confounding factor: there are no cells in which the exposure is present and the confounder is absent, and vice versa.

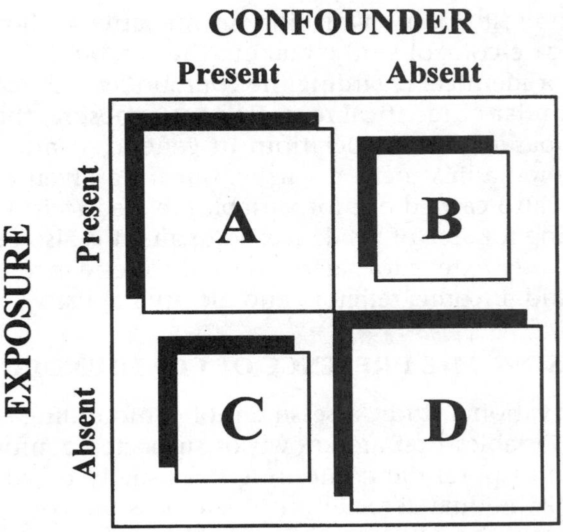

CONFOUNDER

Present   **Absent**

Figure 5–7 Correlation between an exposure of interest and a confounding factor: all four cells for a cross-tabulation of dichotomous categories are represented. In this schematic representation, the larger sizes of cells A and D denote the magnitude of the positive correlation between the exposure and the confounder.

cholesterol/triglycerides and race/SES. A similar situation is when components of the same exposure variable are strongly correlated, making it difficult to adjust for one while looking at the "independent" contribution of the other. For example, it may be difficult, if not impossible, to examine smoking duration while simultaneously finely controlling for age of smoking initiation.

As a corollary of the preceding discussion, it is important to underscore that it is only possible to adjust for a confounder while examining the relationship between exposure and outcome when levels of the confounder and those of the exposure overlap, a situation not always encountered in observational epidemiology studies. For example, it would be impossible to adjust for age if there were no overlap in ages between exposed and unexposed individuals (eg, if all those exposed were over 45 and all those unexposed were less than 45 years old).

A related issue is *overadjustment* (or *overmatching,* see Chapter 7, Section 7.6), which occurs when adjustment (or matching, see Chapter 1, Section 1.4.5) is carried out for a variable so closely related to the variable of interest that no variability in the latter is allowed. For example, in a case-control study, making the case and control groups very similar or identical regarding the confounder results in their also being very similar or identical regarding the exposure, thereby resulting in an apparent null association. In general, it must be kept in mind that when adjustment is carried out for a given confounding variable, it is also carried out for variables related to it. For example, when adjusting for area of residence, adjustment is also carried out to a greater or lesser extent for factors related to residence, such as ethnic background, income, religion, and dietary habits.

5.3 ASSESSING THE PRESENCE OF CONFOUNDING

In an observational study, assessment of confounding effects is carried out for variables that are known or suspected confounders. The identification of potential confounders is usually based on a priori knowledge of the dual association of the possible confounder with the exposure and the outcome, the two poles of the study hypothesis. In addition to the a priori knowledge about these associations, it is important to verify whether confounding is present in the study. There are several approaches to assess the presence of confounding, which are related to the following questions:

1. Is the confounding variable related to both the exposure and the outcome in the study?
2. Does the exposure-outcome association seen in the crude analysis have the same direction as and similar magnitude to the associations seen within strata of the confounding variable?
3. Does the exposure-outcome association seen in the crude analysis have the same direction as and similar magnitude to the associations seen after controlling (adjusting) for the confounding variable?

These different approaches to assess the presence and magnitude of confounding effects are illustrated using an example based on a hypothetical case-control study of male gender as a possible risk factor for malaria infection. The crude analysis shown in Exhibit 5–2 suggests that males are at a higher risk of malaria than females (odds ratio [OR] = 1.7; 95% confidence limits, 1.1–2.7). A "real" association between male gender and malaria can be inferred if these results are free of random (sampling) and systematic (bias) errors: that is, males do have higher risk of malaria in this particular population setting. The next

Exhibit 5–2 Example of Confounding: Hypothetical Study of Male Gender as a Risk Factor for Malaria Infection

	Cases	Controls	Total	
Males	88	68	156	**Odds ratio = 1.71**
Females	62	82	144	
Total	150	150	300	

question is whether the association is *causal*—ie, whether there is something inherent to gender that would render males more susceptible to the disease than females (eg, a hormonal factor). Alternatively, a characteristic that is associated with both gender and an increased risk of malaria may be responsible for the association. One such characteristic is work environment, in the sense that individuals who primarily work outdoors (eg, in agriculture) are more likely to be exposed to the mosquito bite that results in the disease than those who work indoors (Figure 5–8). Thus, if the proportion of individuals with mostly outdoor occupations were higher in males than in females, working environment might explain the observed association between gender and malaria.

5.3.1   Is the Confounding Variable Related to Both the Exposure and the Outcome?

The associations of the confounder with both the exposure and work environment in this hypothetical example are shown in Exhibit 5–3.

- 43.6% (68/156) of males, compared with only 9% (13/144) of females, have mostly outdoor occupations, yielding an odds ratio of 7.8.
- 42% (63/150) of the malaria cases, but only 12% (18/150) of controls have mostly outdoor occupations, yielding an odds ratio of 5.3.

The strong positive associations of the confounder (work environment) with both the risk factor of interest (male gender) and the outcome ("caseness") suggest that work environment may indeed have a strong confounding effect.

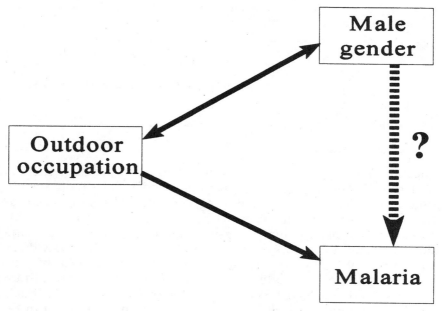

Figure 5–8 Work environment as a possible confounder of the association between male gender and malaria risk.

5.3.2   Does the Exposure-Outcome Association Seen in the Crude Analysis Have the Same Direction as and Similar Magnitude to Associations Seen Within Strata of the Confounding Variable?

Stratification according to the confounder represents one of the strategies to *control for* its effect (see Chapter 7, Section 7.2). When there is a confounding effect, the associations seen across strata of the potentially confounding variable are of similar magnitude to each other but are all different from the crude estimate. In the above example, the data can be stratified by the confounder (work environment) to verify whether the association between the exposure (male gender) and the outcome (malaria) is present *within* the relevant strata (mostly outdoors or mostly indoors). As shown in Exhibit 5–4, the estimated odds ratios in both strata are very close to one and are different from the crude value (1.71), thus suggesting that work environment is a confounder that explains virtually all of the association between male gender and the presence of malaria. If the association seen in the unadjusted analysis had persisted within strata of the sus-

Exhibit 5–3 Association of the Putative Confounder (Mostly Outdoor Occupation) with the Exposure of Interest (Male Gender) and the Outcome (Malaria) in the Hypothetical Study in Exhibit 5–2 and Figure 5–8.

Confounder versus exposure		Mostly Outdoor	Mostly Indoor	Total	
	Males	68	88	156	**Odds ratio = 7.8**
	Females	13	131	144	
				300	

Confounder versus outcome		Cases	Controls		
	Mostly Outdoor	63	18		**Odds ratio = 5.3**
	Mostly Indoor	87	132		
	Total	150	150	300	

pected confounder, it would have been appropriate to conclude that a confounding effect of work environment did not explain the association observed between male gender and malaria.

With regard to using stratification as a means to verify presence of confounding, it must be emphasized that, as demonstrated by Miettinen and Cook[10] for odds ratios (and subsequently by Greenland[11] for rate ratios and absolute differences between rates), the unadjusted odds ratio is sometimes different from the stratum-specific odds ratios *even if confounding is absent*. Therefore, the strategy of comparing stratum-specific odds ratios with the pooled (unadjusted) odds ratio for the assessment of confounding should be confirmed through the use of the previous strategy and that which follows.

5.3.3 Does the Exposure-Outcome Association Seen in the Crude Analysis Have the Same Direction and Magnitude as That Seen after Controlling (Adjusting) for the Confounding Variable?

Perhaps the most persuasive approach to determine whether there is a confounding effect is the comparison between adjusted and crude associations. The gender/malaria infection example is also

Exhibit 5–4 Stratified Analyses of the Association Between Gender and Malaria (from Exhibit 5–2), According to Whether Individuals Work Mainly Outdoors or Indoors

Mostly outdoor occupation		Cases	Controls	
	Males	53	15	**Odds ratio = 1.06**
	Females	10	3	
	Total	63	18	
Mostly indoor occupation		Cases	Controls	
	Males	35	53	**Odds ratio = 1.00**
	Females	52	79	
	Total	87	132	

used in Chapter 7, Section 7.3.3, to illustrate the use of the Mantel-Haenszel approach to calculate an adjusted odds ratio. As described in that section, the Mantel-Haenszel adjusted odds ratio in this example is 1.01. (This odds ratio is merely a weighted average of the stratum-specific odds ratios shown in Exhibit 5–4.) The comparison between the crude (1.71) and the work environment–adjusted (1.01) odds ratios is consistent with and confirms the inference based on the previous strategies that the increased risk of malaria in males (odds increased by 71%) resulted from their being more likely to work outdoors (Exhibit 5–3).

Another example to illustrate the different approaches to assess confounding is given by a cohort study of employed middle-aged men (Western Electric Company study) that assessed the relationship of vitamin C and beta carotene intakes to risk of death.[12] For the tables that follow, the suspected risk factor is defined on the basis of a summary index that takes both vitamin C and beta carotene intakes into consideration. For simplification purposes, this intake index defining the exposure of interest is classified as "low," "moderate," or "high." The potential confounder for these examples is current smoking, categorized as absent or present. In this example, the question of interest is whether there is an inverse relationship between intake index and the outcome, all-cause death rate, and, if so, whether it can be partly or totally explained by the confounding effect of smoking.

The first approach to assess whether confounding can explain the graded unadjusted relationship found in this study (Table 5–1)—that is, whether the confounder is associated with both exposure and outcome—is illustrated in Tables 5–2 and 5–3. An inverse relationship between current smoking and the exposure, intake index, was observed in this study, with a higher percentage of the low-intake and a lower percentage of the high-intake categories seen in current smokers, than in nonsmokers (Table 5–2). Current smoking was also found to be associated with a 72% increase in all-cause mortality (Table 5–3). Because of its dual association with both intake index (exposure) and mortality (outcome), smoking can be regarded as a confounder of the association of the composite vitamin C/beta carotene intake index with all-cause mortality.

The second approach to examine confounding (stratification according to categories of the potential confounder) is illustrated in Table 5–4, which shows that the rate ratios in the strata formed by current smoking categories are similar to the unadjusted rate ratios. The results of the third approach (adjustment) are presented in Table 5–5, which shows the rate ratios adjusted using the direct method (see Chapter 7, Section 7.3.1). Though slightly weakened, the inverse graded relationship of intake index with all-cause mortality remained after adjustment for current smoking. Thus, it can be concluded that although current smoking (categorized dichotomously as "no" or "yes") fulfilled both criteria needed to define it as a confounder (strategy 1, Tables 5–2 and 5–3), it acted only as an extremely weak con-

---

Table 5–1 Unadjusted Mortality Rates and Corresponding Rate Ratios in the Western Electric Company Study Population According to Intake Index

Intake Index	No. of Person-Years of Observation	No. of Deaths	Mortality/1000 Person-Years	Rate Ratio
Low	10,707	195	18.2	1.00
Moderate	10,852	163	15.0	0.82
High	11,376	164	14.4	0.79

Source: Data from DK Pandey et al, Dietary Vitamin C and β-Carotene and Risk of Death in Middle-Aged Men. The Western Electric Study, *American Journal of Epidemiology,* Vol 142, pp 1269–1278, © 1995, The Johns Hopkins University School of Hygiene & Public Health.

Table 5–2 Percentage Distribution of Person-Years of Observation in the Western Electric Company Study Population, According to Vitamin C/Beta Carotene Intake Index and Current Smoking

| | | | Percentage Distribution | | |
| | | | Intake Index | | |
Current Smoking	No. of Individuals	Person-Years	Low	Moderate	High
No	657	14,534 (100.0%)	29.3	35.3	35.4
Yes	899	18,401 (100.0%)	35.0	31.1	33.9

Source: Data from DK Pandey et al, Dietary Vitamin C and β-Carotene and Risk of Death in Middle-Aged Men. The Western Electric Study, *American Journal of Epidemiology,* Vol 142, pp 1269–1278, © 1995, The Johns Hopkins University School of Hygiene & Public Health.

founder in this study. This weak confounding effect may be explained by the relatively weak relationship between smoking and intake index (Table 5–2) coupled with a total mortality rate ratio for the current smoking category of only 1.72 (Table 5–3). This is probably due to the lack of specificity of the outcome, which included both smoking-related and nonsmoking-related deaths. (It could also be argued that adjustment for only two categories of smoking, which does not take into account either duration or amount of smoking, leaves room for substantial residual confounding; see Section 5.4.3.)

Table 5–3 Mortality Rates and Corresponding Rate Ratios in the Western Electric Company Study Population by Current Smoking

Current Smoking	No. of Person-Years	No. of Deaths	Mortality/1000 Person-Years	Rate Ratio
No	14,534	165	11.3	1.00
Yes	18,401	357	19.4	1.72

Source: Data from DK Pandey et al, Dietary Vitamin C and β-Carotene and Risk of Death in Middle-Aged Men. The Western Electric Study, *American Journal of Epidemiology,* Vol 142, pp 1269–1278, © 1995, The Johns Hopkins University School of Hygiene & Public Health.

Table 5–4 Mortality Rates and Corresponding Rate Ratios Associated with Vitamin C/Beta Carotene Intake Index, According to Current Smoking, Western Electric Company Study

Current Smoking	Vitamin C/Beta Carotene Intake Index	No. of Person-Years	Mortality/1000 Person-Years	Rate Ratio
No	Low	4260	13.4	1.0
	Moderate	5131	10.7	0.80
	High	5143	10.3	0.77
Yes	Low	6447	21.4	1.0
	Moderate	5721	18.9	0.88
	High	6233	17.8	0.83
Total (unadjusted)	Low	10,707	18.2	1.0
	Moderate	10,852	15.0	0.82
	High	11,376	14.4	0.79

Source: Data from DK Pandey et al, Dietary Vitamin C and β-Carotene and Risk of Death in Middle-Aged Men. The Western Electric Study, *American Journal of Epidemiology*, Vol 142, pp 1269–1278, © 1995, The Johns Hopkins University School of Hygiene & Public Health.

5.4 ADDITIONAL ISSUES RELATED TO CONFOUNDING

5.4.1 The Importance of Using Different Strategies to Assess Confounding

Although, as discussed above, the best evidence supporting presence of confounding is the demonstration that the crude and the adjusted estimates differ, it is useful to consider the other strategies discussed in this chapter to evaluate confounding. For example, observation of the directions of the associations of the confounder with the exposure and the outcome permits an a priori expectation as to whether removal of confounding would lead to an increase or a decrease in the strength of the association (see Section 5.4.4). Should the adjusted estimate be inconsistent with the expectation, the adjustment procedure must be verified for a possible error. For example, in a case-control study where cases are younger than controls and age is directly (positively) related to the exposure of interest, confounding is expected to result in an unadjusted relative risk estimate closer to 1.0. Thus, it would be against expectation—and consequently requiring verification—if the unadjusted estimate were found to be further away from the null hypothesis than the adjusted estimate.

Table 5–5 Unadjusted and Smoking-Adjusted All-Cause Mortality Ratios Rate in the Western Electric Company Study

	Vitamin C/Beta Carotene Intake Index Rate Ratios		
Rate Ratios	Low	Moderate	High
Unadjusted	1.00	0.82	0.79
Adjusted*	1.00	0.85	0.81

*Adjusted using the direct method and the total cohort (sum of the person-years of observation for the three intake index categories) as standard population (see Chapter 7, Section 7.3.1).

Source: Data from DK Pandey et al, Dietary Vitamin C and β-Carotene and Risk of Death in Middle-Aged Men. The Western Electric Study, *American Journal of Epidemiology,* Vol 142, pp 1269–1278, © 1995, The Johns Hopkins University School of Hygiene & Public Health.

Stratification is also a useful step when analyzing epidemiologic data, as it constitutes another strategy allowing the formulation of an a priori expectation of the effects of confounding on the association, and thus of the effects of adjustment on the association (notwithstanding the caveat, previously referred to, that even when confounding is absent the pooled measure of association may be different from the stratum-specific ones). For example, when the estimates in the strata formed by the confounder are closer to the null hypothesis than the pooled unadjusted value, the relative risk should be closer to 1.0 after adjustment. (Exceptions include certain situations in which multiple variables confound each other.) Furthermore, as discussed in Chapters 6 and 7, stratification allows the assessment of interaction.

5.4.2   Confounding Is Not an "All or None" Phenomenon

In the example illustrated in Exhibits 5–2 through 5–4, the confounding variable (work environment) is responsible for the entirety of the relationship between the exposure of interest (male gender) and the outcome (malaria). Another example of a confounding effect that explains away the whole relationship is given in Table 5–6, which shows both the unadjusted and the adjusted results of the study on calcium channel blockers and gastrointestinal bleeding discussed earlier in this chapter (see example 3 in Section 5.1).[3] Because the rate ratio decreased from 1.8 to 1.5 with adjustment for demographic characteristics and use of other drugs, it can be concluded that these variables were only partial confounders of the association

Table 5–6 Unadjusted and Adjusted Relative Risks of Upper Gastrointestinal Hemorrhage According to Calcium Channel Blocker Use, Tennessee Medicaid Recipients, Aged 65 Years or Older, 1984 to 1986

	*Relative Risk**	*95% CI*
Unadjusted	1.8	1.2–2.7
Adjusted for demographic characteristics[†]		
and for use of other drugs[‡]	1.5	1.0–2.2
Above plus comorbidity indicators[§]	1.1	0.7–1.7

*Based on incidence rates (per person-time) and Poisson regression multivariate models (see Chapters 2 and 7).

[†]Age, race, gender, and residence.

[‡]Nonsteroidal anti-inflammatory agents, oral corticosteroids, oral anticoagulants, and anti-neoplastic drugs.

[§]Recent use of medical care (hospitalizations and oral nitrate use).

Source: Data from WE Smalley et al, No Association Between Calcium Channel Blocker Use and Confirmed Bleeding Peptic Ulcer Disease, *American Journal of Epidemiology,* © 1998, The Johns Hopkins University School of Hygiene & Public Health.

between calcium channel blockers and gastrointestinal bleeding. However, when other comorbidities were taken into account, the association disappeared almost completely. In many instances, however, the confounding effect is only partial. In the example shown in Tables 5–1 through 5–5, adjustment for smoking had only a slight effect on the association between vitamin C/beta carotene intake index and mortality.

5.4.3   Residual Confounding

Residual confounding, which will be discussed in more detail in Chapter 7 (Section 7.5), occurs when either the categories of the confounder controlled for are too broad, resulting in an imperfect adjustment, or when some confounding variables remain unaccounted for. Thus, in one of the examples discussed above (Table 5–5), the use of only two categories of smoking ("present" or "absent") may explain the similarity between the crude and the smoking-adjusted relative risks expressing the relationship between vitamin C/beta carotene intake index and mortality. If the confounding effect of smoking were a function of other exposure components, such as amount, duration, or time since quitting, marked residual confounding might have remained after adjusting for only two smoking categories.

Another example is the study of the association between sexual activity and mortality discussed previously.[2] Aware of the possibility of confounding, the authors of this study used multiple logistic regression (see Chapter 7, Section 7.4.3) to adjust for several health-related variables. Data on these variables were collected at the baseline examination, including presence of prevalent coronary heart disease, total serum cholesterol, smoking, systolic blood pressure, and occupation (manual vs nonmanual). The lower mortality of study participants with a higher frequency of sexual intercourse persisted when these variables were adjusted for. The authors, nevertheless, aptly concluded that "despite this, confounding may well account for our findings," pointing out that in an observational study, unaccounted-for variables may confound the observed association even after adjustment has been attempted. For example, in this study, other diseases affecting both sexual activity and mortality (eg, diabetes, perhaps psychiatric conditions) were not taken into account. Furthermore, subtle health status differences that are not captured by the presence or absence of known diseases and risk factors (eg, psychological profile or general "well-being") remained unaccounted for, thus underscoring the difficulties of taking fully into consideration the confounding effects of general health status in observational epidemiologic studies.

Another type of residual confounding occurs when the variable used for adjustment is an imperfect marker of the true variable one wishes to adjust for. Thus, the appropriateness of educational level as a proxy for social class has been questioned, particularly when comparing whites and blacks in the United States.[13]

Another cause of residual confounding (ie, errors in the measurement of the confounding variable) is discussed in Chapter 7, Section 7.5.

5.4.4 Types of Confounding Effects: Negative, Positive, and "Qualitative" Confounding

Confounding may lead to an overestimation of the true strength of the association (*positive* confounding) or its underestimation (*negative* confounding). In other words, in positive confounding, the magnitude of the unadjusted (vis-à-vis the adjusted) association is exaggerated; in negative confounding, it is attenuated. Note that the terms *overestimation* and *underestimation* are used in relation to the null hypothesis. Thus, for example, an adjusted odds ratio of 0.7 is (in absolute terms) "greater" than an unadjusted odds ratio of 0.3; however, the fact that the former is closer than the latter to the odds ratio denoting no association (1.0) defines the confounding effect as "positive."

In Table 5–7, hypothetical examples showing relative risk estimates illustrate the effect of confounding. The first three examples show unadjusted associations, which either disappear or become weaker when confounding is adjusted for. Examples of positive confounding are abundant, including most of the examples used above in this chapter (eg, gender/malaria vis-à-vis occupation, which would be analogous to example no. 1 in Table 5–7, or the example of vitamin C intake/colon cancer vis-à-vis healthy lifestyle, possibly comparable to example no. 3 in Table 5–7).

Examples no. 4 through 6 in Table 5–7 show the reverse situation—namely, negative confounding, in which the unadjusted is an "underestimate"of the adjusted relative risk (vis-à-vis the null hypothesis). Adjustment reveals or strengthens an association that was rendered either absent (example no. 4) or weakened (examples no. 5 and 6) because of confounding. An example of negative confounding, in which the adjusted relative risk is further away from 1.0 when compared with the unadjusted value, is a study by Barefoot et al.[14] Using the Cook-Medley Hostility scale, a subscale of the widely used Minnesota Multiphasic Personality Inventory (MMPI) to measure psychological constructs, the authors examined the relationship of hostility to the incidence of acute myocardial infarction. Although the completely unadjusted results were not given, the relative risk was reported to change from 1.2 when only age and sex were adjusted for to about 1.5 when systolic blood pressure, smoking, triglycerides, sedentary work, and sedentary leisure were also included in the Cox proportional hazard regression model (see Chapter 7, Section 7.4.4). Thus, it can be concluded that one or more of these additional covariates (blood pressure, smoking, triglycerides, seden-

Table 5–7 Hypothetical Examples of Unadjusted and Adjusted Relative Risks According to Type of Confounding (Positive or Negative)

Example No.	Type of Confounding	Unadjusted Relative Risk	Adjusted Relative Risk
1	Positive	3.5	1.0
2	Positive	3.5	2.1
3	Positive	0.3	0.7
4	Negative	1.0	3.2
5	Negative	1.5	3.2
6	Negative	0.8	0.2
7	Qualitative	2.0	0.7
8	Qualitative	0.6	1.8

tary lifestyle) were negative confounders of the association between hostility and myocardial infarction incidence.

An extreme case of confounding is when the confounding effect results in an inversion of the direction of the association (Table 5–7, examples no. 7 and 8), a phenomenon that can be properly designated as *qualitative* confounding. For instance, in example no. 1 in Section 5.1, the US/Venezuela ratio of crude mortality rates is 8.7/4.4 = 1.98; however, when the age-adjusted rates are used, it becomes 3.6/4.6 = 0.78. The opposite patterns of the adjusted and crude rate ratios can be explained by the striking difference in the age distribution between these two countries.

As a summary, Figure 5–9 shows schematic representations of negative, positive, and qualitative confounding effects.

The direction of the confounding effect (positive or negative) can be inferred from the directions of the associations of the confounder

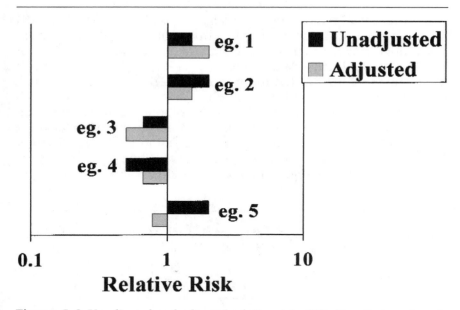

Figure 5–9 Unadjusted and adjusted relative risks (RR): Negative confounding is seen in examples no. 1 and 3 (adjusted RRs are further away from the null value of 1.0 than unadjusted RRs); positive confounding is seen in examples no. 2 and 4 (adjusted RRs are closer to the null value of 1.0 than unadjusted RRs). Example no. 5 denotes confounding in which the direction of the association changes (qualitative confounding).

with exposure and outcome, if known. Table 5–8 summarizes the expectations of the changes brought about by the adjustment, resulting from the directions of these associations. Thus, positive confounding is to be expected when the confounder-exposure association is in the same direction as the confounder-outcome association. When these associations are in divergent directions, there will be negative confounding (or qualitative confounding in extreme cases).

5.4.5 Statistical Significance in Assessing Confounding

It is inappropriate to rely on statistical significance to identify confounding, especially when either the exposure (in case-control studies) or the outcome (in cohort studies) varies markedly according to the confounding variable. For example, in a hypothetical case-control study examining the relationship of the occurrence of menopause to disease Y in women aged 45 to 54 years, small, statistically nonsignificant differences in age between cases and controls may cause an important confounding effect in view of the strong relationship between age and presence of menopause in this age range. Thus, even if

Table 5–8 Directions of the Associations of the Confounder with the Exposure and the Outcome, and Expectation of Change of Estimate with Adjustment (Assume a Direct Relationship Between Exposure and Outcome, ie, for Exposed/Unexposed, RR, or Odds Ratio > 1.0)

Association of Confounder with Exposure Is	Association of Confounder with Outcome Is	Type of Confounding	Expectation of Change from Unadjusted to Adjusted Estimate
Direct*	Direct*	Positive‡	Unadjusted > Adjusted
Direct*	Inverse†	Negative§	Unadjusted < Adjusted
Inverse†	Inverse†	Positive‡	Unadjusted > Adjusted
Inverse†	Direct*	Negative§	Unadjusted < Adjusted

*Direct association: presence of the confounder is related to an increased probability of the exposure or the outcome.

†Inverse association: presence of the confounder is related to a decreased probability of the exposure or the outcome.

‡Positive confounding: when the confounding effect results in an unadjusted measure of association (eg, relative risk) further away from the null hypothesis than the adjusted estimate.

§Negative confounding: when the confounding effect results in an unadjusted measure of association closer to the null hypothesis than the adjusted estimate.

there is no association whatsoever between occurrence of menopause and disease, if for each year of age the odds of menopause hypothetically increased from 1:1 to 1.5:1 (for an increase in menopause prevalence from 50% to 60%), a case-control age difference as small as 1 year (which might not be statistically significant if the study sample was not large) would result in an age-unadjusted menopause relative odds of 1.5 (Figure 5–10).

For those who choose to use the *p* value as a criterion to identify confounding, it may be wiser to use more "lenient" (conservative) *p* values as a guide to identify confounders—for example, 0.20. Doing so allows for the possibility of accepting the presence of confounding even when there are small differences between cases and controls in case-control studies, or between exposed and unexposed subjects in cohort studies. This strategy, however, should not replace the investigator's consideration of the *strength* of the associations of the sus-

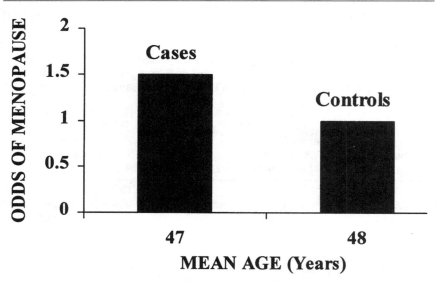

Figure 5–10 Odds of menopause occurrence in a hypothetical case-control study. The menopause odds increases by 50% for each year of age, corresponding to an absolute difference of 10% in the prevalence of menopause (in this example 60% and 50% in cases and controls, respectively). Cases and controls have a 1-year difference in age. Thus, the relative odds of 1.5 (1.5/1.0) reflects entirely the age difference and does not result from an association between menopause and disease.

pected confounder(s) with the exposure and outcome as a means to identify confounding.

5.4.6 Conditional Confounding

A presumed confounding variable may be confounded by other variables. Thus, univariate evaluation may suggest that a given variable Z is a confounder, but the same variable may not act as a confounder when other variables are adjusted for. Similarly, Z may not appear to be a confounder univariately because it is negatively confounded by other variables, in which case a confounding effect of Z may become evident upon adjustment.

5.4.7 Confounding and Bias

Should confounding be regarded as a type of selection bias? Some epidemiology textbooks suggest that confounding is one more type of bias (eg, Rothman and Greenland[15]), essentially because a confounded association can be considered as a "biased estimate" of the

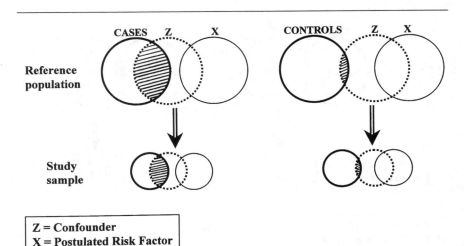

Z = Confounder
X = Postulated Risk Factor

Figure 5–11 Schematic representation of confounding. In the reference population, confounding factor Z is truly more common in cases than in controls. Assuming no random variability, the higher frequency of Z in cases (represented by the shaded overlapping areas of the circles) is reflected in the study samples, and as a result, the frequency of the exposure of interest X (which, by definition, is related to Z) is higher in cases than in controls.

causal association (that which is expressed by the adjusted estimate—assuming that the adjustment procedure is appropriate and not subject to residual confounding). In contrast, other textbooks (eg, Lilienfeld and Stolley[16] and Gordis[17]), differentiate between "spurious" associations due to bias and "indirect" (or "statistical") associations due to confounding, thus suggesting that confounding is distinct from bias. The rationale for keeping confounding conceptually distinct from bias can be described as follows. Assuming no random variability, schematic representations of confounding and bias are shown in Figures 5–11 and 5–12, respectively. In these figures, circles represent cases or controls, the confounding or selection factor Z and the exposure of interest X. Larger and smaller circles denote the reference population and study sample subsets, respectively. In Figure 5–11, the proportion of Z (eg, smoking) in the reference population is truly greater in cases than in controls; thus, any factors related to Z, such as X (eg, alcohol intake), are more frequent in cases. In confounding, the study samples accurately reflect the fact that X (via Z) is more common in cases than in controls. On the other hand, in Figure 5–12, the proportion of cases and controls in whom Z is present is the same

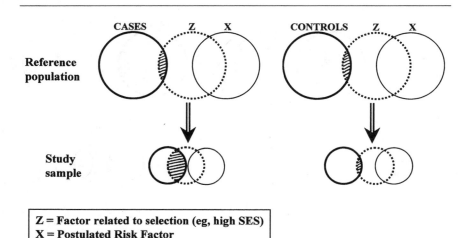

Z = Factor related to selection (eg, high SES)
X = Postulated Risk Factor

Figure 5–12 Schematic representation of selection bias. In the reference population, the proportion of factor Z is the same in cases and controls. Assuming no random variability, the higher frequency of Z in the study sample of cases (represented by the shaded area of overlap between the circles denoting cases and Z) is the result of selection bias whereby the selection of cases is influenced by the presence of Z. SES, socioeconomic status.

in the reference population; however, in the study samples, selection bias has resulted in cases' having a (spuriously) higher proportion of Z (and thus X) than controls. Consider, for example, a case-control study in which cases are ascertained in hospitals that preferentially admit upper SES patients, and controls are sampled from noncases in the reference population. As a result of this type of selection bias, positive associations will be observed for exposures related to high SES.

This conceptual distinction between confounding and bias, perhaps of only intellectual interest when assessing causal relationships (because, for accepting a relationship as causal, both confounding and bias must be deemed unlikely explanations), nevertheless becomes important when epidemiologic findings are considered in the context of public health practice. Whether or not confounding is labeled as a bias, there is a clear-cut role for true, yet confounded associations, as they allow identification of markers that may be useful to define high-risk groups for secondary prevention.

Exhibit 5–5 The Relationship Between Type of Evidence Needed in Epidemiologic Studies and Type of Prevention Carried Out (Primary or Secondary)

GOAL	TYPE OF EVIDENCE NEEDED
Primary prevention: Prevention or cessation of risk factor exposure (eg, saturated fat intake and atherosclerosis).	Causal association *must* be present; otherwise, intervention on risk factor will not affect disease outcome. For example, if fat did not cause atherosclerosis, a lower fat intake would not affect atherosclerosis risk.
Secondary prevention: Early diagnosis via selective screening of "high risk" subjects (eg, identification of individuals with high triglyceride levels).	Association may be *either* causal or statistical (the latter must not be biased): that is, the association may be *confounded*. For example, even if hypertriglyceridemic individuals had a higher probability of developing atherosclerotic disease because of the confounding effect of low high-density lipoprotein levels, atherosclerosis is *truly* more common in these individuals.

As summarized in Exhibit 5–5, for primary prevention purposes a causal association between the risk factor and the disease outcome must exist; otherwise, modification of the former will not lead to a reduction of the risk of the latter. However, for secondary prevention, it is sufficient that there be a statistical association between the risk factor and the disease, regardless of whether this association is also causal. An example is the relationship of high serum triglyceride (TG) levels to atherosclerotic disease. For years, there has been uncertainty regarding the independent role of high serum TG levels on the development of atherosclerosis, as this relationship could be a mere reflection of the strong inverse relationship between high TG and low HDL levels known to be causally linked to the development of atherosclerosis (Figure 5–13). Whether or not the causal link between high TG levels and atherosclerosis exists, there is no doubt that individuals with high TG levels are more likely to develop atherosclerosis. Thus, unlike a spurious relationship resulting from bias, a confounded, yet true relationship allows identification of individuals with a higher likelihood of disease occurrence.

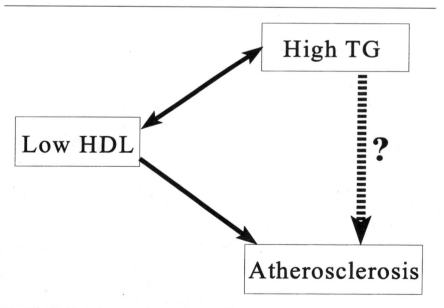

Figure 5–13 Relationship between hypertriglyceridemia, low high-density cholesterol levels, and atherosclerosis.

5.5 CONCLUSION

Confounding, along with bias, constitutes a formidable threat to the evaluation of causal relationships. In this chapter, issues related to the definition of confounding effects as well as some approaches to verify the presence of confounding were discussed. The assessment of confounding before adjustment was underscored as a means of predicting the magnitude and direction of possible changes (if any) in the measure of association brought about by adjustment. The concept of residual confounding (which is also discussed in Chapter 7), was introduced in this chapter, as was the notion that statistical significance testing should not be used as a criterion to evaluate confounding. Finally, the rationale for not classifying confounding as a type of bias was discussed in the context of the usefulness of confounded, yet true associations as a way to identify high-risk groups for secondary prevention purposes.

REFERENCES

1. Organizacion Panamericana de la Salud/Pan American Health Organization. *Las condiciones de salud en las Americas*. Washington, DC: OPS/PAHO; 1990. Publicacion Cientifica no. 524.
2. Davey Smith G, Frankel S, Yarnell J. Sex and death: are they related? Findings from the Caerphilly Cohort Study. *Br Med J*. 1997;315:1641–1644.
3. Smalley WE, Ray WA, Daugherty JR, et al. No association between calcium channel blocker use and confirmed bleeding peptic ulcer disease. *Am J Epidemiol*. 1998; 148:350–354.
4. Heilbrun LK, Nomura A, Hankin JH, et al. Diet and colorectal cancer with special reference to fiber intake. *Int J Cancer*. 1989;44:1–6.
5. Broda G, Davis CE, Pajak A, et al. Poland and United States Collaborative Study on Cardiovascular Epidemiology: A comparison of HDL cholesterol and its subfractions in populations covered by the United States Atherosclerosis Risk in Communities study and the Pol-MONICA project. *Arterioscler Thromb Vasc Biol*. 1996;16:339–349.
6. Manson JE, Stampfer MJ, Hennekens CH, et al. Body weight and longevity: a reassessment. *JAMA*. 1987;257:353–358.
7. Rush D. A correction by the author: "Maternal smoking: a reassessment of the association with perinatal mortality." *Am J Epidemiol*. 1973;97:425.
8. Breslow NE, Day NE. *Statistical Methods in Cancer Research. Vol. 1. The Analysis of Case-Control Studies*. Lyon, France: International Agency for Research on Cancer Scientific Publications; 1980.
9. Shimakawa T, Sorlie P, Carpenter MA, et al. Dietary intake patterns and sociodemographic factors in the Atherosclerosis Risk in Communities (ARIC) study. *Prev Med*. 1994;23:769–780.

10. Miettinen OS, Cook EF. Confounding: essence and detection. *Am J Epidemiol.* 1981; 114:593–603.
11. Greenland S. Absence of confounding does not correspond to collapsibility of the rate ratio or rate difference. *Epidemiology.* 1996;7:498–501.
12. Pandey DK, Shekelle R, Selwyn BJ, et al. Dietary vitamin C and β-carotene and risk of death in middle-aged men. The Western Electric study. *Am J Epidemiol.* 1995; 142:1269–1278.
13. Krieger N, Williams DR, Moss NE. Measuring social class in US public health research: concepts, methodologies, and guidelines. *Annu Rev Public Health.* 1997;18: 341–378.
14. Barefoot JC, Larsen S, von der Lieth L, et al. Hostility, incidence of acute myocardial infarction, and mortality in a sample of older Danish men and women. *Am J Epidemiol.* 1995;142:477–484.
15. Rothman KJ, Greenland S. *Modern Epidemiology.* 2nd ed. Philadelphia, Pa: Lippincott-Raven Publishers; 1998.
16. Lilienfeld DE, Stolley PD. *Foundations of Epidemiology.* New York, NY: Oxford University Press; 1994.
17. Gordis L. *Epidemiology.* Philadelphia, Pa: WB Saunders; 1996.

CHAPTER 6

Defining and Assessing Heterogeneity of Effects: Interaction

6.1   INTRODUCTION

The term *interaction* is used in epidemiology to describe a situation in which two or more risk factors modify the effect of each other with regard to the occurrence or level of a given outcome. This phenomenon is also known as *effect modification* and is distinguished from the phenomenon of confounding. As discussed in detail in Chapter 5, *confounding* refers to a situation in which a variable that is associated with both the exposure and the outcome of interest is responsible for the entirety or part of the statistical association between the exposure and the outcome. Interaction between a given variable (*effect modifier*) and a given exposure is a different phenomenon, as detailed in the following sections.

For dichotomous variables, *interaction* means that the effect of the exposure on the outcome differs depending on whether another variable (the effect modifier) is present. If the presence of the effect modifier potentiates (accentuates) the effect of the exposure of interest, this variable and the exposure are said to be *synergistic* (*positive interaction*); if the presence of the effect modifier diminishes or eliminates the effect of the exposure of interest, it can be said that the effect modifier and the exposure are *antagonistic* (*negative interaction*). This concept can be extended to continuous variables. In this context, the phenomenon of interaction means that the effect of the exposure on

211

the outcome differs depending on the level of another variable (the effect modifier).

A minimum of three factors are needed for the phenomenon of interaction to occur. For this chapter, the main putative risk factor will be designated as factor A, the outcome variable as Y, and the third factor (potential effect modifier) as Z. In addition, although it is recognized that there are differences between absolute or relative differences in risk, rate, and odds, the generic terms *risk, attributable risk*, and *relative risk* will be mostly used. In this chapter, the term *homogeneity* indicates that the effects of a risk factor A are homogeneous or similar in strata formed by factor Z. *Heterogeneity* of effects, therefore, implies that these effects are dissimilar.

The discussion that follows is largely based on the simplest situation involving interaction between two variables with two categories each—a discrete outcome (eg, disease present or absent) and positive associations (ie, those characterized by a relative risk greater than 1.0). Other types of interaction that can be assessed but are not discussed in detail in this textbook include those based on more than two "independent" variables, or on continous variables. Finally, the word *effect*, which should be used with caution when inferring etiologic relationships from observational studies,[1] is often referred to in this chapter in a somewhat loose sense, so as to allow use of the term *effect modification*.

Interaction can be defined in two different, yet compatible ways. Each definition leads to a specific strategy for the evaluation of interaction.

1. *Definition based on homogeneity or heterogeneity of effects:* Interaction occurs when the effect of a risk factor A on the risk of an outcome Y is not homogeneous in strata formed by a third variable Z. When this definition is used, variable Z is often referred to as an *effect modifier*.
2. *Definition based on the comparison between observed and expected joint effects of risk factor A and third variable Z:* Interaction occurs when the observed joint effect of A and Z differs from that expected on the basis of the independent effects of A and Z.

6.2   HOW IS EFFECT MEASURED?

An important decision in the evaluation of interaction using either definition is how to measure "effect." "Effect" can be measured either by the attributable risk (*additive model*) or by the relative difference—

for example, the relative risk (*multiplicative model*). The conceptual basis for the evaluation of interaction is the same for both models.

6.3 STRATEGIES TO EVALUATE INTERACTION

6.3.1 Assessment of Homogeneity of Effects

Variability in susceptibility to an outcome given exposure to a risk factor, reflected as between-individual heterogeneity of the effect of the risk factor, seems to be a universal phenomenon for both infectious and noninfectious diseases. For example, even for a strong association, such as that between smoking and lung cancer, not every exposed person develops the disease. Assuming that chance does not play a role in determining which smokers develop lung cancer, this suggests that smoking by itself is not a sufficient cause. Thus, smokers who develop lung cancer are likely to differ from smokers who do not in that another component cause[2] must be present in smokers who develop lung cancer to make them susceptible to smoking-induced disease. Presence of this necessary component cause can be thought of generically as a susceptibility factor, which could be either genetically or environmentally determined.

A simplistic representation of the conceptual framework for interaction defined as heterogeneity of effects is shown in Figure 6–1. After it is observed that a statistical association exists between a risk factor A and a disease outcome Y and it is reasonably certain that the association is not due to confounding or bias, the key question in evaluating interaction is: Does the magnitude or direction of the effect of A on Y vary according to the occurrence of some other variable Z in the study population? A positive answer suggests the presence of interaction. For example, because diabetes is a stronger risk factor for coronary heart disease (CHD) in women than in men, it can be concluded that there is interaction: that is, that gender modifies the effect of diabetes on CHD risk.[3]

The conceptualization of interaction as the occurrence of heterogeneous effects of A (eg, asbestos exposure) according to the presence or absence of Z (eg, smoking) explains why the expression, *effect modification* is used as a synonym for *interaction*. For example, the proper language when describing the interaction between smoking and asbestos in regard to the risk of respiratory cancer is that "the *effect* of asbestos exposure on respiratory cancer risk is *modified* by cigarette smoking in that it is much stronger in smokers than in nonsmokers." The expression *effect modifier* suggests that the investigator has cho-

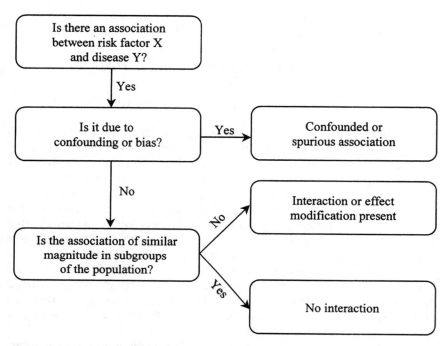

Figure 6–1 Conceptual framework for the definition of interaction based on the homogeneity concept.

sen some kind of hierarchical level in approaching the two independent variables: A is the "main" variable of interest and Z is the effect modifier. From the preventive standpoint, the variable not amenable to intervention (eg, a gene) is usually regarded as the effect modifier, in contrast to an exposure that can be prevented or eliminated.

As mentioned previously, a key issue in the evaluation of interaction is that it involves at least three variables: the main factor of interest A (eg, diabetes), the potential effect modifier Z (eg, gender), and a given outcome Y (eg, coronary heart disease). There may, however, be more than two interacting independent variables: for instance, if diabetes is a more important risk factor for women than for men only among older subjects. In this hypothetical example, the simultaneous presence of two variables would be needed to modify the effect of diabetes: gender and age.

Detection of Additive Interaction: The Absolute Difference or Attributable Risk Model

Additive interaction is considered to be present when the attributable risk in those exposed to factor A (AR $_{exp}$, ie, the absolute difference in risks between those exposed and those not exposed to A; see Chapter 3, Equation 3.4) varies (is heterogeneous) as a function of a third variable Z.

The easiest way to evaluate interaction in this instance is to calculate the attributable risks for those exposed to risk factor A for each stratum defined by levels of the potential effect modifier Z. Hypothetical examples of this strategy to evaluate additive interaction are shown in Tables 6–1 and 6–2. In Table 6–1, the absolute excess risks of Y attributable to A do not differ according to exposure to Z. In Table 6–2, the attributable risk for A is larger for those exposed than for those not exposed to Z, denoting heterogeneity of the absolute effects of A. Note that, in these tables, there are two different reference categories for the attributable risks associated with A: for the stratum in which Z is absent, the reference category is Z absent, A absent; for the stratum in which Z is present, the reference category is Z present, A absent.

The patterns shown in Tables 6–1 and 6–2 can be examined graphically (Figure 6–2A). A graph with arithmetic scales is used to assess additive interaction. The risks for each category of the risk factor A are plotted separately for individuals exposed and those not exposed to the third variable Z. In this type of graph (arithmetic), the steepness of the slopes is a function of the absolute differences. Thus, when the absolute difference in risk of the outcome (attributable risk in those exposed to A) is the same regardless of exposure to Z, the two lines are

Table 6–1 Hypothetical Example of Absence of Additive Interaction

Z	A	Incidence Rate (per 1000)	Attributable Risk (per 1000)*
No	No	10.0	0
	Yes	20.0	10.0
Yes	No	30.0	0
	Yes	40.0	10.0

*Attributable risk for A within strata of Z.

Table 6–2 Hypothetical Example of Presence of Additive Interaction

Z	A	Incidence Rate (per 1000)	Attributable Risk (per 1000)*
No	No	5.0	0
	Yes	10.0	5.0
Yes	No	10.0	0
	Yes	30.0	20.0

*Attributable risk for A within strata of Z.

parallel. When the absolute differences differ, denoting additive interaction, the lines are not parallel.

Detection of Multiplicative Interaction: The Relative Difference or Ratio Model

Multiplicative interaction is considered to be present when the relative difference (ratio) in the risk of an outcome Y between subjects exposed and those not exposed to a putative risk factor A differs (is heterogeneous) as a function of a third variable Z. Hypothetical examples of the evaluation of multiplicative interaction are shown in Tables 6–3 and 6–4. (Note that, consistently with Tables 6–1 and 6–2, there are two different reference categories for the relative risks associated with A: for the stratum in which Z is absent, the reference category is Z absent, A absent; for the stratum in which Z is present, the reference category is Z present, A absent.) In Table 6–3, the relative risk for A is the same for those exposed and those not exposed to Z. In Table 6–4, the relative risk for A is larger for those exposed than for those not exposed to Z, indicating that the effects of A measured by the relative risk are heterogeneous according to Z.

As for additive interaction, multiplicative interaction can be evaluated graphically by plotting the rates for each category of A according to the strata defined by Z (Figure 6–2B). For multiplicative interaction assessment, however, a log scale is used in the ordinate. Thus, the steepness of the slopes is a function of the relative differences: when the risk ratios for A are the same in those exposed or not exposed to Z, the Z-specific curves are parallel, indicating absence of multiplicative interaction. Nonparallel lines suggest the presence of multiplicative interaction.

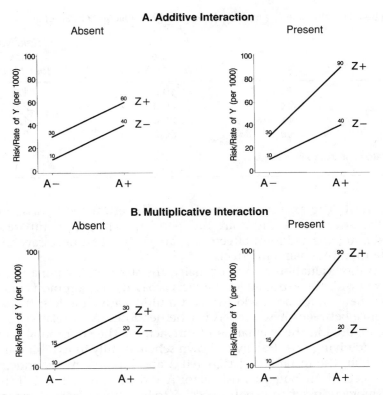

Figure 6–2 Assessment of interaction by means of graphs. For additive interaction (**A**), use arithmetic scale on ordinate (slopes represent absolute differences). Interaction is absent on the left panel because the absolute difference
between A$^+$ and A$^-$ is the same regardless of the presence of Z (60 − 30 = 40
− 10 = 30 per 1000). Interaction is present on the right panel because the absolute difference between A$^+$ and A$^-$ is higher when Z is present (90 − 30 =
60 per 1000) than when Z is absent (40 − 10 = 30 per 1000). For multiplicative interaction (**B**), use logarithmic scale on ordinate (slopes represent relative difference). Interaction is absent on the left panel because the relative
difference between A$^+$ and A$^-$ is the same regardless of the presence of Z
(30/15 = 20/10 = 2). Interaction is present on the right panel because the relative difference between A$^+$ and A$^-$ is higher when Z is present (90/15 = 6)
than when Z is absent (20/10 = 2).

6.3.2 Comparing Observed and Expected Joint Effects

As discussed previously, an alternative definition of interaction is
when the observed joint effect of A and Z differs from the expected

Table 6–3 Hypothetical Example of Absence of Multiplicative Interaction

Z	A	Incidence Rate (per 1000)	Relative Risk (per 1000)*
No	No	10.0	1.0
	Yes	20.0	2.0
Yes	No	25.0	1.0
	Yes	50.0	2.0

*Relative risk for A within strata of Z

joint effect. The expected joint effect can be estimated by assuming that the effects of A and Z are independent. Thus, to compare observed and expected joint effects of A and Z, it is first necessary to estimate their independent effects.

As in the evaluation of homogeneity, the strategy of comparing the observed with the expected joint effects is based on a common conceptual framework for both additive and multiplicative models; the only difference between these models is whether absolute or relative differences are used in the evaluation of interaction. The conceptual framework underlying this strategy is shown schematically in Exhibit 6–1. In the exhibit, the rectangles designated A and Z represent the independent effects of the potential risk factor A and effect modifier Z. If there is no interaction, when exposure occurs to both these factors, the joint effect is expected to be merely the sum of the independent effects, as denoted by the rectangle A + Z in Exhibit 6–1A. (The term *sum* is not used here in the context of a simple (arithmetic) sum, which would make it limited to the additive model; rather, it implies the combined

Table 6–4 Hypothetical Example of Multiplicative Interaction

Z	A	Incidence Rate (per 1000)	Relative Risk (per 1000)*
No	No	10.0	1.0
	Yes	20.0	2.0
Yes	No	25.0	1.0
	Yes	125.0	5.0

*Relative risk for A within strata of Z

Exhibit 6–1 Conceptual Framework of the Definition of Interaction Based on Comparing Expected and Observed Joint Effects

A. When there is *no* interaction, the joint effect of risk factors A and Z equals the sum of their independent effects:

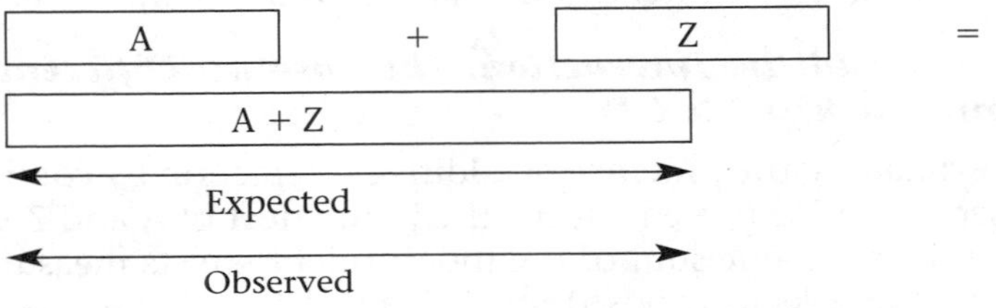

| A | + | Z | = |

| A + Z |

←————————————————————→
              Expected

←————————————————————→
              Observed

B. When there is *positive* interaction (*synergism*), the *observed* joint effect of risk factors A and Z is greater than that *expected* on the basis of summing the independent effects of A and Z:

| A | + | Z | = |

| A + Z | † |

←————————————————————→
              Expected

←——————————————————————————————→
              Observed

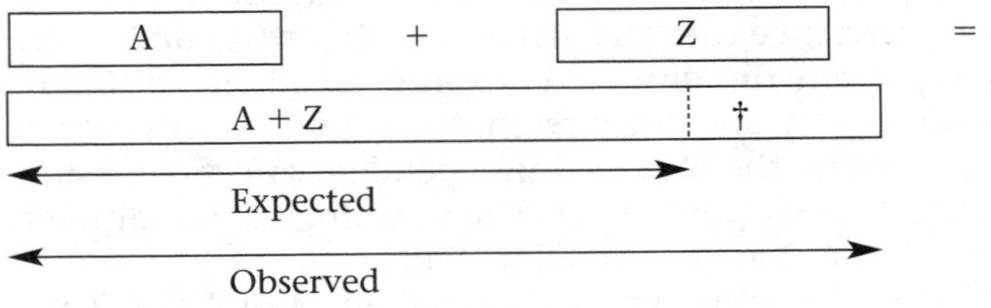

† Excess due to positive interaction.

C. When there is *negative* interaction (*antagonism*), the *observed* joint effect of risk factors A and Z is smaller than that *expected* on the basis of summing the independent effects of A and Z:

| A | + | Z | = |

| A + Z | * |

←——————————————————————————————→
              Expected

←————————————————————→
              Observed

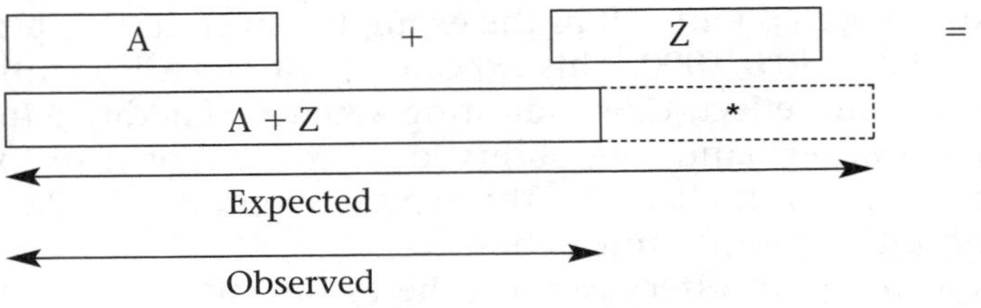

*"Deficit" due to negative interaction.

effects of A and Z.) In Exhibit 6–1B, the observed joint effect exceeds the expected joint effect. The area to the right of the dotted line represents the excess due to interaction. As the observed joint effect is greater than expected, there is positive interaction or synergism. However, if the observed joint effect of A and Z is smaller than that expected, there is negative interaction or antagonism (Exhibit 6–1C).

Detection of Additive Interaction: The Absolute Difference or Attributable Risk Model

When evaluating the presence of additive interaction by comparing joint observed and expected effects, the joint effect of A and Z is estimated as the arithmetic sum of the independent effects measured by the attributable risks in exposed individuals (AR_{exp}). Exhibit 6–2 presents two hypothetical examples showing the absence (A) and presence (B) of additive interaction. The first step is to calculate incidence rates for each of the four table cells defined by the two factors A and Z. The cell representing the absence of both exposures ($-/-$) is designated as the reference category. The observed attributable risks in Exhibit 6–2 represent the observed absolute incidence differences between each category and the reference category. In this manner, it is possible to separate the observed independent effects of A and Z and thus to estimate their joint effect. The meanings of the different categories in Exhibit 6–2 are described in Table 6–5.

Estimation of the joint expected (Expd) effect of A and Z measured by the attributable risk (AR) is carried out by a simple sum of their independent observed (Obs) attributable risks, as follows:

[Equation 6.1]

$$\text{Expd } AR_{A+Z+} = \text{Obs } AR_{A+Z-} + \text{Obs } AR_{A-Z+}$$

Thus, the expected joint AR in the example shown in Exhibit 6–2A is $20.0 + 10.0 = 30.0/1000$. This expected joint effect is identical to the observed joint effect, thus indicating absence of additive interaction. On the other hand, the observed joint AR shown in Exhibit 6–2B of $50.0/1000$ is higher than the expected joint AR of $30.0/1000$, denoting positive additive interaction.

The expected joint effect can also be estimated by an expected (Expd) joint incidence (Inc), as follows:

[Equation 6.2]

$$\text{Expd } Inc_{A+Z+} = \text{Obs } Inc_{A-Z-} + (\text{Obs } Inc_{A+Z-} - \text{Obs } Inc_{A-Z-}) + (\text{Obs } Inc_{A-Z+} - \text{Obs } Inc_{A-Z-})$$

$$= \text{Obs } Inc_{A-Z-} + \text{Obs } AR_{A+Z-} + \text{Obs } AR_{A-Z+}$$

Exhibit 6–2 Detection of Interaction Through the Comparison of
Expected and Observed Joint Effects: Additive Interaction

A. No Additive Interaction

Z	Observed Incidence Rates/1000 A	
	−	+
−	10.0	30.0
+	20.0	40.0

Z	Observed Attributable Risks/1000 A	
	−	+
−	0.0	20.0
+	10.0	30.0

Joint expected AR = 10.0 + 20.0 = 30.0
Joint observed AR = 30.0

B. Additive Interaction Present

Z	Observed Incidence Rates/1000 A	
	−	+
−	10.0	30.0
+	20.0	60.0

Z	Observed Attributable Risks/1000 A	
	−	+
−	0.0	20.0
+	10.0	50.0

Joint expected AR = 10.0 + 20.0 = 30.0
Joint observed AR = 50.0

For example, for Exhibit 6–2B,

$$\text{Expd Inc}_{A+Z+} = 10.0 + (30.0 - 10.0) + (20.0 - 10.0) = 40.0/1000$$

which is less than the joint observed incidence of 60.0/1000, thus
again denoting positive additive interaction.

Detection of Multiplicative Interaction: The Relative Difference or Ratio Model

The strategy for detecting multiplicative interaction is analogous to
that for detecting additive interaction; however, in the evaluation of
multiplicative interaction, the expected joint effect is estimated by
multiplying the independent relative effects of A and Z:

Table 6–5 Assessment of Interaction: Additive Model

Factor Z	Factor A	Observed Attributable Risks Represent
Absent	Absent	Reference category = 0.0
Absent	Present	Independent effect of A (ie, in the absence of Z) (eg, in Exhibit 6–2A, 30.0 − 10.0 = 20.0)
Present	Absent	Independent effect of Z (ie, in the absence of A) (eg, in Exhibit 6–2A, 20.0 − 10.0 = 10.0)
Present	Present	Joint effect of A and Z (eg, in Exhibit 6–2A, 40.0 − 10.0 = 30.0)

[Equation 6.3]

$$\text{Expd RR}_{A+Z+} = \text{Obs RR}_{A+Z-} \times \text{Obs RR}_{A-Z+}$$

Independent and joint effects expressed by relative risks (RR) are shown in Exhibit 6–3, with interpretations akin to those for additive interaction based on Exhibit 6–2. In Exhibit 6–3A, the expected (3.0 × 2.0 = 6.0) and the observed joint effects are equal, suggesting no multiplicative interaction. In Exhibit 6–3B, the expected joint relative risk is also 6.0, but the observed joint relative risk is 9.0, denoting positive multiplicative interaction.

6.3.3 Examples of Interaction Assessment in a Cohort Study

Data from a cohort study conducted in Washington County, Maryland, allow evaluation of additive and multiplicative interactions between father's educational level and maternal smoking on the risks of neonatal and postneonatal deaths[4] (Tables 6–6 and 6–7). As shown in Table 6–6A, both the relative risks and the attributable risks for the maternal smoking/neonatal mortality associations are heterogeneous according to the educational level of the father, thus denoting both multiplicative and additive interactions, which express the magnification of the smoking effect on neonatal mortality when father's educational level is low. (Note that the heterogeneity in Table 6–6 may be due to residual confounding resulting from the use of broad educational and smoking categories; see Chapter 5, Section 5.4.3 and Chapter 7, Section 7.5. For the purposes of this example, however, it is assumed that the heterogeneity is not due to residual confounding.) The interaction on both scales is confirmed when the joint observed and expected effects are compared in Table 6–6B. For the additive

Exhibit 6–3 Detection of Interaction Through the Comparison of Expected and Observed Joint Effects: Multiplicative Interaction

A. No Multiplicative Interaction

Z	Observed Incidence Rates/1000 A	
	−	+
−	10.0	30.0
+	20.0	60.0

Z	Observed Relative Risks A	
	−	+
−	1.0	3.0
+	2.0	6.0

Joint expected RR = 2.0 × 3.0 = 6.0
Joint observed RR = 6.0

B. Multiplicative Interaction Present

Z	Observed Incidence Rates/1000 A	
	−	+
−	10.0	30.0
+	20.0	90.0

Z	Observed Relative Risks A	
	−	+
−	1.0	3.0
+	2.0	9.0

Joint expected RR = 2.0 × 3.0 = 6.0
Joint observed RR = 9.0

model, the observed joint attributable risk is 31.2/1000 live births, whereas the expected is only 3.7/1000 (ie, 1.5 + 2.2). For the multiplicative model, joint observed and expected relative risks are 3.1 and 1.2, respectively. Little or no interaction on either scale is apparent when assessing the association of maternal smoking and father's education with *post*neonatal mortality (Tables 6–7A and B). The small differences between observed and expected joint effects (or the slight heterogeneity of effects) are probably due to random variability.

6.4 ASSESSMENT OF INTERACTION IN CASE-CONTROL STUDIES

The preceding discussion of the assessment of interaction has relied on absolute and relative measures of risk (incidence rates, attributable

Table 6–6 Neonatal Death Rates per 1000 Live Births According to Smoking Status of the Mother and Education of the Father, Washington County, 1953 to 1963

A. Homogeneity Strategy

Father's Education	Mother's Smoking	Estimated No. of Live Births	Rate/1000 Live Births	RR*	AR†/1000 Live Births (Exposed)
0–8 grades	No	1967	16.4	1.0	0
	Yes	767	46.1	2.8	29.7
9+ grades	No	5967	14.9	1.0	0
	Yes	3833	17.1	1.1	2.2

B. Comparison of Joint Observed and Expected Effects

Father's Education	Incidence/1000 Live Births Mother's Smoking		AR†/ 1000 Live Births (Exposed) Mother's Smoking		RR* Mother's Smoking	
	No	Yes	No	Yes	No	Yes
9+ grades (unexposed)	14.9	17.1	0	2.2	1.0	1.1
0–8 grades (exposed)	16.4	46.1	1.5	31.2	1.1	3.1

Expected joint effects:
  Additive → AR = 1.5 + 2.2 = 3.7/1000 live births
  Multiplicative → RR = 1.1 × 1.1 = 1.2

Observed joint effects:
  Additive → AR = 31.2/1000 live births
  Multiplicative → RR = 3.1

*Relative risk.

†Attributable risk.

Source: Data from GW Comstock and FE Lundin, Parental Smoking and Perinatal Mortality, *American Journal of Obstetrics and Gynecology*, Vol 98, pp 708–718, © 1967.

risks, and relative risks) obtained in cohort studies. What follows is a discussion of the same concepts and strategies applied to the analysis of case-control data. It should be noted that because case-control studies merely provide an efficient approach to analyze cohort data, the concept of interaction does not have a special meaning in these studies. Thus, the discussion that follows merely aims at facilitating the application of the concept of interaction to the analysis of case-

Table 6–7 *Postneonatal Death Rates per 1000 Live Births According to Smoking Status of the Mother and Education of the Father, Washington County, 1953 to 1963*

A. Homogeneity Strategy

Father's Education	Mother's Smoking	Estimated No. of Live Births	Rate/1000 Live Births	RR*	AR†/1000 Live Births (Exposed)
0–8 grades	No	1967	12.3	1.0	0
	Yes	767	19.8	1.6	7.5
9+ grades	No	5967	6.1	1.0	0
	Yes	3833	11.1	1.8	5.0

B. Comparison of Joint Observed and Expected Effects

Father's Education	Incidence/1000 Live Births Mother's Smoking		AR†/ 1000 Live Births (Exposed) Mother's Smoking		RR* Mother's Smoking	
	No	Yes	No	Yes	No	Yes
9+ grades (unexposed)	6.1	11.1	0	5.0	1.0	1.8
0–8 grades (exposed)	12.3	19.8	6.2	13.7	2.0	3.2

Expected joint effects:
  Additive → AR = 6.2 + 5.0 = 11.2/1000 live births
  Multiplicative → RR = 2.0 × 1.8 = 3.6

Observed joint effects:
  Additive → AR = 13.7/1000 live births
  Multiplicative → RR = 3.2

*Relative risk.

†Attributable risk.

Source: Data from GW Comstock and FE Lundin, Parental Smoking and Perinatal Mortality, *American Journal of Obstetrics and Gynecology*, Vol 98, pp 708–718, © 1967.

control data. The formulas presented in this section are equally applicable to cohort and case-control studies.

6.4.1   Assessment of Homogeneity of Effects

In a case-control study, the homogeneity strategy can be used only to assess the presence or absence of multiplicative interaction. The reason for this is that absolute measures of disease risk are usually not available in case-control studies; thus, it is not possible to measure the absolute difference between exposed and unexposed—that is, the attributable risk (absolute excess risk) in those exposed to the main risk factor. As a result, the homogeneity of attributable risks (in exposed subjects) in strata formed by the potential effect modifier Z cannot be readily assessed in case-control studies. However, as shown in the next section, it is possible to assess additive interaction in a case-control study by using the strategy of comparing observed and expected joint effects.

In most case-control studies, the assessment of the homogeneity of effects is based on the odds ratio. This assessment, as illustrated in Table 6–8, is analogous to the assessment of the homogeneity of relative risks. In the table, cases and controls are stratified according to categories of both the putative risk factor of interest, A, and the potential effect modifier, Z. Different reference categories are used for the comparison of the odds ratios associated with A in the strata formed by Z: when Z is absent, the reference category—denoted by an odds ratio of 1.0—is that in which A is also absent. On the other hand, for the individuals exposed to Z, the reference category with an odds ratio of 1.0 is formed by subjects exposed to Z but unexposed to A. Thus, each odds ratio derived in Table 6–8 refers to the effect of A, first in the absence (upper half) and then in the presence (lower half) of Z.

It is important to emphasize that the odds ratio for A when Z is present does not represent the independent effect of A, but rather the effect of A in the presence of Z. This point should be kept in mind

---

Table 6–8 Outline of Table Illustrating the Homogeneity Strategy for Assessing Multiplicative Interaction in Case-Control Studies

	Exposed to A?	Cases	Controls	Odds Ratio	What Does It Mean?
Z absent	No			1.0	Reference category
	Yes				= Effect of A in the absence of Z
Z present	No			1.0	Reference category
	Yes				= Effect of A in the presence of Z

when contrasting this strategy with that described in the section that follows, of comparing observed and expected joint effects.

The interpretation of results in Table 6–8 is straightforward: when multiplicative interaction is present, odds ratios will be dissimilar; when absent, they will be similar. For example, in the study by Shapiro et al[5] examining the interaction between use of oral contraceptives and heavy smoking on the odds of myocardial infarction (Table 6–9), the odds ratios were only somewhat heterogeneous (4.5 vs 5.6), indicating that multiplicative interaction, if present, was not strong. (Shapiro et al examined three smoking categories: none, 1 to 24 cigarettes/day, and $\geq$ 25 cigarettes/day. For simplification purposes, however, only the nonsmoking and heavy smoking categories are discussed in this and subsequent sections.) In contrast, in the study by Coughlin[6] on the relationship between asthma and idiopathic dilated cardiomyopathy (Table 6–10), notwithstanding small numbers, the odds ratios appeared to be fairly heterogeneous, thus suggesting the presence of multiplicative interaction.

It has been pointed out by Morabia et al[7] that the odds ratios may be heterogeneous when relative risks are not, a phenomenon that these authors designated as *interaction fallacy*. Morabia et al argued that although the likelihood of this "fallacy" is usually negligible in most real-life instances in chronic disease epidemiology, it may increase when the risk of the outcome is expected to be high—for example, in an epidemic situation, or when studying population groups in which there is a strong genetic susceptibility to the risk factor–induced disease.

Table 6–9 The Relationship of Smoking and Oral Contraceptive (OC) Use to the Odds of Myocardial Infarction in Women

Heavy Smoking*	OC Use	Odds Ratio	What Does It Mean?
No	No	1.0	Reference category
	Yes	4.5	Effect of OC in nonsmokers
Yes	No	1.0	Reference category
	Yes	5.6	Effect of OC in heavy smokers

* $\geq$ 25 cigarettes/day

Source: Data from S. Shapiro et al, Oral-Contraceptive Use in Relation to Myocardial Infarction, *Lancet*, Vol i, pp 743–747, © 1979.

Table 6–10 The Relationship of Hypertension and Asthma to Idiopathic Dilated Cardiomyopathy

Hypertension	Asthma	Odds Ratio	What Does It Mean?
No	No	1.0	Reference category
	Yes	2.4	Effect of asthma in normotensives
Yes	No	1.0	Reference category
	Yes	13.4	Effect of asthma in hypertensives

Source: Data from SS Coughlin, *A Case-Control Study of Dilated Cardiomyopathy,* Doctoral Dissertation, p 109, © 1987, Johns Hopkins University School of Hygiene and Public Health.

6.4.2   Comparing Observed and Expected Joint Effects

The strategy of comparing observed and expected joint effects in case-control studies is similar to the technique used when incidence data are available. That is, the independent effects of A and Z are estimated in order to compute the expected joint effect, which is then compared to the observed joint effect. When the expected and observed joint effects differ, interaction is said to be present.

Table 6–11 shows schematically how assessment of both additive and multiplicative interactions can be carried out in case-control studies. In this table, independent effects (measured by odds ratios) of A and Z can be estimated by using a single reference category formed by individuals unexposed to both A and Z. The effect of A alone—that is, the independent effect of A in absence of Z—is estimated by the odds of the category A_+Z_- relative to that of the reference category,

Table 6–11 Outline of Table to Assess Both Additive and Multiplicative Interaction in Case-Control Studies Using the Strategy of Comparing Expected and Observed Joint Effects

What Is Measured	Exp. to Z?	Exp. to A?	Cases	Control	Odds Ratio
Reference category	No	No			$OR_{A-Z-} = 1.0$
Indep. effect of A	No	Yes			OR_{A+Z-}
Indep. effect of Z	Yes	No			OR_{A-Z+}
Observed joint effect	Yes	Yes			OR_{A+Z+}

A_ Z_. Similarly, the independent effect of Z is estimated by the ratio of the odds of the category A_Z_+ to that of the reference category.

Detection of Additive Interaction

As mentioned previously, in case-control studies it is not possible to use Equation 6.1 (or 6.2) (Section 6.3.2), as it requires incidence data usually not available when using this design. Thus, it is important to rewrite this equation in terms of relative risks or odds ratios so that it can be applied to the case-control data shown schematically in Table 6–11. Figure 6–3 allows an intuitive derivation of a formula based on odds ratios that is equivalent to Equations 6.1 and 6.2. In the figure, the baseline value (OR = 1.0) shown in column 1 represents the odds for individuals unexposed to both A and Z. The absolute excesses due to A (column 2) and Z (column 3) are depicted by the parts of the columns above the baseline. The expected joint effect (column 4) is

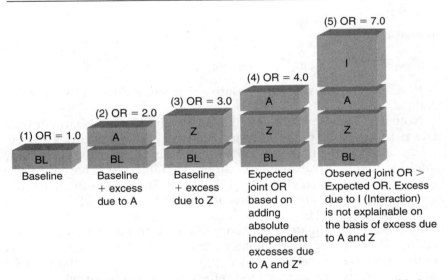

*Note that when the independent relative odds for A and Z are added, the baseline is added twice; thus, it is necessary to subtract 1.0 from the joint expected OR: that is, Expected OR_{A+Z+} = (Excess due to A + baseline) + (Excess due to Z + baseline) − baseline = OR_{A+Z-} + OR_{A-Z+} − 1.0.

Figure 6–3 Schematic representation of the meaning of the formula, Expected OR_{A+Z+} = Observed OR_{A+Z-} + Observed OR_{A-Z+} − 1.0.

then the baseline odds ratio plus the independent excess due to A plus the independent excess due to Z, as follows:

[Equation 6.4]

$$\text{Expd OR}_{A+Z+} = 1.0 + (\text{Obs OR}_{A+Z-} - 1.0) + (\text{Obs OR}_{A-Z+} - 1.0) =$$
$$\text{Obs OR}_{A+Z-} + \text{Obs OR}_{A-Z+} - 1.0$$

The formal derivation of Equation 6.4 is demonstrated as follows. Starting with Equation 6.2, in which Expd Inc and Obs Inc denote expected incidence and observed incidence, respectively (Section 6.3.2),

$$\text{Expd Inc}_{A+Z+} = \text{Obs Inc}_{A-Z-} + (\text{Obs Inc}_{A+Z-} - \text{Obs Inc}_{A-Z-}) +$$
$$(\text{Obs Inc}_{A-Z+} - \text{Obs Inc}_{A-Z-})$$

and dividing every term in this formula by Inc_{A-Z-}, it can be expressed in terms of relative risk as

$$\text{Expd RR}_{A+Z+} = 1.0 + (\text{Obs RR}_{A+Z-} - 1.0) + (\text{Obs RR}_{A-Z+} - 1.0)$$

and thus,

[Equation 6.5]

$$\text{Exp RR}_{A+Z+} = \text{Obs RR}_{A+Z-} + \text{Obs RR}_{A-Z+} - 1.0$$

In a case-control study, the relative risks are estimated by the odds ratios.

Note that Equations 6.4, and 6.5, although using odds ratio or relative risks, are based on positive and negative absolute excesses, respectively (attributable risks in exposed) and thus estimate expected joint *additive* effects. An example is shown in Table 6–12, based on the same study used as an example in Table 6–9. The data in the table suggest that there is a strong additive interaction, as $\text{Expd OR}_{A+Z+} = 10.5 \ll \text{Obs OR}_{A+Z+} = 39.0$.

Also note that Equation 6.4 cannot be used to assess additive interaction when one of the variables (A or Z) has been matched for, as its odds ratio has been set at 1.0 by design (see Chapter 1, Section 1.4.5); in other words, the independent effect of a variable for which cases and controls have been matched cannot be determined. Because the homogeneity strategy cannot be used to examine additive interaction

Table 6–12 Example of How To Assess Interaction on Both Scales in a Case-Control Study Using the Formulas Expd OR_{A+Z+} = Obs OR_{A+Z-} + Obs OR_{A-Z+} − 1.0 (Additive) and Expd Obs OR_{A+Z+} = Obs OR_{A+Z-} × Obs OR_{A-Z+} (Multiplicative): The Relationship of Heavy Smoking and Oral Contraceptive (OC) Use to the Odds of Myocardial Infarction in Women

Heavy Smoking (Z)*	OC Use (A)	Odds Ratio
No	No	1.0
No	Yes	4.5
Yes	No	7.0
Yes	Yes	**39.0**

Observed OR_{A+Z+}: 39.0
Expected OR_{A+Z+}:
  Additive model: 4.5 + 7.0 − 1.0 = 10.5
  Multiplicative model: 4.5 × 7.0 = 31.5

*≥ 25 cigarettes/day

Source: Data from S. Shapiro et al, Oral-Contraceptive Use in Relation to Myocardial Infarction, *Lancet*, pp 743–747, © 1979.

in case-contol studies either, it follows that it is not possible to evaluate additive interaction between a matched factor and other factors in (matched) case-control studies.

Detection of Multiplicative Interaction

In case-control studies, the evaluation of multiplicative interaction based on comparing observed and expected joint effects is analogous to the strategy used in the context of a cohort study. Evaluation of multiplicative interaction comparing expected and observed joint effects is based on the same type of table as that used for assessing additive interaction (eg, Table 6–12). The expected joint odds ratio is estimated as merely the product of the multiplication of the independent odds ratio.

[Equation 6.6]

$$\text{Expd } OR_{A+Z+} = \text{Obs } OR_{A+Z-} \times \text{Obs } OR_{A-Z+}$$

which is the analogue of Equation 6.3. (These equations also can be used to assess multiplicative interaction when the odds ratio/relative risks are below 1.0.) Using Table 6–12's findings, it is possible to estimate the expected joint odds ratio as Expd OR_{A+Z+} = 4.5 × 7.0 = 31.5. As the expected joint odds ratio (31.5) is fairly close to the observed (39.0), interaction, if present, is weak on the multiplicative scale, which is the same conclusion derived previously from using the homogeneity strategy (Section 6.4.1).

Note that as for additive interaction, this strategy cannot be used to evaluate multiplicative interaction between a matched variable and another factor, as the independent effect of the former cannot be measured. However, the homogeneity strategy can be applied to assess multiplicative interaction in matched case-control studies. This is done by stratifying the matched sets according to the levels of the matched variables and evaluating homogeneity of the odds ratios across the strata. Thus, in the schematic example shown in Table 6–13, the heterogeneity of odds ratios for alcohol use (based on discrepant case-control pairs) in strata formed by smoking (yes vs no) suggests presence of multiplicative interaction. A summary of the issues related to the evaluation of interaction between the matched variable and another factor in matched case-control studies is given in Table 6–14.

As stated at the beginning of this section, Equations 6.4 and 6.6 can be also used when assessing interaction in cohort studies. For example, using the relative risks from Table 6–6, it is possible to construct a table similar to Table 6–11 (Table 6–15). Note that in Tables 6–6 and 6–15, father's educational level of 0 to 8 grades was categorized as "exposed." The expected joint effects are expressed by relative risks of $(1.1 + 1.1 - 1.0) = 1.2$ in an additive scale and $(1.1 \times 1.1) = 1.2$ in a

---

Table 6–13 Hypothetical Example of Evaluation of Interaction in a Case-Control Study Between Smoking and Alcohol Use, in Which Cases and Controls Are Matched by Current Smoking ("Yes" Versus "No")

Pair No.	Smoking	Case	Control	Odds Ratio for Alcohol Use by Smoking*
1	No	+	−	
2	No	−	+	OR = 2/1 = 2.0
3	No	−	−	
4	No	+	−	
5	No	+	+	
6	Yes	+	−	
7	Yes	+	−	OR = 4/1 = 4.0
8	Yes	−	+	
9	Yes	+	−	
10	Yes	+	−	

Note: The signs (+) and (−) denote alcohol users and non-users, respectively.
*Using the ratio of discrepant pairs

Table 6–14 Summary of Issues Related to the Evaluation of Interaction in Matched Case-Control Studies Using as an Example Smoking as the Matched Variable and Alcohol as the Exposure of Interest

Scale	Strategy	Information Needed	Is This Strategy Feasible?	Why?
Additive	Homogeneity of effects	ARs for alcohol use according to smoking	No	Because incidence rates for alcohol according to smoking are unavailable in case-control studies.
Additive	Observed vs expected joint effects	ORs expressing independent effects of smoking and of alcohol use	No	The OR expressing the independent effect of smoking is unavailable because cases and controls have been matched for smoking.
Multiplicative	Homogeneity of effects	ORs for alcohol use according to smoking	Yes	ORs for alcohol use are available for case-control pairs according to smoking.
Multiplicative	Observed vs expected joint effects	ORs expressing independent effects of smoking and of alcohol use	No	The OR expressing the independent effect of smoking is unavailable because cases and controls have been matched for smoking.

Note: AR = attributable risks in exposed subjects; OR = odds ratio.

multiplicative scale (Table 6–15). The difference between these expected values and the observed joint relative risk of 3.1 leads to the same conclusion reached previously using incidence rates (Table 6–6) that there is interaction in both scales.

6.5 MORE ON THE INTERCHANGEABILITY OF THE DEFINITIONS OF INTERACTION

It can be easily shown mathematically that the two definitions of interaction (ie, based on homogeneity of effects or on the comparison between joint observed and expected effects) are completely inter-

234

234 EPIDEMIOLOGY

Table 6–15 Neonatal Death Rates per 1000 Live Births According to Smoking Status of the Mother and Education of the Father, Washington County, 1953 to 1963

Father's Education (Grades)	Mother's Smoking	Rate/1000 Live Births	Relative Risk
Higher (9+) ("unexposed")	No	14.9	1.0
Higher (9+) ("unexposed")	Yes	17.1	1.1
Lower (0–8) ("exposed")	No	16.4	1.1
Lower (0–8) ("exposed")	Yes	46.1	3.1

Source: Data from GW Comstock and FE Lundin, Parental Smoking and Perinatal Mortality, *American Journal of Obstetrics and Gynecology,* Vol 98, pp 708–718, © 1967.

changeable: that is, if the effects are heterogeneous (ie, there is inter-action), then the observed is different from the expected joint effect, and vice versa. Consider, for example, two variables, A and Z, and their potential effects with regard to a given outcome. To evaluate joint additive effects, under the hypothesis of no interaction:

[Equation 6.7]

$$\text{Expd } RR_{A+Z+} = \text{Obs } RR_{A+Z+} = \text{Obs } RR_{A+Z-} + \text{Obs } RR_{A-Z+} - 1.0.$$

The equation can be rewritten as

[Equation 6.8]

$$\text{Obs } RR_{A+Z+} - \text{Obs } RR_{A-Z+} = \text{Obs } RR_{A+Z-} - 1.0$$

As shown previously (Section 6.4.2), to derive relative risks from the formula for assessing the expected joint additive effect, all incidence terms in the equation are divided by the incidence when both factors are absent (ie, Inc_{A-Z-}). Working backwards, the incidence when both factors are absent times the relative risk for a given exposed category equals the incidence in that exposed category (eg, $\text{Inc}_{A+Z-} = \text{Inc}_{A-Z-} \times RR_{A+Z-}$). Thus, Equation 6.8 is equivalent to

[Equation 6.9]

$$\text{Inc}_{A+Z+} - \text{Inc}_{A-Z+} = \text{Inc}_{A+Z-} - \text{Inc}_{A-Z-}$$

Thus, when the joint observed additive effect of A and Z is the same as the expected effect (Equation 6.7), the effect of A in the presence of Z will be the same as the effect of A in the absence of Z (Equation 6.9). Alternatively, when the joint observed effects are different from the joint expected effects (ie, interaction is present), the effects of A will vary according to the presence or absence of Z.

The same reasoning applies to the assessment of multiplicative interaction. For example, under the assumption of no interaction on a multiplicative scale,

[Equation 6.10]

$$\text{Expd RR}_{A+Z+} = \text{Obs RR}_{A+Z+} = \text{Obs RR}_{A+Z-} \times \text{Obs RR}_{A-Z+}$$

Equation 6.10 can be rewritten as

[Equation 6.11]

$$\text{Obs RR}_{A+Z+}/\text{Obs RR}_{A-Z+} = \text{Obs RR}_{A+Z-}/1.0$$

The equivalence of Equations 6.10 and 6.11 means that when the observed joint effects are equal to the multiplication of the independent effects (Equation 6.10), then the relative risk for one factor does not vary as a function of the level of the other factor (Equation 6.11), and vice versa.

6.6   WHICH IS THE RELEVANT MODEL: ADDITIVE VERSUS MULTIPLICATIVE INTERACTION?

The popularity of the Mantel-Haenszel adjustment approach (Chapter 7, Section 7.3.3) and of multiple regression methods based on multiplicative models (Chapter 7, Sections 7.4.3 through 7.4.6) has often led to equating interaction almost exclusively with multiplicative interaction. If the odds ratios or relative risks are homogeneous across strata of a potential effect modifier, it may be concluded that there is no interaction in general, even though this conclusion applies exclusively to multiplicative interaction. Yet, as discussed later in this chapter, additive interaction may be of greater interest if disease prevention is being contemplated. Thus, even when using the odds ratio or the relative risk to describe study data, it is often important to also explore the presence of additive interaction. Evaluation of additive interaction can be carried out even in the context of inherently multiplicative models, such as the logistic regression model.[8]

In the biological sciences, the notion of interaction has been closely related to the mechanisms underlying a causal relationship. A discussion of the limits of inferring biologic mechanisms from the observation of interactions in epidemiologic studies can be found in the literature[9] and is beyond the scope of this textbook. Thompson[10] has aptly pointed out that epidemiology can detect mostly macro associations and that its sensitivity to identify intermediate variables tends to be limited, thus making it difficult to interpret interactions using results of epidemiologic research. Usually, interaction detected in epidemiologic studies may merely represent the joint effect of exposures occurring soon before the development of clinical disease (Figure 6–4). An interaction detected by epidemiologic observation does not take into account the usually long causal chain. This chain could be characterized by either multiplicative or additive joint effects of other causal components, which are needed to create causal constellations[2] responsible for the earlier progression of the disease from one phase (eg, metabolically altered cells) to another (eg, abnormal cell multiplication). The inability to describe the physiologic and anatomic cell abnormalities in the pathogenetic sequence leading to the disease outcome severely limits epidemiology's ability to select the best model(s) for interaction. As a consequence, choice of a model by epidemiologists is usually dictated by pragmatism—for example, when selecting the statistical model for adjustment purposes or when considering the possible application of findings in setting up public health policy and prevention.

From the viewpoint of translating epidemiologic findings into public health practice, presence of additive interaction is important, even if multiplicative interaction is absent.[11] A hypothetical example is

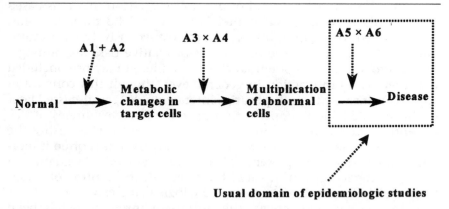

Usual domain of epidemiologic studies

Figure 6–4 Schematic representation of a causal chain in which both additive and multiplicative interactive effects occur. Causes A1 and A2 interact in an additive fashion to produce metabolic changes in the target cells. For multiplication of abnormal cells and progression to clinical disease, additional risk factors are required (A3 and A4, A5 and A6, respectively), which interact in a multiplicative fashion.

given in Table 6–16, which examines the relationship of familial history of disease Y and smoking to the incidence of Y. Although relative risks describing the relationship between smoking and incidence are homogeneous in those with and without a family history, the attributable risks differ markedly according to family history: 20/100 in those with and only 5/100 in those without a positive family history. Thus, there is strong additive interaction but no multiplicative interaction. Depending on the prevalence of the combination of family history and smoking in the target population, prevention or elimination of smoking in those with a positive, compared to those with a negative, family history could lead to a greater reduction of the number of incident cases in the reference population.* Positive additive interaction may even occur in the presence of negative multiplicative interaction (Table 6–17), and takes precedence over the latter in terms of defining high-risk groups, which should be the target of preventive action. For additional discussion of negative multiplicative and positive additive interaction, see Section 6.10 of this chapter.

6.7 THE NATURE AND RECIPROCITY OF INTERACTION

6.7.1 Quantitative Versus Qualitative Interaction

When the association between factor A and outcome Y exists and is of the same direction in each stratum formed by Z but the strength of

---

Table 6–16 Hypothetical Example of Additive Interaction ("Public Health Interaction") Without Multiplicative Interaction: Incidence of Disease Y by Smoking and Family History of Y

Family History	Smoking	Incidence/100	Attributable Risk (Exposed)	Relative Risk
Absent	No	5.0	Reference	1.0
	Yes	10.0	5.0	2.0
Present	**No**	20.0	Reference	1.0
	Yes	40.0	20.0	2.0

---

*The impact of the elimination of smoking in those with a family history is best estimated by means of the population attributable risk, which takes into account the strength of the association between smoking and disease in each stratum of family history, as well as the prevalence of the joint presence of these factors (see Chapter 3, Section 3.2.2).

Table 6–17 Hypothetical Example of Negative Multiplicative and Positive Additive Interactions: Incidence of Disease Y by Family History of Y and Smoking

Family History	Smoking	Incidence/100	Attributable Risk (Exposed)	Relative Risk
Absent	No	10	Reference	1.0
	Yes	40	30/1000	4.0
Present	No	40	Reference	1.0
	Yes	100	60/1000	2.5

the association varies from stratum to stratum, *quantitative* interaction is said to exist. On the other hand, *qualitative* interaction is regarded as present either when the effects of A on the outcome Y are in opposite directions (*crossover*) according to the presence of the third variable Z or when there is an association in one of the strata formed by Z but not in the other (Figure 6–5).

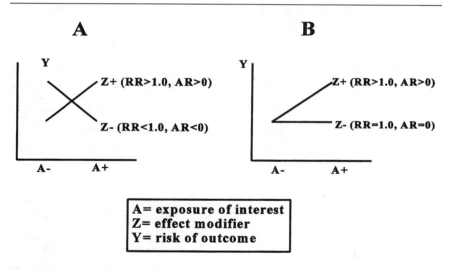

Figure 6–5 Qualitative interaction is always seen in both scales (additive and multiplicative) because when the relative risk (RR) > 1.0, the attributable risk (AR) > 0; when RR < 1.0, the AR < 0; and when RR = 1.0, the AR = 0. In **A**, there is crossover: that is, $RR_{A+/A-} > 1.0$ and $AR_{A+/A-} > 0$ when Z (effect modifier) is present, and RR < 1.0 and AR < 0 when Z is absent. In **B**, RR > 1.0 and AR > 0 when Z is present, and RR = 1.0 and AR = 0 when Z is absent.

An example of qualitative interaction is given by a study by Stanton and Gray.[12] To examine the effects of caffeine consumption on waiting time to conception, the authors obtained information retrospectively on pregnancies occurring from 1980 through 1990 in 1430 noncontracepting, parous women. The main exposure of interest was daily caffeine intake, estimated from the consumption of caffeinated beverages during the first month of pregnancy. Information on delayed conception was analyzed as a dichotomous variable ($\leq$1 year versus >1 year) for the purpose of calculating relative risks. Whereas relative risks were below 1 for caffeine consumption among smoking women, an increase in delayed conception risk was seen in nonsmoking women with a high ($\geq$300 mg/day) caffeine consumption (Table 6–18). According to the authors, the qualitative interaction found in their study supports the notion that smoking increases the rate of caffeine metabolism and that, in contrast, cessation of smoking results in slower caffeine elimination.

In the example shown in Table 6–18, the effects of high caffeine consumption appear to cross over as a function of smoking (ie, there is a positive association of high caffeine intake and delayed conception in nonsmokers and a negative association in smokers). Qualitative interaction can be expressed either by this type of crossover (Figure 6–5A) or by an association between the factor of interest and the outcome in the presence but not in the absence of an effect modifier (or vice versa) (Figure 6–5B). An example of the latter type of interaction is given by the results of the Health Insurance Plan randomized clinical trial of the effectiveness of mammography.[13] In this study,

Table 6–18 Relationship Between Caffeine Consumption and Risk of Delayed Conception (>1 Year) According to Smoking among 2465 Pregnancies Occurring in Noncontracepting Women Between 1980 and 1990

Caffeine Consumption (mg/Day)	Nonsmoking Women			Smoking Women		
	Pregnancies	Delayed Conception	RR	Pregnancies	Delayed Conception	RR
None	575	47	1.0	76	15	1.0
1–150	975	69	0.9	233	33	0.7
151–300	290	26	1.1	166	18	0.5
$\geq$ 300	90	17	2.3	83	11	0.7

Source: Data from CK Stanton and RH Gray, The Effects of Caffeine Consumption on Delayed Conception, *American Journal of Epidemiology,* Vol 142, pp 1322–1329, © 1995, The Johns Hopkins University School of Hygiene & Public Health.

menopausal status seemed to modify the effect of mammography in that a lower breast cancer death rate in the group undergoing mammography compared with the control group was seen only in post-menopausal women. In premenopausal women, no difference in rates was found between the experimental and the control groups. Both the caffeine/smoking/delayed conception and the menopause/mammography/breast cancer examples underscore the notion that when qualitative interaction is present, it is always present in both the additive and the multiplicative models and is thus independent of the measurement scale (Figure 6–5). Consider, for example, the data shown in Table 6–18: because the relative risk in nonsmoking women with a caffeine consumption of ≥300 mg/day is greater than 1.0, the attributable risk by definition must be greater than 0; in smokers, on the other hand, the relative risk is less than 1.0; thus, by definition, the attributable risk has to be less than 0. Note that although Table 6–18 presents only relative risks and therefore on a first glance may be regarded as suitable only for assessing multiplicative interaction, the occurrence of qualitative interaction indicates that interaction is present in both scales; in other words, when there is qualitative interaction, the scale does not need to be specified.

6.7.2   Reciprocity of Interaction

Interaction is completely reciprocal in the case of two variables A and Z, in that if Z modifies the effect of A, then A modifies the effect of Z. As mentioned previously, the choice of A as the suspected risk factor of interest and Z as the potential effect modifier is arbitrary and a function of the hypothesis being evaluated. For example, because the effect of cigarette smoking on lung cancer is strong and has been firmly established, it may be of interest to explore its role as an effect modifier when assessing other potential lung cancer risk factors.

The concept of interaction reciprocity is illustrated in Table 6–19, which rearranges the data from Table 6–18 such that smoking becomes the risk factor of interest and caffeine consumption becomes the effect modifier (for simplification purposes, only two caffeine consumption categories are used). As seen, smoking is positively associated with delayed conception in mothers who drink no caffeine, but it seems to be a protective factor in those with a high level of consumption. This pattern is the mirror image of the pattern shown in Table 6–18, again emphasizing that there is no intrinsic hierarchical value when deciding which variable should be treated as the effect modifier and which as the factor of primary interest.

Table 6–19 Relationship Between Maternal Smoking and Risk of Delayed Conception (>1 Year) According to Heavy Caffeine Consumption (≥300 mg/Day) among 824 Pregnancies Occurring in Noncontracepting Women Between 1980 and 1990

	No Caffeine Consumption			Caffeine Consumption ≥300 mg/day		
Smoking	Pregnancies	Delayed Conception	RR	Pregnancies	Delayed Conception	RR
No	575	47	1.0	90	17	1.0
Yes	76	15	2.4	83	11	0.7

Source: Data from CK Stanton and RH Gray, The Effects of Caffeine Consumption on Delayed Conception, *American Journal of Epidemiology,* Vol 142, pp 1322–1329, © 1995, The Johns Hopkins University School of Hygiene & Public Health.

6.8 INTERACTION, CONFOUNDING EFFECT, AND ADJUSTMENT

Although on occasion the same variable may be both a confounder and an effect modifier, confounding and interaction are generally distinct phenomena. Confounding effects are undesirable, as they make it difficult to evaluate whether a statistical association is also causal. Interaction, on the other hand, if true, is part of the web of causation[14] and may have important implications for prevention, as in the example of smoking and caffeine consumption illustrated in Tables 6–18 and 6–19.

When a variable is found to be both a confounding variable and an effect modifier, adjustment for this variable is contraindicated. When additive interaction is found, it is not appropriate to adjust for the effect modifier to obtain an adjusted attributable risk, and when there is multiplicative interaction, it is inappropriate to obtain an effect modifier–adjusted relative risk. This is because when there is interaction the notion of an overall adjusted (weighted) mean value (main effect) makes little sense. For example, if odds ratios are found to be 2.0 for men and 25.0 for women, an "average" that summarizes the increase in odds for all individuals regardless of gender is meaningless. This notion is even more important in qualitative interaction; if the odds ratios for a given exposure are 0.3 in men and 3.5 in women, an "average, gender-adjusted" odds ratio may denote no association whatsoever—an illogical inference given that strong associations, albeit in opposite directions, exist in both sexes (for additional examples, see Chapter 7, Section 7.3.1).

Because some heterogeneity is usually found, the epidemiologist is often faced with the dilemma as to whether to adjust for the possible effect modifier. One solution is to carry out statistical testing and not to adjust if the homogeneity null hypothesis is rejected (see Section 6.9 and Appendix C). But if, for example, the two odds ratios are 2.3 and 2.6, it is foolish not to adjust and obtain an average adjusted effect, regardless of the p value. (If the sample size is very large, an interaction of small magnitude may be statistically significant even if devoid of medical or public health significance.) On the other hand, if the odds ratios are 12.0 and 1.5, even if the heterogeneity is not found to be statistically significant, adjustment may be contraindicated. Although no clear-cut rule exists regarding whether to adjust in presence of heterogeneity, consideration of the following question may be helpful: "Given heterogeneity of this magnitude, am I willing to report an average (adjusted) effect that is reasonably representative of all strata of the study population formed on the basis of the suspected effect modifier?" Some examples and possible answers to this question are shown in Table 6–20 and may help in the pragmatic evaluation of this issue. Regardless of

Table 6–20 Relative Risks (RR) for Factor A in Relation to Outcome Y, Stratified by Potential Effect Modifier Z

Suspected Effect Modifier (Z)		Given a Heterogeneity of This Magnitude, Should a Weighted Average (Z-Adjusted) Effect That Applies to All Z Strata of the Study Population Be Reported?
Absent	Present	
2.3	2.6	Yes. Even if the difference in RRs is statistically significant, it makes sense to say that, on the average—that is, regardless of Z—the relative risk has a value somewhere between 2.3 and 2.6.
2.0	20.0	Even if this difference is not statistically significant, presentation of a Z-adjusted, "average" RR may not be appropriate in view of the great difference in the magnitude of the RRs. It is recommended that Z-specific RRs be presented.
0.5	3.0	No. When there is a suggestion of qualitative interaction, Z-specific RRs should be presented.
3.0	4.5	Perhaps. Although this quantitative interaction may be of interest, effects are in the same direction, and it *may* be appropriate to present a Z-adjusted RR. In addition, it is wise to present Z-specific RRs.

whether a "Z-adjusted" effect is reported, it is often informative to report the stratum-specific values as well.

6.9 STATISTICAL MODELING AND STATISTICAL TESTS FOR INTERACTION

The examples given in this chapter refer to risk of disease as the outcome, but interaction may be studied in relation to any outcome—for example, the mean value of a physiologic variable such as glucose level. As mentioned previously, it is also possible to examine interaction for continuous variables, as when assessing homogeneity of effects of continuous blood pressure levels on stroke between men and women or between blacks and whites. In this situation, the investigator often uses more complex statistical models to evaluate interaction—for example, by including "interaction terms" in the regression equation (see Chapter 7, Section 7.4.2). These models can also be used to evaluate interaction between categorical variables as an alternative to the stratification methods presented in the previous sections.

Another question with important practical implications is whether the observed heterogeneity is produced by chance. When using regression models to evaluate interaction, the answer to this question is simply indicated by the statistical significance of the interaction term in the regression equation (see Chapter 7, Section 7.4.8, and Appendix A, Section A.9). When evaluating interaction using the stratification techniques described in the previous sections, formal statistical tests are available to assess whether an observed heterogeneity is statistically significant. These tests, including tests for additive interaction in case-control studies, have been described in detail in other textbooks (see, eg, Schlesselman[15] or Selvin[16]) and are illustrated in Appendix C.

It should be emphasized again that statistical tests of homogeneity, although helpful, are not sufficient to fully evaluate interaction. When sample sizes are large, as in multicenter studies, even a slight heterogeneity of no practical value may be statistically significant. On the other hand, although not statistically significant, relative risk point estimates markedly different from each other suggest the possibility of true heterogeneity. Ideally, such nonstatistically significant, yet marked heterogeneity should be confirmed by a study with sufficient statistical power to detect it.

6.10 INTERPRETING INTERACTION

There are many reasons why an observed effect of an exposure may differ according to the level or the presence of a third variable. The apparent heterogeneity may be due to chance, selective confounding, or bias. It could in addition result from a heterogeneous exposure dose (often unbeknownst to the investigator). Differential susceptibility at different levels in the pathogenesis of the disease in question is yet another explanation for heterogeneity of effects. A succinct practical guide to the main issues involved in interpreting an observed interaction follows.

6.10.1   Heterogeneity Due to Random Variability

Heterogeneity may result from random variability produced by the stratification according to a suspected effect modifier. Random variability may occur in spite of an a priori specification of interaction in the context of the hypothesis to be evaluated. A more common situation, however, is when interaction is not specified a priori, but the investigator decides to carry out subgroup analysis. The decision to examine subgroups is often motivated by "negative" findings in the study. The investigator may decide to pursue more specific hypotheses once the original postulated association did not meet expectations. Post hoc questions posed by the frustrated epidemiologist may, for example, include: "Since I cannot find an association when studying all study participants, will I be able to find it in men only? In older men? In older men with a high educational level?" And so on.

Sample size inevitably decreases as more strata are created in subgroup analysis, making it likely that heterogeneity would occur by chance alone. Thus, subgroup analysis should be regarded as an exploratory strategy. The detection of heterogeneity should be assessed vis-à-vis its plausibility. An example is provided by the Multiple Risk Factor Intervention Trial (MRFIT) study, a randomized clinical trial that assessed the efficacy of multiple cardiovascular risk factor cessation strategies. An increased mortality was found in hypertensive participants with electrocardiographic changes undergoing the experimental interventions.[17] Although not predicted when the study was planned, the harmful effect of the intervention limited to this subset of study participants led to the hypothesis that potassium-depleting drugs may be contraindicated in hypertensives with cardiac abnormalities. Once observed by means of subgroup analysis, interaction has to be confirmed in a study especially designed to evaluate it.

6.10.2   Heterogeneity Due to Confounding

When associations between A and Y in strata formed by Z are being explored, differential confounding effects according to strata may be responsible for the heterogeneity of effects. As a hypothetical example, let us consider a case-control study assessing the relationship between coffee intake and cancer Y (Table 6–21). The investigator wishes to assess gender as an effect modifier and accordingly stratifies cases and controls by coffee intake (yes/no) and gender. In this hypothetical example, smoking is a cause of cancer Y, female cases and controls include only nonsmokers, smoking is associated with coffee drinking, and male cases include a higher proportion of smokers than controls. As smoking is related to coffee intake and cancer Y, it acts as a positive confounder in males. Assuming that coffee intake is not causally related to cancer Y, in females (who are all nonsmokers) a relative odds of 1.0 is found. The confounding effect of smoking in males, on the other hand, results in male cases' having a higher odds of coffee intake than controls, and as a consequence the relative odds is found to be markedly higher than 1.0. There is, therefore, a statistical interaction due to confounding by smoking limited to males.

The possibility that interaction may be explained partially or entirely by a confounding effect makes it essential to adjust for potential confounders when assessing interaction. In the example shown in Table 6–21, the confounding effect of smoking explains the entire apparent heterogeneity of coffee intake by sex. Most real-life instances of confounding do not completely explain the heterogeneity of effect but may either exaggerate or decrease it. An example is given by Yu et al,[18] who examined the interaction of cigarette smoking and alcohol

Table 6–21 Apparent Interaction Due to Confounding (Hypothetical Example)

Gender/Smoking	Coffee Intake	Cases	Controls	Odds Ratio
Female/nonsmoker	Yes	10	10	
	No	90	90	1.0
	Total	100	100	
Male/total	Yes	38	22	
	No	62	78	2.2
	Total	100	100	
Male/smoker	Yes	35	15	
	No	35	15	1.0
	Total	70	30	
Male/nonsmoker	Yes	3	7	
	No	27	63	1.0
	Total	30	70	

Note: Assume that smoking causes cancer Y; 50% of smokers but only 10% of nonsmokers drink coffee; coffee intake is not independently related to cancer Y; all females are nonsmokers; and 70% of male cases and 30% of male controls are smokers.

drinking in chronic hepatitis B surface antigen (HBsAg) carriers with regard to the risk of liver cirrhosis (Table 6–22). An unadjusted heterogeneity for smoking according to drinking could be detected, which became more marked for heavy smokers ($\geq$ 20 cigarettes/day) versus nonsmokers (but less so for moderate smokers) when the relative risk was simultaneously adjusted for five confounding factors using a Cox proportional hazards model (see Chapter 7, Section 7.4.4).

6.10.3 Heterogeneity Due to Bias

As for confounding, the observed heterogeneity may also result from differential bias across strata. For example, in a study of the incidence of medically treated miscarriage in a county in North Carolina, Savitz et al[19] found that, overall, blacks appeared to have a lower risk of miscarriage than whites. The authors interpreted this finding as probably resulting from bias due to underascertainment of miscarriage among blacks. As shown in Table 6–23, when stratification according to educational status was undertaken, the apparent decreased risk of miscarriage in blacks was seen only in the lower educational strata. This pattern of an apparent modification of the race effect by

Table 6–22 Relative Risks of Liver Cirrhosis According to Alcohol Drinking and Cigarette Smoking in Chronic HBsAg Carriers

			Relative Risk	
Variable	Total No.	No. of Incident Cases	Without Adjustment	With Multivariate Adjustment*
Nondrinker				
Nonsmoker	744	31	1.0	1.0
<20 cigarettes/day	267	19	1.7	1.5
$\geq$20 cigarettes/day	167	14	2.0	1.9
Drinker				
Nonsmoker	111	1	1.0	1.0
<20 cigarettes/day	100	6	6.7	3.9
$\geq$20 cigarettes/day	105	7	7.4	9.3

*Simultaneously adjusted for age, HBsAg carrier status at recruitment, elevation of serum aminotransferase concentration for at least 6 months, educational level, and blood type, using a Cox proportional hazards model (see Chapter 7, Section 7.4.4).

Source: Data from MW Yu et al, A Prospective Study of Liver Cirrhosis in Asymptomatic Chronic Hepatitis B Virus Carriers, *American Journal of Epidemiology,* Vol 145, pp 1039–1047, © 1997, The Johns Hopkins University School of Hygiene & Public Health.

Table 6–23 Risk of Miscarriages per 100 Pregnancies, Corrected for Induced Abortions in Relation to Maternal Years of Education: Alamance County, North Carolina, 1988 to 1991

	White		*Black*		*Black/White Ratio*
	No.	*Risk/100*	*No.*	*Risk/100*	
Total	325	7.7	93	5.5	0.7
Mother's years of education:					
<9	12	10.4	0	—	—
10–11	52	8.0	15	4.5	0.6
12	111	6.3	44	4.7	0.7
≥13	150	9.2	33	9.5	1.0

Source: Data from DA Savitz et al, Medically Treated Miscarriage in Alamance County, North Carolina, 1988–1991, *American Journal of Epidemiology,* Vol 139, pp 1100–1106, © 1994, The Johns Hopkins University School of Hygiene & Public Health.

educational level is probably due to the underascertainment bias operating only in less educated blacks.

6.10.4 Heterogeneity Due to Differential Intensity of Exposure

An apparent interaction can occur when there is heterogeneity in the levels of exposure according to the alleged effect modifier. For example, in a recent study of epidemic asthma, White et al[20] investigated the role of airborne soy dust originating from vessel cargo from the New Orleans harbor. The association was stronger when the maximum wind speed was below 12 miles per hour (relative odds = 4.4) than when wind speeds were higher (relative odds = 1.7). This heterogeneity was probably due to a heavier exposure to soy dust resulting from slower wind speeds and would thus not represent "true" interaction using the narrow criterion of differential biologic susceptibility to the same environmental exposure intensity. For practical purposes, however, there are important public health implications of establishing this kind of heterogeneity.

6.10.5 Interaction and Host Factors

Facilitation and, ultimately, intensity of exposure can also occur because of anatomic or pathophysiologic characteristics of the host. For example, a qualitative interaction has been found in a case-control study by Reif et al[21] between the shape of the skull in pet dogs and passive smoking in relation to lung cancer: the increase in odds of lung cancer was limited to dogs with a short nose (brachy- and mesocephalic), presumably because of the mechanical barrier to carcinogenic particles represented by the ciliae of the long-nosed (dolichocephalic) dogs. (An alternative explanation is that there are genetic differences in susceptibility to smoking-induced lung cancer between these types of dogs.) In a subsequent study by the same authors, a qualitative interaction was again found between passive smoking and skull shape with regard to nasal cancer, except that a higher odds of cancer was found for the long-nosed than for the shorter-nosed dogs,[22] leading the authors to speculate that "an increased risk of nasal cancer among long-nosed dogs may be explained by enhanced filtration, and impaction of particles in the mucosa."

These examples underscore the importance of considering the intensity and/or facilitation of exposure when attempting to explain heterogeneity of effects. Effective exposure dose is obviously a function of the net result of the amount of "exposure" in the individual's environment (the example of soy dust), the dose absorbed into the organism, and the dose that reaches the cellular levels (the examples of canine lung and nasal cancers).

From the host viewpoint, effect modifiers can act on different portals of entry (skin, gastrointestinal, respiratory). For example, it is well known that exposure to the same intensity of a skin pathogen (eg, streptococci) is related to a higher probability of infection in individuals with an existing skin rash than in those with a normal skin. Thus, factors that produce skin lesions (eg, skin allergens, mechanical trauma) interact with infectious agents in increasing risk of infection.

The biological mechanism of effect modifiers can also vary at the metabolic or cellular level. Interaction between metabolic pathways and exposure to risk factors is exemplified by genetic disorders such as phenylketonuria. In this disorder, the inability to oxidize a metabolic product of phenylalanine found in many food items may result in severe mental deficiency. Genetic differences among individuals may be also responsible for the differential individual susceptibility in relation to risk factor–induced disease. For example, judging from experiments in mice, it is possible that humans, too, have a differential genetic susceptibility to salt-induced hypertension.[23] At the immunological level, the interactions between certain drugs (eg, steroids, immunosuppressants) and infectious agents in relation to risk and/or severity of infections are well known. The relatively low risk of coronary heart disease in white women at similar levels of exposure to traditional cardiovascular risk factors as men in the United States suggests that hormones may play a role in modifying the effects of these risk factors.[24]

6.11 INTERACTION AND SEARCH FOR NEW RISK FACTORS IN LOW-RISK GROUPS

The strength of an association measured by a relative difference (eg, a relative risk) is a function of the relative prevalence of other risk factors.[15,25] This concept seems to have been first recognized by Cornfield et al,[26(p194)] who stated:

> If two uncorrelated agents, A and B, each increases the risk of a disease, and if the risk of the disease in the absence of either agent is small . . . then the apparent relative risk for A . . . is less than the (relative) risk for A in the absence of B.

This notion is readily understood when considering a situation in which a risk factor is strongly associated with the disease, as in the case of smoking and lung cancer: to examine the role of a weaker factor A, it would be intuitively logical to study nonsmokers, as otherwise the vast majority of cases would be explained by smoking. In other words, a magnification of the relative risk for A in those unexposed to smoking (vis-à-vis smokers) is expected—that is, a negative multiplicative interaction.[15] The tendency toward a negative multiplicative interaction when examining the joint effect of a strong risk factor Z and a weak risk factor A can be intuitively understood by considering two facts: (1) the maximum absolute risk associated with the exposure to any risk factor cannot surpass 100%, and (2) the higher the independent relative risk associated with exposure to Z, the more the risk in those exposed to Z approximates 100%.

For illustration purposes, let us assume an extremely simplistic hypothetical example involving risk factors Z and A, shown in Table 6–24, in which the baseline incidence of the disease (ie, the incidence in those unexposed to both risk factors) is about 10% and the independent relative risk for Z (ie, in the absence of A) is 9.0 (reflecting an incidence in those unexposed to A but exposed to Z of 90%). As the incidence in those exposed to A in the stratum exposed to Z cannot surpass the 100% mark, the maximum possible relative risk for A if Z is present is 100% ÷ 90% = 1.1. A similar absolute difference of 10% due to exposure to A in those unexposed to Z would result in a relative risk of 20% ÷ 10% = 2.0. A similar reasoning can be applied to a

Table 6–24 Example of Negative Interaction Between a Stronger and a Weaker Risk Factor

Factor Z	Factor A	Population Size	Incidence/ 100	Attributable Risk for A/ 100	Relative Risk for A	Relative Risk for Z
Absent	Absent	1000	10.0	0	1.0	1.0
	Present	1000	20.0	10.0	2.0	1.0
Present	Absent	1000	90.0	0	1.0	9.0*
	Present	1000	100.0	10.0	1.1	5.0**

*Relative risk of Z in persons unexposed to A.
**Relative risk of Z in persons exposed to A.

situation in which Z is a constellation of risk factors, rather than a single variable: for example, when studying cardiovascular disease outcomes, Z can be defined as the simultaneous presence of hypertension, hypercholesterolemia, smoking, diabetes, and so forth.

An example is given by the known gender difference with regard to the prevalence of gallstones. It is estimated that in the population at large, 80% of women and 8% of men have gallbladder disease.[27] Thus, the relative risks for risk factors other than gender would have a tendency to be larger in men than in women.

Because of its intuitive appeal, the idea of studying "emergent" risk factors in individuals with no known risk factors is on occasion considered in the design of a study. For example, in a recent study of the putative protective effect of antibiotics on coronary heart disease (CHD), Meier et al[28] compared prior antibiotic use (obtained from pharmacy records) in CHD cases and controls; in selecting these groups, the authors excluded all individuals with a known prior history of CHD or other cardiovascular diseases, as well as individuals with evidence of hypertension, hypercholesterolemia, or diabetes. It is important to realize, however, that use of this strategy may limit the generalizability of the study findings to the general population, which includes both low- and high-risk individuals. Furthermore, associations that rely on synergism between risk factors may be missed altogether. For example, if infections are not sufficient or necessary causes for atherosclerosis but rather are involved in atherogenesis because of their synergism with other cardiovascular risk factors (eg, hypercholesterolemia, diabetes), as suggested elsewhere,[29] the "low-risk" approach may underestimate the potential impact of infections (or, by analogy, antibiotics) on atherosclerosis.

6.12 INTERACTION AND "REPRESENTATIVENESS" OF ASSOCIATIONS

An important assumption when generalizing results from a study is that the study population should have an "average" susceptibility to the exposure under study with regard to a given outcome. When susceptibility is unusual, results cannot be easily generalized. For example, results of a study on the effectiveness of a vaccine in African children may not be applicable to Swiss children, as inadequate nutrition in the former may significantly alter the immune system and thus the production of antibodies to the killed or inactivated agent.

Consider, for example, the findings in Table 6–10, with regard to the influence of interaction on the ability to generalize. Assuming that hypertensives are indeed susceptible to asthma-induced cardiomyopathy, results in hypertensives are obviously not generalizable to nonhypertensives. It follows that the so-called "average" effect of asthma on cardiomyopathy is a function of the prevalence of hypertensives in the population to which one wishes to generalize results. Assuming that the relative odds from Coughlin's[6] study (Table 6–10) represented the true estimates, in populations in which most individuals are hypertensive, the odds ratio would approximate 13.4; on the other hand, in populations with a low proportion of hypertensives the relative odds would be closer to 2.4. Whereas the example of hypertension and asthma is based on an easily measurable effect modifier (hypertension), differences in the strength of an association from population to population may also be due to between-population differences in the prevalence of unmeasured environmental or genetic effect modifiers.

Although it is difficult to establish to which extent the susceptibility of a study population differs from the "average" susceptibility, the assessment of its epidemiological profile (based on well-known risk factors) may indicate how "usual" or "unusual" that population is. Thus, in studies of breast cancer, assuming no bias, a study population in which the well-known association with age at first pregnancy was not found would suggest that it might not be a population of "average" susceptibility. However, this strategy is limited because level of susceptibility to a known risk factor may not be representative of the level of susceptibility regarding the exposure under study.

REFERENCES

1. Petitti DB. Associations are not effects. *Am J Epidemiol.* 1991;133:101–102.
2. Rothman KJ, Greenland S. *Modern Epidemiology.* 2nd ed. Philadelphia, Pa: Lippincott-Raven Publishers, 1998.
3. Kannel WB. Lipids, diabetes and coronary heart disease: insights from the Framingham study. *Am Heart J.* 1985;110:1100–1107.
4. Comstock GW, Lundin FE. Parental smoking and perinatal mortality. *Am J Obstet Gynecol.* 1967;98:708–718.
5. Shapiro S, Slone D, Rosenberg L, et al. Oral-contraceptive use in relation to myocardial infarction. *Lancet.* 1979;1:743–747.
6. Coughlin SS. A case-control study of dilated cardiomyopathy. Doctoral dissertation, Johns Hopkins University School of Hygiene and Public Health, 1987.
7. Morabia A, Ten Have T, Landis JR. Interaction fallacy. *J Clin Epidemiol.* 1997; 50:809–812.
8. Thompson WD. Statistical analysis of case-control studies. *Epidemiol Rev.* 1994; 16:33–50.
9. Darroch J. Biologic synergism and parallelism. *Am J Epidemiol.* 1997;145:661–668.
10. Thompson WD. Effect modification and the limits of biological inference from epidemiologic data. *J Clin Epidemiol.* 1991;44:221–232.
11. Rothman KJ, Greenland S, Walker AM. Concepts of interaction. *Am J Epidemiol.* 1980;112:467–470.
12. Stanton CK, Gray RH. The effects of caffeine consumption on delayed conception. *Am J Epidemiol.* 1995;142:1322–1329.
13. Shapiro S, Venet W, Strax P. Selection, follow-up, and analysis in the Health Insurance Plan study: a randomized trial with breast cancer screening. *Natl Cancer Inst Monogr.* 1985;67:65–74.
14. MacMahon B, Pugh TE. *Epidemiology: Principles and Methods.* Boston, Mass: Little, Brown & Co.; 1970.
15. Schlesselman JJ. *Case-Control Studies: Design, Conduct, Analysis.* New York, NY: Oxford University Press; 1982.
16. Selvin S. *Statistical Analysis of Epidemiologic Data.* New York, NY: Oxford University Press; 1991.
17. Cohen JD. Abnormal electrocardiograms and cardiovascular risk: role of silent myocardial ischemia. *Am J Cardiol.* 1992;70:14F–18F.
18. Yu MW, Hsu FC, Sheen IS, et al. A prospective study of liver cirrhosis in asymptomatic chronic hepatitis B virus carriers. *Am J Epidemiol.* 1997;145:1039–1047.
19. Savitz DA, Brett KM, Evans LE, Bowes W. Medically treated miscarriage in Alamance County, North Carolina, 1988–1991. *Am J Epidemiol.* 1994;139:1100–1106.
20. White MC, Etzel RA, Olson DR, et al. A re-examination of epidemic asthma in New Orleans, Louisiana, in relation to the presence of soy at the harbor. *Am J Epidemiol.* 1997;145:432–438.
21. Reif JS, Dunn K, Ogilvie GK, et al. Passive smoking and canine lung cancer risk. *Am J Epidemiol.* 1992;135:234–239.

22. Reif JS, Bruns C, Lower KS. Cancer of the nasal cavity and paranasal sinuses and exposure to environmental tobacco smoke in pet dogs. *Am J Epidemiol.* 1998; 147:488–484.

23. Szklo M. Epidemiologic patterns of blood pressure in children. *Epidemiol Rev.* 1979;1:143–169.

24. Szklo M. Epidemiology of coronary heart disease in women. In: Gold EB, ed. The changing risk of disease in women. Lexington, Mass: Collamore Press; 1984: 233–241.

25. Rothman KJ, Poole C. A strengthening programme for weak associations. *Int J Epidemiol.* 1988;17:955–959.

26. Cornfield J, Haenszel W, Hammond EC, et al. Smoking and lung cancer: Recent evidence and a discussion of some questions. *J Natl Cancer Inst.* 1959;22:173–203.

27. Greenberger NJ, Isselbacher KJ. Diseases of the gallbladder and bile ducts. In: Isselbacher KJ, Braunwald E, Wilson JD, et al, eds. *Harrison's Principles of Internal Medicine.* 13th ed. New York, NY: McGraw-Hill Inc; 1994:1504–1516.

28. Meier CR, Derby LE, Jick SS, et al. Antibiotics and risk of subsequent first-time acute myocardial infarction. *JAMA.* 1999;281:427–431.

29. Nieto FJ. Infections and atherosclerosis: new clues from an old hypothesis? *Am J Epidemiol.* 1998;148:937–948.

Dealing with Threats to Validity

CHAPTER 7

Stratification and Adjustment: Multivariate Analysis in Epidemiology

7.1 INTRODUCTION

Analytic epidemiologic studies are designed to evaluate the association between environmental exposures or other subject characteristics (eg, demographic variables, genetic polymorphisms) and disease risk. Even if the epidemiologist's interest is focused on a single exposure, there are usually several other factors that need to be considered in the analysis, either because they may distort (confound) the exposure-disease relationship (see Chapter 5) or because the magnitude of the association between exposure and disease may vary across levels of these variables (effect modification; see Chapter 6). *Stratification* and *multivariate analysis (modeling)* are the analytical tools used to control for confounding effects, to assess effect modification, and to summarize the association of several predictor variables with disease risk in an efficient fashion.

The simplest method to analyze the possible presence of confounding is stratification; this is frequently a very informative method because (1) it allows a straightforward and simultaneous examination of the possible presence of both confounding and effect modification and (2) examining stratified results is often useful when choosing the appropriate statistical technique for adjustment (see below).

Multivariate analysis refers to a series of analytical techniques, each based on a more or less complex mathematical model, which are used to carry out *statistical adjustment*; that is, the estimation of a certain measure of association between an exposure and an outcome while "controlling" for one or more possible confounding variables. Effect modification can be also assessed in the context of multivariate analysis. The next section presents an example to illustrate the basic idea of stratification and adjustment as two often complementary alternatives to discern and control for confounding variables. The following sections discuss in more detail some of the adjustment techniques frequently used in epidemiology. Note that because it can be seen as both an "adjustment" technique and a study design feature, matching (including individual and frequency matching) has been previously addressed in Chapter 1 of this book, in which the main observational design strategies were discussed (Section 1.4.5). In the present chapter, the issue of individual matching is taken up again, but only insofar as it relates to the application of this strategy in adjusting for follow-up length in cohort studies (Section 7.4.6) and to demonstrate its analytic convergence with the Mantel-Haenszel approach when matched sets are treated as strata for the adjustment of the odds ratio (OR) (Section 7.3.3).

7.2   STRATIFICATION AND ADJUSTMENT TECHNIQUES TO DISENTANGLE CONFOUNDING

Table 7–1 shows an example of a case-control study of male gender as a possible risk factor for malaria infection. This example was used in Chapter 5 to illustrate how to assess whether a variable is a confounder (Section 5.3). The crude analysis shown at the top of the table suggests that males are at higher risk of malaria (OR = 1.71). If random and systematic errors (bias) are deemed to be unlikely explanations for the observed association, the possibility of confounding needs to be considered; that is, whether the association may be explained by characteristics related to both gender and increased odds of malaria. One such characteristic is occupation: individuals who work mostly outdoors (eg, agricultural workers) are more likely to be exposed to mosquito bites than those who work indoors and are thus at a higher risk of malaria. Thus, the observed association could be explained if the likelihood of working outdoors differed between genders. In Section 5.3, occupation was shown to be related to both gender (the "exposure") and malaria (the "outcome") (strategy no. 1 for the assessment of confounding, see Exhibit 5–3); it was also shown that when the data were stratified by type of occupation (strategy

Table 7–1 Example of Stratified Analysis: Hypothetical Study of Male Gender as a Risk Factor for Malaria Infection

Crude Analysis

All Cases and Controls

	Cases	Controls	Total	
Males	88	68	156	OR = 1.71
Females	62	82	144	
Total	150	150	300	

Stratified Analysis: By Occupation

Cases and Controls with Mostly Outdoor Occupations

	Cases	Controls	Total	
Males	53	15	68	OR = 1.06
Females	10	3	13	
Total	63	18	81	

Cases and Controls with Mostly Indoor Occupations

	Cases	Controls	Total	
Males	35	53	88	OR = 1.00
Females	52	79	131	
Total	87	132	219	

no. 2 to assess confounding), the stratified estimates were different from the pooled (crude) estimate. These results are presented in the lower part of Table 7–1. The estimated odds ratios in both strata are very close to 1. By stratifying the study results according to the potential confounder, it is possible to *control for* its effect; that is, it is possible to assess the association between the risk factor of interest (male gender) and the disease (malaria) separately for those whose work is mostly outdoors (OR = 1.06) and for those who work mostly indoors (OR = 1.00). The fact that these stratum-specific odds ratios are similar to each other and fairly different from the crude estimate suggests that occupation is a confounder of the association between male gender and the presence of malaria. In contrast to the crude estimate (OR = 1.71), the stratified odds ratios are very close to 1, suggesting that once occupation is taken into account, there is *no* association between gender and the presence of malaria—in other words, that the crude association can be "explained" by the confounding effect of occupation. (As discussed in Chapter 5, Section 5.3, unadjusted odds ratios, rate ratios, and absolute differences can be different from the stratum-specific estimates even if confounding is not present.[1,2] Thus, the assessment of potential confounding effects by means of stratification must be confirmed by the use of the other strategies discussed in Chapter 5 and in this chapter.)

The stratified data shown in the two-by-two tables in the lower part of Table 7–1 allow a closer examination of why occupation is a confounder in this hypothetical example: (1) 43.6% (68/156) of males have mostly outdoor occupations, compared with only 9% (13/144) of females (OR = 7.8); and (2) 42% (63/150) of the malaria cases have mostly outdoor occupations, compared with 12% (18/150) of controls (OR = 5.3). The strong positive associations of the confounder (occupation) with both the risk factor of interest (male gender) and case-control status explain the (positive) confounding effect.

The stratified analysis also allows the assessment of the possible presence of interaction. In the example above, the fact that stratum-specific odds ratios are very similar (homogeneous) (Table 7–1) indicates that no interaction is present (see Chapter 6), and thus an overall occupation-adjusted odds ratio can be calculated. As described later in this chapter, this can be done by calculating a *weighted average* of the stratum-specific estimates, eg, using the Mantel-Haenszel weighted odds ratio, OR_{MH}, which turns out to be 1.01 in this particular example; see Section 7.3.3. Compared with the examination of the stratum-specific results, the calculation of this weighted average (ie, this adjusted odds ratio) requires the assumption that the association is *homogeneous* across strata. In view of the similarity of the stratified odds ratios, it is easy to accept the homogeneity assumption for the results shown in Table 7–1. On the other hand, when the odds ratios are not too similar (eg, 1.4 and 2.0), it may be difficult to decide whether the observed heterogeneity is real; that is, whether there is actual effect modification, as opposed to its being the result of random variability caused by the small size of the strata (see Chapter 6, Section 6.10.1), in which case it can be ignored. In other words, the issue is whether presence of interaction should be accepted by the investigator. As discussed in Chapter 6, Section 6.9, in addition to the statistical significance of the observed heterogeneity, its magnitude should be considered when deciding whether interaction is present; thus, stratum-specific odds ratios of 1.4 and 20.0 are more likely to reflect a true interaction than odds ratios of 1.4 and 2.0. Other factors that should be considered are whether the interaction is quantitative (eg, stratum-specific odds ratios of 1.4 and 2.0) or qualitative (eg, odds ratios of 1.4 and 0.3) and, most importantly, its perceived biological plausibility.

If interaction is judged to be present, adjustment (eg, obtaining a combined odds ratio) is unwarranted, for in this case the "adjusted" odds ratio has no relevance, as it will be a weighted average of heterogeneous stratum-specific odds ratios. Consider, for example, the study by Reif et al,[3] cited in Chapter 6, showing that an association between environmental tobacco smoke and lung cancer in pet dogs was present in short-nosed dogs (OR = 2.4) and virtually absent (OR= 0.9) in long-nosed dogs. The biological plausibility of this possible qualitative interaction was discussed in Section 6.10.5. Assuming that this interaction is real, adjustment for skull shape (nose length) is obviously not warranted, since an adjusted odds ratio, representing the weighted average of the stratum-specific odds ratios of 2.4 and 0.9, has no useful interpretation.

Another example is provided in Table 7–2, which summarizes the results from a case-control study of oral contraceptive use as a possible risk factor for myocardial infarction among women of reproductive ages.[4] As shown in the upper part of the table, the odds of disease among women who used oral contraceptives was estimated to be about 70% higher than the odds in those who did not use oral contraceptives. The possibility of confounding by age, however, was considered by the authors of this study. Because age was known to be directly related to the outcome (risk of myocardial infarction) and inversely related to the exposure (increased oral contraceptive use among younger women), it could act as a *negative* confounder (see Chapter 5, Section 5.4.4).

In a stratified analysis by age, also shown in Table 7–2, all but one of the strata had estimated odds ratios further away from 1.0 than the overall crude estimate, confirming the expectation of negative confounding (ie, age driving the estimated crude association toward the null). The adjusted odds ratio (see Section 7.3.3) of the five age-specific odds ratios in Table 7–2 was found to be 4.0, thus more than twice the crude estimate. As mentioned previously, implicit when calculating any average, this adjusted odds ratio estimate requires assuming that the odds ratios are homogeneous; that is, that the observed between-strata differences in odds ratios result from random variation. In this example, this assumption is probably reasonable,

Table 7–2 Example of Stratified Analysis: Case-Control Study of Oral Contraceptives (OC) and Myocardial Infarction in Women

Crude Analysis

All Cases and Controls

	Cases	Controls	
OC	29	135	
No OC	205	1607	OR = 1.7
	234	1742	

Stratified Analysis: By Age

Age 25–29

	Cases	Controls	
OC	4	62	OR = 7.2
No OC	2	224	

Age 30–34

	Cases	Controls	
OC	9	33	OR = 8.9
No OC	12	390	

Age 35–39

	Cases	Controls	
OC	4	26	OR = 1.5
No OC	33	330	

Age 40–44

	Cases	Controls	
OC	6	9	OR = 3.7
No OC	65	362	

Age 45–49

	Cases	Controls	
OC	6	5	OR = 3.9
No OC	93	301	

Source: Data from S Shapiro et al, Oral-Contraceptive Use in Relation to Myocardial Infarction, *Lancet,* pp 743–747, © 1979.

given the small number of cases in some of the cells and the fact that all odds ratios are in the same direction (denoting absence of qualitative interaction; see Chapter 6, Section 6.7.1). On the other hand, it could be argued that the quantitative differences among odds ratios in Table 7–2 are too large and thus that the estimation of a single average (adjusted) odds ratio supposedly "representative" of all age strata is not warranted. In other words, it could be argued that the effect seems to be stronger in women younger than 35 years (odds ratios of 7.2 and 8.9) than in older women (odds ratios ranging from 1.5 to 3.9). Acceptance of this heterogeneity of odds ratios suggests an alternative approach that consists of calculating two age-adjusted odds ratios: one for women 25 to 34 years old—that is, the weighted average odds ratio for the two younger groups—and another for women 35 to 49 years old—that is, the weighted average odds ratio for the three older groups. (These calculations yield OR_{MH} values of 8.3 and 2.7, respectively; see Section 7.3.3.) This example illustrates the advantages of stratification for assessing the presence of confounding and/or interaction and for deciding when adjustment is appropriate and how it should be carried out. It also illustrates a common situation in epidemiologic analysis: the exposure of interest seems to have heterogeneous effects according to a certain grouping of a third variable, sometimes not considered prior to the analysis of the data. Given the large number of possibilities for grouping variables when conducting stratified analysis and the potential random variability of apparent subgroup effects (Section 6.10.1), this type of analysis, if not based on biologically plausible a priori hypotheses, should be considered exploratory.

Because the previous examples were based on the assessment of odds ratios, they were used to illustrate the evaluation of multiplicative interaction. It is, however, important to bear in mind that if the measure of association of interest is the attributable risk (Section 3.2.2), it is additive interaction that should be considered (see Section 6.6), as discussed in the context of the direct method of adjustment in Section 7.3.1.

7.2.1 Stratification and Adjustment: Assumptions

Compared to adjustment, stratification is virtually (but not completely) assumption-free. It does require assuming that the strata are meaningful and properly defined. This means that there should be homogeneity *within* each stratum. For example, for the strata in Table 7–1, it must be implicitly assumed that there is uniformity regarding the association of gender with malaria in each of the two occupational strata (mostly outdoors or mostly indoors); similarly, in Table 7–2, it is assumed that the association of oral contraceptives with myocardial infarction is homogeneous within each 5-year age group. If this assumption were not appropriate in each of these examples, other, more precisely defined categories (eg, more specific occupational categories, or finer age intervals, respectively) would have to be chosen for the stratified analysis. This assumption is equivalent to the assumption of *lack of residual confounding*, described later in this chapter (Section 7.5).

For adjustment, further assumptions must be met. As described in the next section, all adjustment techniques are based on assuming some kind of *statistical model* that summarizes the association between the variables under investigation. Sometimes the statistical model is a simple one, as in the case of *adjustment methods based on stratification*, namely direct and indirect adjustment (Sections 7.3.1 and 7.3.2) or the Mantel-Haenszel method (Section 7.3.3). As discussed above, for the calculation of a (weighted) mean of a number of stratum-specific odds ratios, it is assumed that these are homogeneous across strata; that is, that there is no (multiplicative) interaction. These simpler stratification-based adjustment methods are most often used when controlling for a limited number of potential confounders that are categorical or that can be categorized (see Section 7.3.4). On the other hand, more mathematically complex models are the basis for *multivariate adjustment methods based on regression methods*.* As described more extensively in Section 7.4, these more complex models are used as tools for epidemiologic inferences about the relationships between a number of factors and a disease, while simultaneously controlling (or adjusting) for the potentially mutual confounding effects of all these factors. These multiple-regression methods can also handle continuous covariates.

In the following paragraphs, some of the most frequently used techniques for adjustment and multivariate analysis of epidemiologic data are briefly described. Sections 7.3 and 7.4 describe the techniques based on stratification and those based on multiple-regression methods, respectively. Each of these analytical techniques is based on both a conceptual and a mathematical model; that is, something we could refer to as a "statistical model." Sections 7.5 and 7.6 discuss some potential limitations of multivariate adjustment (residual confounding and overadjustment), and the final section of this chapter (Section 7.7) presents a summary and overview of common uses of multivariate statistical modeling techniques in epidemiologic practice.

---

*The term *multivariate analysis,* commonly used in the epidemiology literature, is in contrast with "crude" analysis, which assesses the relationship between one variable and one outcome. Most often, the term *multivariate* is used when simultaneously controlling for more than one variable (in contrast to *bivariate analysis*). It is, however, used in a different way in the field of biostatistics, where *multivariate analysis* usually refers to the multiple-regression techniques involving more than one *dependent* variable.

7.3 ADJUSTMENT METHODS BASED ON STRATIFICATION

7.3.1 Direct Adjustment

Direct adjustment has been traditionally used for age adjustment when comparing morbidity and mortality rates across countries or regions or across different time periods, although age adjustment is by no means its only application. The popularity of more mathematically sophisticated statistical methods (such as those presented in the following sections) has limited the use of direct adjustment in epidemiology research in recent years, but the method remains a straightforward technique that is particularly useful to illustrate the basic principles of statistical adjustment.

The direct method is described in most introductory epidemiologic textbooks (eg, Gordis[5]). Table 7–3 outlines the procedure when comparing incidence rates between two groups, A and B (eg, exposed and unexposed), stratified according to the suspected confounding variable (strata i = 1 to *k*).

1. For each stratum of the suspected confounding variable, the incidence is calculated in the two study groups (columns 4 and 7).
2. A standard population with a specific number of individuals in each stratum is identified (column 8).
3. The *expected* number of cases in each stratum of the standard population is calculated by multiplying the corresponding stratum-specific rates observed in study group A (column 9) and in study group B (column 10) times the number of subjects in the standard population stratum.
4. The overall sums of expected cases in the standard population (based on the rates of A and B) divided by the total number of individuals in the standard population are the *adjusted* or *standardized* incidence rates; that is, the incidence rates that would be observed in groups A and B if these populations had exactly the same age distribution as the standard population or, conversely, the incidence that would be observed in the standard population if it had the stratum-specific rates of the study group A (I^*_A) or the stratum-specific rates of the study group B (I^*_B).

It should be evident from looking at the formula for the calculation of the adjusted rates that these are *weighted averages* of the stratum-specific rates in each study group, using as weights the corresponding number of subjects in each stratum of the standard population. The

Table 7–3 Direct Adjustment for Comparison of Incidence (I) in Two Study Groups

Suspected Confounding Variable (1)	Study Group A			Study Group B			Standard Population		
	No. (2)	Cases (3)	Incidence (4) = (3)/(2)	No. (5)	Cases (6)	Incidence (7) = (6)/(5)	No. (8)	Expected Cases Using I of A (9) = (4) × (8)	Expected Cases Using I of B (10) = (7) × (8)
Stratum 1	n_{A1}	x_{A1}	I_{A1}	n_{B1}	x_{B1}	I_{B1}	W_1	$I_{A1} \times W_1$	$I_{B1} \times W_1$
Stratum 2	n_{A2}	x_{A2}	I_{A2}	n_{B2}	x_{B2}	I_{B2}	W_2	$I_{A2} \times W_2$	$I_{B2} \times W_2$
Stratum 3	n_{A3}	x_{A3}	I_{A3}	n_{B3}	x_{B3}	I_{B3}	W_3	$I_{A3} \times W_3$	$I_{B3} \times W_3$
—								—	—
Stratum k	n_{Ak}	x_{Ak}	I_{Ak}	n_{Bk}	x_{Bk}	I_{Bk}	W_k	$I_{Ak} \times W_k$	$I_{Bk} \times W_k$
Total	N_A	X_A	I_A	N_B	X_B	I_B	$\sum_i W_i$	$\sum_i [I_{Ai} \times W_i]$	$\sum_i [I_{Bi} \times W_i]$

Adjusted Incidence

$$I^{\star}_A = \frac{\sum_i [I_{Ai} \times W_i]}{\sum_i W_i}$$

$$I^{\star}_B = \frac{\sum_i [I_{Bi} \times W_i]}{\sum_i W_i}$$

fact that both averages are calculated using the same weights allows their comparison. The resulting adjusted rates can then be used to calculate either the adjusted attributable risk (AR) in those exposed (for standard error of this estimate, see Appendix A, Section A.6) or the relative risk (RR):

$$\text{Adjusted AR} = I^*_A - I^*_B$$

$$\text{Adjusted RR} = \frac{I^*_A}{I^*_B}$$

As discussed in the previous section, the main assumption implicit in the calculation of adjusted attributable risks or relative risks obtained by direct adjustment is that *effects are homogeneous* across the strata of the confounding variable(s): that is, if an overall summary measure of effect across strata of a given variable is calculated, it is assumed that this *average* is reasonably representative of each and all the involved strata. Further specification of this assumption is necessary, namely whether the homogeneity refers to an absolute scale (additive model) or a relative scale (multiplicative model). This concept is simplistically illustrated by the hypothetical situations shown in Tables 7–4 and 7–5, in which there is strong confounding by age: that is, the outcome is more frequent in older than in younger subjects, and the study groups are quite different with regard to their age distributions.

In Table 7–4, the attributable risks are homogeneous across the two age strata (stratum-specific ARs = 10%), and both are different from the crude overall attributable risk (20%), denoting a confounding effect by age. Because the stratum-specific attributable risks are homogeneous (identical in this hypothetical example), the weighted average of these differences (ie, the adjusted attributable risk) does not vary with the choice of the standard population (lower half of Table 7–4). However, the same is not true when calculating an adjusted relative risk in this example: because relative risks vary by age, the adjusted relative risk (ie, the weighted average of the nonhomogeneous age-specific relative risks) depends on which stratum is given more weight when choosing the standard population. For example, because the relative risk is higher in the younger (2.0) than in the older (1.25) stratum, the use of a younger standard population results in a higher age-adjusted relative risk (1.67) than that obtained when using an older standard population (1.29). In conclusion, because there is homogeneity of attributable risks (ie, no additive interaction), it is appropriate to use directly adjusted rates for the purpose of calculating an age-adjusted attributable risk. However, given the heterogeneity of relative risks by age, it is not appropriate to estimate an age-adjusted

Table 7–4 Hypothetical Example of Direct Adjustment When Stratum-Specific Absolute Differences (Attributable Risks) Are Homogeneous

Age (yrs)	Study Group A			Study Group B			AR (%)	RR
	N	Cases	Rate (%)	N	Cases	Rate (%)		
<40	100	20	20	400	40	10	**10**	2.00
≥40	200	100	50	200	80	40	**10**	1.25
Total	300	120	40	600	120	20	20	2.00

Calculation of the adjusted estimates:

Age (yrs)	Younger Standard Population			Older Standard Population		
	N	Expected Cases if A Rates	Expected Cases if B Rates	N	Expected Cases if A Rates	Expected Cases if B Rates
<40	500	100	50	100	20	10
≥40	100	50	40	500	250	200
Total	600	150	90	600	270	210
Adjusted rate (%)		25	15		45	35
AR			10%			10%
RR			1.67			1.29

Note: AR, attributable risk; RR, relative risk.

---

relative risk in this case. Note that in this situation, the adjusted relative risk may vary depending on the standard chosen. This is a matter of special concern in situations in which there is qualitative or strong quantitative interaction.

A situation opposite to that depicted in Table 7–4 is shown in Table 7–5. In the hypothetical example given in Table 7–5, the stratum-specific relative risks are homogeneous; however, the same is not true for the attributable risks. Thus, the adjusted relative risks are identical regardless of the choice of the standard population, but the value of the adjusted attributable risk estimate depends on which stratum is given more weight. For instance, the older standard population yields a higher adjusted attributable risk because the attributable risk is greater for the older (15%) than for the younger (3%) stratum. Thus, given the heterogeneity of stratum-specific attributable risks, it may not be appropriate to calculate an age-adjusted attributable risk. On the other hand, an age-adjusted relative risk accurately reflects the homogeneity of multiplicative effects by age when comparing groups A and B.

Other practical considerations about the direct method of adjustment are as follows:

Table 7–5 Hypothetical Example of Direct Adjustment When Stratum-Specific Relative Differences (Relative Risks) Are Homogeneous

Age (yrs)	Study Group A			Study Group B			AR (%)	RR
	N	Cases	Rate (%)	N	Cases	Rate (%)		
<40	100	6	6	400	12	3	3	**2.00**
≥40	200	60	30	200	30	15	15	**2.00**
Total	300	66	22	600	42	7	15	3.14

Calculation of the adjusted estimates:

Age (yrs)	Younger Standard Population			Older Standard Population		
	N	Expected Cases if A Rates	Expected Cases if B Rates	N	Expected Cases if A Rates	Expected Cases if B Rates
<40	500	30	15	100	6	3
≥40	100	30	15	500	150	75
Total	600	60	30	600	156	78
Adjusted rate (%)		10	5		26	13
AR		5%			13%	
RR		**2.00**			**2.00**	

Note: AR, attributable risk; RR, relative risk.

- This method is used for the *comparison* of rates in two or more study groups; the *absolute* value of an adjusted rate is usually not the main focus because it depends on the choice of the standard population, which is often arbitrary.
- Several options are available for the choice of the standard population, including
  1. An entirely artificial population (eg, 1000 subjects in each stratum).
  2. One of the study groups. This will make calculations simpler and save time, for the observed rate in the group chosen to be the standard population is, by definition, "standardized."*

---

*When one of the study groups is particularly small, it should be used as the standard, so as to minimize random variability. This is because when the smaller group is used as the standard, there is no need to use its statistically unstable stratum-specific rates to estimate expected numbers of events, as its total observed rate *is* the adjusted rate. In addition, more precise age-specific rates of the other (larger) population(s) produce a stabler expected number of events and thus more precise adjusted rate(s).

3. The sum of the study populations or groups.
4. A population that may be either a reference population or an "external" population, such as the population of the state, province, or country from which the study groups originate (or the whole world when the focus is on comparing several countries). When comparing occupational groups in residents of a metropolitan area, for example, it would be reasonable to select the total metropolitan area working population as the standard. Although this choice is still arbitrary, the resulting adjusted rates will be at least somewhat representative of the "true" study group rates.
5. The so-called *minimum-variance* standard population, which produces the most statistically stable adjusted estimates and is thus particularly useful when sample sizes are small. When two groups are compared using the same notation as in Table 7–3, for each stratum (i), the stratum-specific minimum-variance standard population is calculated as

[Equation 7.1]

$$W_i = \frac{1}{\dfrac{1}{n_{Ai}} + \dfrac{1}{n_{Bi}}} = \frac{n_{Ai} \times n_{Bi}}{n_{Ai} + n_{Bi}}$$

For the example shown in Table 7–4 , the minimum-variance standard population would therefore be

Stratum age under 40 years:

$$\text{Standard population} = \frac{100 \times 400}{100 + 400} = 80$$

Stratum age greater than or equal to 40 years:

$$\text{Standard population} = \frac{200 \times 200}{200 + 200} = 100$$

Note that if one of the groups (eg, population A) is much smaller than the other—that is, if $n_{Ai} \ll n_{Bi}$—then $(1/n_{Ai}) \gg (1/n_{Bi})$, and thus Equation 7.1 reduces to $w_i \approx n_{Ai}$, which formally supports the recommendation mentioned previously that when one of the groups is small, it should be used as the standard.

- Although, as mentioned previously, the direct method of adjustment has been traditionally used for age-adjusted comparisons of mortality and morbidity rates by time or place, it is an appropriate method to carry out adjustment for any categorical variables. It can also be used to simultaneously adjust for more than one variable (see layout in Table 7–6). Obviously, the latter application will be limited if there are too many strata and data are sparse.

- The direct method can be used for the adjustment of any rate or proportion (mortality, case fatality rate, incidence per person-time, prevalence). Thus, this method can also be used in the context of a case-control study to obtain the *adjusted* proportions of exposed cases and controls, which in turn could be used to calculate an adjusted odds ratio.

7.3.2 Indirect Adjustment

Like the direct adjustment method, indirect adjustment has been traditionally used for age adjustment of mortality and morbidity data. In the indirect method of adjustment, which has been particularly popular in the field of occupational epidemiology, the expected number of events (eg, deaths) in a study group (eg, an occupational cohort) is calculated by applying reference rates ("standard" rates) to the number of individuals in each stratum of the study group(s). For each study group, the ratio of the total number of observed events to the number of expected events (if the rates in the study group were the "standard" rates) provides an estimate of the factor-adjusted relative risk or rate ratio *comparing the study group with the population that served as the source of the reference rates* (Table 7–7). When used in the context of mortality data, this ratio is known as the *standardized mor-*

Table 7–6 Example of Layout for Using the Direct Method for Simultaneous Adjustment for Gender, Race, and Education (Categorically Defined)

Gender	Race	Education (yrs)	Stratum (i)	Study Group A Rate	Study Group B Rate	Standard Population (Weights)
Male	Black	<12	1	–	–	–
		≥12	2	–	–	–
	White	<12	3	–	–	–
		≥12	4	–	–	–
Female	Black	<12	5	–	–	–
		≥12	6	–	–	–
	White	<12	7	–	–	–
		≥12	8	–	–	–

Table 7–7 Indirect Adjustment: Comparing the Observed Mortality in a Study Population with That of an External Reference Population

	Study Population A			Reference Population
Suspected Confounding Variable (1)	No. (2)	Observed Deaths (3)	Mortality Rate (4)	Expected Deaths in A if It Had Rates of Reference Population (5) = (4) × (2)
Stratum 1	n_{A1}	x_{A1}	M_1	$M_1 \times n_{A1}$
Stratum 2	n_{A2}	x_{A2}	M_2	$M_2 \times n_{A2}$
Stratum 3	n_{A3}	x_{A3}	M_3	$M_3 \times n_{A3}$
. . .	. . .	. . .	. . .	. . .
Stratum k	n_{Ak}	x_{Ak}	M_k	$M_k \times n_{Ak}$
Total		$\sum_i x_{Ai}$		$\sum_i [M_i \times n_{Ai}]$

Standardized Mortality Ratio
$$\text{SMR} = \frac{\text{Observed deaths}}{\text{Expected deaths}} = \frac{\sum_i x_{Ai}}{\sum_i [M_i \times n_{Ai}]}$$

tality ratio (SMR), with similar terms used for morbidity data, such as *standardized incidence ratio (SIR)* and *standardized prevalence ratio (SPR)*.

The so-called indirect method is considered to be particularly useful either when stratum-specific risks or rates are missing in one of the groups under comparison or when the study group(s) is(are) small, so that the stratum-specific rates are considered too unstable, thus resulting in statistically unreliable expected numbers when using the direct method (columns 9 and 10 in Table 7–3).

When carrying out indirect adjustment, it is not appropriate to define the population serving as the source of the rates as a "standard population," the reason being that the true standard population is actually the study group(s) to which the external reference ("standard") rates are applied. As the calculation of the SMRs or SIRs is based on applying the rates of a reference population to each study group's distribution, *when comparing more than one study group to the source of reference rates* the SMRs are in fact adjusted to different standards (ie, the study groups themselves). As a corollary, the comparison of SMRs for different study groups may be inappropriate, as illustrated in the hypothetical example in Table 7–8. In this example, the two study groups have identical age-specific rates; however, because of their different age distributions, crude overall rates are different (18.3% and 11.7%). Application of the "stan-

Table 7–8 Hypothetical Example of Two Study Groups with Identical Age-Specific Rates but Different Age Distributions: Use of the Indirect Method Using External Reference Rates Results in Different SMRs

Age (yrs)	Study Group A			Study Group B			External Reference Rates
	N	Deaths	Rate	N	Deaths	Rate	
<40	100	10	**10%**	500	50	**10%**	12%
≥40	500	100	**20%**	100	20	**20%**	50%
Total	600	**110**	18.3%	600	**70**	11.7%	

Age (yrs)	Expected No. of Deaths Obtained by Applying the Reference Rates to Groups A and B	
	Study Group A	Study Group B
<40	12% × 100 = 12	12% × 500 = 60
≥40	50% × 500 = 250	50% × 100 = 50
Total number expected	**262**	**110**
SMR (oberved/expected)	110/262 = **0.42**	70/110 = **0.64**

dard" (reference) rates to each of these study groups results in expected numbers that are unevenly weighted and, consequently, in different SMRs (0.42 and 0.64). As discussed in detail by Armstrong,[6] this situation arises when the ratios of rates in study groups and in the reference population are not homogeneous across strata.

Thus, although the use of SMRs to compare study groups is a relatively common practice in the epidemiologic literature, it is not always appropriate. SMRs are obviously appropriate when the comparison of interest is that between each study group and the reference population. Note, however, that when the SMR is obtained for only a pair of populations (eg, an occupational group vs the total area population serving as the source of "standard" rates, or any study group vs a reference population), the direct and indirect methods converge: in this situation, the calculation of the SMR can be also thought of as a *direct* method, with one of the groups under comparison (eg, an occupational group) serving as the "standard population" (Figure 7–1).

7.3.3 Mantel-Haenszel Method for Estimating an Adjusted Measure of Association

When the measure of association of interest is the odds ratio (eg, when one is analyzing results of a case-control study), the method de-

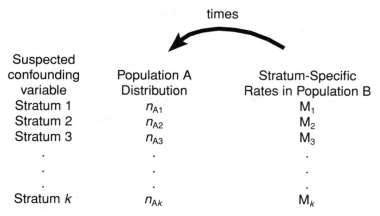

Figure 7–1 When only two populations are compared, the direct and indirect methods converge. The approach can be regarded as a direct method in which one of the populations (A) is the standard or as an indirect method using the other population (B) as the source of the reference ("standard") rates.

scribed by Mantel and Haenszel[7] to calculate an overall adjusted odds ratio is frequently used for adjusting for one or more categorically defined potential confounders. Table 7–9 shows the notation for the formulation of the Mantel-Haenszel adjusted odds ratio for data stratified into k strata:

$$OR_{MH} = \frac{\sum\limits_i \dfrac{a_i d_i}{N_i}}{\sum\limits_i \dfrac{b_i c_i}{N_i}}$$

which is equivalent to a *weighted average of the stratum-specific odds ratios.** For standard error and confidence interval estimate, see Appendix A, Section A.8.

---

*Note that this formula is algebraically identical to the following formula:

$$OR_{MH} = \frac{\sum\limits_i \dfrac{b_i c_i}{N_i} \times \dfrac{a_i d_i}{b_i c_i}}{\sum\limits_i \dfrac{b_i c_i}{N_i}} = \frac{\sum\limits_i w_i\, OR_i}{\sum\limits_i w_i}$$

Thus, the OR_{MH} is a weighted average of the stratum-specific odds ratio (OR_i), with weights equal to each stratum's ($b_i c_i / N_i$).

Table 7–9 Notation for the Calculation of the Mantel-Haenszel Adjusted Odds Ratio in a Case-Control Study, Stratified According to a Potential Confounding Variable

Stratum i		*Cases*	*Controls*	*Total*
Exposed		a_i	b_i	m_{1i}
Unexposed		c_i	d_i	m_{2i}
Total		n_{1i}	n_{2i}	N_i

The calculation of the OR_{MH} is straightforward, as illustrated by the following examples. In Table 7–1 the crude association between the presence of malaria and gender suggested that males were at a higher risk of the disease; however, when the association was examined by strata of occupation, no association with gender was observed in either occupational category. In addition to inspecting the occupation-specific odds ratios, a summary odds ratio can be calculated, expressing the occupation-adjusted association between gender and malaria. The adjusted OR_{MH} (the weighted average of the occupational stratum-specific odds ratio) is calculated as follows:

$$OR_{MH} = \frac{\sum_i \frac{a_i d_i}{N_i}}{\sum_i \frac{b_i c_i}{N_i}} = \frac{\frac{53 \times 3}{81} + \frac{35 \times 79}{219}}{\frac{10 \times 15}{81} + \frac{52 \times 53}{219}} = 1.01$$

Note that the estimate of OR_{MH} lies between the stratum-specific estimates (1.06 and 1.00). However, it is closer to the stratum "mostly indoor occupation" because of the larger sample size in that stratum, for which the estimate is consequently given more "weight" ($b_i c_i / N_i$) when calculating the average adjusted OR_{MH}.

In the example in Table 7–2, the age-adjusted estimate of the OR_{MH} is

$$OR_{MH} = \frac{\sum_i \frac{a_i d_i}{N_i}}{\sum_i \frac{b_i c_i}{N_i}} = \frac{\frac{4 \times 224}{292} + \frac{9 \times 390}{444} + \frac{4 \times 330}{393} + \frac{6 \times 362}{442} + \frac{6 \times 301}{405}}{\frac{2 \times 62}{292} + \frac{12 \times 33}{444} + \frac{33 \times 26}{393} + \frac{65 \times 9}{442} + \frac{93 \times 5}{405}} = 4.0$$

The statistical model implicit in the Mantel-Haenszel procedure for the calculation of an adjusted odds ratio is that there is homogeneity of effects (expressed by odds ratios in this case) across the categories of the stratifying variable. In other words, it is assumed that there is no multiplicative interaction between the exposure and the stratifying variable (see Section 6.3.1). Specifically in the example from Table 7–2, when calculating an overall adjusted odds ratio, it is assumed that the odds ratio of myocardial infarction in relation to oral contraceptive use is approximately 4 (the calculated weighted average) for all age strata. As discussed previously (Section 7.2), in this example the observed differences in the stratum-specific odds ratio values are assumed to result from random variation; if the observed heterogeneity is considered excessive, an option is to calculate separate age-adjusted odds ratios for younger and older women (see Section 7.2), as follows:

$$OR_{MH, 25-34y} = \frac{\sum_i \frac{a_i a_i}{N_i}}{\sum_i \frac{b_i c_i}{N_i}} = \frac{\frac{4 \times 224}{292} + \frac{9 \times 390}{444}}{\frac{2 \times 62}{292} + \frac{12 \times 33}{444}} = 8.3$$

$$OR_{MH, 35-49y} = \frac{\sum_i \frac{a_i d_i}{N_i}}{\sum_i \frac{b_i c_i}{N_i}} = \frac{\frac{4 \times 330}{393} + \frac{6 \times 362}{442} + \frac{6 \times 301}{405}}{\frac{33 \times 26}{393} + \frac{65 \times 9}{442} + \frac{93 \times 5}{405}} = 2.7$$

Mantel-Haenszel Adjusted Rate Ratio

The Mantel-Haenszel method has been extended to the calculation of an adjusted rate ratio (RR) in the context of a cohort study with incidence data based on person-time.[8(pp219–221)] Table 7–10 shows the general layout of the data from each of the stratum-specific tables. Based on the notation in this table, the Mantel-Haenszel estimate of the adjusted rate ratio is calculated as

$$RR_{MH} = \frac{\sum_i \frac{a_{1i} y_{0i}}{T_i}}{\sum_i \frac{a_{0i} y_{1i}}{T_i}}$$

An example of the application of this formula is presented in Table 7–11, based on data[9] from one of the examples used in Chapter 5 to illustrate the techniques for the assessment of confounding (Section 5.3). Note that the estimated RR_{MH} comparing "high" versus "low" vitamin index intake obtained in Table 7–11 is identical to the corre-

Table 7–10 Notation for the Calculation of the Mantel-Haenszel Adjusted Rate Ratio in a Prospective Study Based on Person-Time Incidence Rates Stratified According to a Potential Confounding Variable

Stratum i	Cases	Person-Time
Exposed	a_{1i}	y_{1i}
Unexposed	a_{0i}	y_{0i}
Total		T_i

sponding smoking status–adjusted rate ratio that was presented in Table 5–5 based on the direct method of adjustment.

Mantel-Haenszel Method and the Odds Ratio for Paired Case-Control Data

As presented in basic textbooks (eg, Gordis[5]) and briefly discussed in Section 3.4.1, in matched paired case-control studies, the odds ratio is calculated by dividing the number of pairs in which the case is exposed and the control is not by the number of pairs in which the case is unexposed and the control is exposed. In Table 7–12, each cell represents the number of pairs for the corresponding category defined by case-control and exposure status. Thus, in the two-by-two cross-tabulation shown on the left-hand side, the odds ratio is estimated as the ratio of discordant pairs, b/c. An example is provided on the right-hand side of the table, from a report from the Atherosclerosis Risk in Communities (ARIC) study on the association between chronic cytomegalovirus (CMV) infection and carotid atherosclerosis (measured by B-mode ultrasound).[10] In this study, atherosclerosis cases and controls were individually matched by age, sex, ethnicity, field center, and date of examination; the paired odds ratio (ie, the odds ratio controlling for all matching variables) is estimated as $65/42 = 1.55$. The rationale for estimating the odds ratio as the ratio of discordant pairs in a matched case-control study is readily grasped by the application of the Mantel-Haenszel method for averaging stratified odds ratios.

The data in Table 7–12 can be rearranged as in Table 7–13, where each of the 340 pairs in this study is now a stratum with a size n of 2. The resulting 340 two-by-two tables can be arranged as in Table 7–13 because the pairs can only be of one of four possible types (each of the cells in Table 7–12): for example, for the first type of pair in which both case and control are CMV+ (cell "a" on the left panel of Table 7–12), there would be a total of 214 identical tables; for the second type (the "b" cell, discordant, with case exposed and control unexposed), there would be 65 tables; and so on. In the last two columns

Table 7–11 Example for the Calculation of the Mantel-Haenszel Adjusted Rate Ratio (RR_{MH}): Data on Mortality in Individuals with High and Low Vitamin C/Beta-Carotene Intake Index, by Smoking Status, Western Electric Company Study

	Vitamin C/Beta Carotene Intake Index	No. of Deaths	Person-Years	Stratified RRs
Nonsmokers	High	53	5143	RR = 0.77
	Low	57	4260	
	Total		9403	
Smokers	High	111	6233	RR = 0.83
	Low	138	6447	
	Total		12,680	

$$RR_{MH} = \frac{\sum_i \frac{a_{1i}y_{0i}}{T_i}}{\sum_i \frac{a_{0i}y_{1i}}{T_i}} = \frac{\frac{53 \times 4260}{9403} + \frac{111 \times 6447}{12,680}}{\frac{57 \times 5143}{9403} + \frac{138 \times 6233}{12,680}} = 0.81$$

Note: The "moderate" vitamin intake index category in Table 5–4 has been omitted for simplicity. All rates ratios in the table compare those with "high" with those with "low" vitamin intake index.

Source: Data from DK Pandey et al, Dietary Vitamin C and β-Carotene and Risk of Death in Middle-Aged Men. The Western Electric Study, *American Journal of Epidemiology,* Vol 142, pp 1269–1278, © 1995, The Johns Hopkins University School of Hygiene & Public Health.

---

of Table 7–13, the contribution to the numerator and denominator of the OR_{MH} of each of the 340 pairs is indicated. Note that the contribution (to either the numerator or the denominator) from all the strata based on concordant pairs is always 0, while the discordant pairs contribute to either the numerator ("b"-type pairs) or the denominator ("c"-type pairs). All these contributions, which are always ½—that is, $(1 \times 1)/2$—cancel out, with the actual number of discordant pairs in the numerator and the denominator resulting in the well-known formula $OR_{MH} = b/c$. Thus, this formula represents a *weighted average odds ratio for stratified data (using the Mantel-Haenszel weighing approach), where the strata are defined on the basis of matched pairs.*

7.3.4 Limitations of Stratification-Based Methods of Adjustment

The techniques described in the previous sections (direct and indirect adjustment, Mantel-Haenszel odds ratio or rate ratio) can be used

Table 7–12 Layout of a Two-by-Two Table for the Calculation of a Paired Odds Ratio and an Example

		NOTATION				EXAMPLE*	
		Controls				Controls	
		Exposed	Unexposed			CMV+	CMV−
Cases	Exposed	a	b	Cases	CMV+	214	65
	Unexposed	c	d		CMV−	42	19

$$\text{Paired OR} = \frac{b}{c}$$ $$\text{Paired OR} = \frac{65}{42} = 1.55$$

Note: Each cell represents the number of pairs for each category defined by case-control and exposure status.

*Cases represent individuals with carotid atherosclerosis defined by B-mode ultrasound; controls are individuals without atherosclerosis, individually match-paired to cases by age group, sex, ethnicity, field center, and date of examination. Cytomegalovirus (CMV) infection status is defined according to the presence or absence of IgG serum antibodies.

Source: Data from PD Sorlie et al, Cytomegalovirus/Herpesvirus and Carotid Atherosclerosis: The ARIC Study, *Journal of Medical Virology,* Vol 42, pp 33–37, © 1994, John Wiley & Sons.

---

for multivariate analysis; that is, for simultaneously controlling for more than one covariate. This can be done simply by constructing the strata based on the basis of all possible combinations of the adjustment variables (eg, see Table 7–6). These stratification-based methods, however, have practical limitations for multivariate adjustment:

1. Although they can be used to adjust for several covariates simultaneously, adjustment is carried out only for the association between one independent variable and an outcome at a time. For example, to assess the association of oral contraceptives with myocardial infarction while controlling for age and educational level, it would be necessary to create two-by-two tables for oral contraceptives vis-à-vis myocardial infarction for each stratum combining age and educational level. However, if the exposure of interest is educational level and the covariates to be adjusted for are age and oral contraceptive use, a new set of two-by-two tables would have to be created (representing education vs myocardial infarction for each stratum defined by categories of age and oral contraceptive use).

2. These methods allow adjustment only for categorical covariates (eg, gender); continuous covariates need to be categorized, as age was in the example shown in Table 7–2. Residual differences within these more or less arbitrarily defined categories may in

Table 7–13 Calculation of the Paired Odds Ratio for the Data in Table 7–12, Based on the Mantel-Haenszel Estimation Approach

Four Possible Pair Types:		Exp	Case	Cont	No. of Pairs in Table 7–12	Each Pair Contributes to OR_{MH}	
						Num $\left(\dfrac{a \times d}{N}\right)$	Den $\left(\dfrac{b \times c}{N}\right)$
Type 1	Concordant	+	1	1			
		−	0	0	2 $a = 214$	0	0
Type 2	Discordant	+	1	0			
		−	0	1	2 $b = 65$	½	0
Type 3	Discordant	+	0	1			
		−	1	0	2 $c = 42$	0	½
Type 4	Concordant	+	0	0			
		−	1	1	2 $d = 19$	0	0

$$OR_{MH} = \frac{(214 \times 0) + (65 \times 1/2) + (42 \times 0) + (19 \times 0)}{(214 \times 0) + (65 \times 0) + (42 \times 1/2) + (19 \times 0)} = \frac{65 \times 1/2}{42 \times 1/2} = \frac{65}{42} = \frac{b}{c}$$

Note: Exp, exposure status; Cont, controls; OR, odds ratio; Num, numerator; Den, denominator.

turn result in residual confounding (Section 7.5 and Chapter 5, Section 5.4.3).

3. Finally, data become sparse when the strata are too numerous. For the direct method, for example, if the sample size of a given stratum is 0, no corresponding stratum-specific rate is available for application to the standard population in that stratum; as a result, the adjusted rate becomes undefined.

Thus, in practice, stratification methods are usually limited to simultaneous adjustment for few categorical confounders (usually one or two), with a small number of categories each. When simultaneous adjustment for multiple covariates (including continuous variables) is needed, methods based on multiple-regression techniques are usually used.

7.4 MULTIPLE REGRESSION TECHNIQUES FOR ADJUSTMENT

Multiple-regression techniques are better suited to address the difficulties related to the application of the simpler techniques discussed heretofore, as they allow the examination of the effects of all exposure variables reciprocally and simultaneously adjusting for all the other variables in the model. In addition, they allow adjusting for continuous covariates, and, within reasonable limits, they are generally more efficient than stratification-based methods for the use of sparse data. Moreover, in addition to multivariate *adjustment*, multiple-regression techniques are useful for *prediction*—that is, for estimating the predicted value of a certain outcome as a function of given values of independent variables, as in the case of the prediction equations of coronary risk that were developed from the Framingham study using logistic regression[11] (see Section 7.4.3).

The sections that follow describe four of the most frequently used regression models for multivariate adjustment in epidemiology: (1) linear regression, used when the outcome is continuous (eg, blood pressure); (2) logistic regression, preferentially used when the outcome is categorical (cumulative incidence, prevalence); (3) proportional hazards (Cox) regression, used in survival analysis; and (4) Poisson regression, used when incidence rate (based on person-time) is the outcome of interest. It is beyond the scope of this chapter to discuss these techniques in detail; for this, the reader is referred to a general statistics textbook (eg, Armitage and Berry[12]) and to the specific references given in each section. Instead, the discussion will focus on the applied aspects of multiple regression.

In spite of their different applications, and even though only one of the models is specifically defined as "linear," the fundamental underpinning of all regression techniques discussed in this chapter is a *linear function*. This can be clearly seen in Table 7–14, in which the right-hand side of all models is exactly the same ($b_0 + b_1x_1 + b_2x_2 + \ldots + b_kx_k$), thus explaining why they are collectively termed *generalized linear models*. Note that the models listed in the table differ only with regard to the type of dependent variable or outcome postulated to be related to predictors in a linear fashion. Consequently, and as underscored in the sections that follow, the interpretation of the multiple-regression coefficients is similar for all these models, varying only with regard to the outcome variable.

In the next section, the concept of linear regression is reviewed in the context of the simplest situation, namely that involving only one predictor variable (one x). The four sections that follow briefly review the basic features of the regression models listed in Table 7–14. Finally, Sections 7.4.6 to 7.4.8 cover issues regarding the application of these models to matched and nested studies and to situations when a "linear" model is not reasonable, as well as issues related to statistical inference based on the parameter estimates.

Table 7–14 Multiple Regression Models and Interpretation of the Regression Coefficients

	Model	Interpretation of b_1
Linear	$y = b_0 + b_1x_1 + b_2x_2 + \ldots + b_kx_k$	Increase in outcome y mean value (continuous variable) per unit increase in x_1, adjusted for all other variables in the model
Logistic	$\log(\text{odds}) = b_0 + b_1x_1 + b_2x_2 + \ldots + b_kx_k$	Increase in the log odds of the outcome per unit increase in x_1, adjusted for all other variables in the model
Cox	$\log(\text{hazard}) = b_0 + b_1x_1 + b_2x_2 + \ldots + b_kx_k$	Increase in the log hazard of the outcome per unit increase in x_1, adjusted for all other variables in the model
Poisson	$\log(\text{rate}) = b_0 + b_1x_1 + b_2x_2 + \ldots + b_kx_k$	Increase in the log rate of the outcome per unit increase in x_1, adjusted for all other variables in the model

7.4.1 Linear Regression: General Concepts

Simple linear regression is a statistical technique usually employed to assess the association between two continuous variables. Figure 7–2, for example, shows a plot of the cross-sectional values of systolic blood pressure (SBP) and the carotid intimal-medial thickness (IMT), a measure of atherosclerosis obtained by B-mode ultrasound imaging, in a subset of 1410 participants from the ARIC study.[13] Each dot in the scatter of points represents an individual, with corresponding SBP and IMT values in the abscissa and ordinate, respectively. It can be seen that although there is a wide scatter, there is a tendency for the IMT values to be higher when SBP is also higher, and vice versa. This pattern warrants the assessment of whether SBP and IMT are *linearly* associated. The hypothesis regarding a possible linear association between these two continuous variables can be expressed as the following questions:

1. Is the average increase in IMT levels associated with a given increase in SBP approximately constant throughout the entire range of SBP values?
2. Can the association between SBP and IMT be assumed to follow a straight-line pattern (the statistical *model*) with the scatter around the line being the consequence of random error?

In addition to visually inspecting the scatter plot (eg, Figure 7–2), assessment of whether the relationship between two continuous variables (eg, SBP and IMT) is *statistically compatible* with a perfect straight line can be done by means of the *Pearson linear correlation coefficient (r)* (see, eg, Armitage and Berry,[12(pp163–165)] as well as an application in Chapter 8, Section 8.4.2). The correlation coefficient values range from -1.0 (when there is a perfect negative correlation—ie, when all

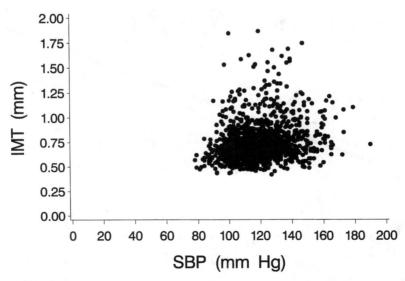

Figure 7–2 Relation between systolic blood pressure (SBP) and carotid intimal-medial thickness (IMT) in a subset of participants in the ARIC study

the points form a perfect straight line with a negative slope) to +1.0 (when there is a perfect positive correlation—ie, when the points form a straight line with a positive slope). A value of 0 indicates no linear correlation. In the example in Figure 7–2, the value of the Pearson correlation coefficient is 0.21, with a corresponding P value of 0.0001. The small P value in this example suggests that there is some kind of linear correlation between SBP and IMT not likely to be explained by chance, even though the magnitude of the coefficient implies that the correlation is only moderate. This conclusion fits the graphical display in Figure 7–2: although there is a tendency of higher SBP values to be associated with higher IMT values, there is a substantial dispersion of values around this hypothetical linear relationship.

Note that the correlation coefficient value contains no information about the strength of the association between the two variables that is represented by the slope of the hypothetical line, such as the amount of increase to be expected in IMT per unit increase in SBP. To estimate the strength of the linear association, it is necessary to find the formula for the regression line that best fits the observed data. In general, this line can be formulated in terms of two parameters (β_0 and

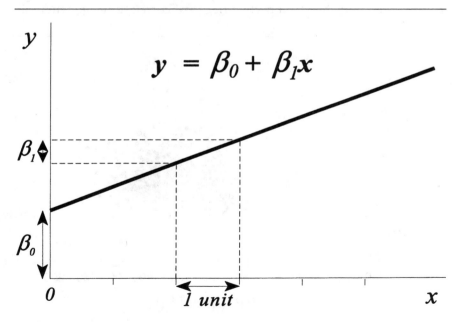

Figure 7–3 Graphical and mathematical representation of a linear model

β_1), which relate the mean (expected) value of the *dependent variable* (conventionally noted as $E(y)$ and placed in the ordinate of the plot) as a function of the *independent* or *predictor variable* (conventionally noted as x, in the abscissa). The general formula for the regression line is

$$E(y) = \beta_0 + \beta_1 x$$

(From this point on, "$E(y)$" is denoted as "y" to simplify the notation.)

Figure 7–3 shows the graphic representation of this general regression line. Inspection of this formula and the figure underscores the fact that the interpretation of each of the two parameters, β_0 and β_1, is straightforward, as follows:

- β_0 is the *intercept*—that is, the estimated value of y when $x = 0$.
- β_1 is the *regression coefficient*—that is, the estimated increase in the dependent variable (y) per unit increase in the predictor variable (x). Thus, when $x = 1$, then $y = \beta_0 + \beta_1$; for $x = 2$, then $y = \beta_0 + \beta_1 \times 2$, and so on. This regression coefficient corresponds to the slope of the regression line; it reflects the *strength* of the association between the two variables—that is, how much increase (or decrease, in the case of a descending line) in y is to be expected as x increases. Note that the absolute value of β_1 depends on the units of measurement for both x and y.

Once this *statistical model* is formulated, the practical question is how to estimate the regression line that *best* fits a given set of data, such as the data in Figure 7–2. (In linear regression, the method usually used to estimate the regression coefficients (or "parameters") is the *least squares method*. This consists in finding the parameter values that minimize the sum of the squares of the vertical distances between each of the observed points and the line. For details on the methods to estimate the regression line see any general statistics textbook, eg, Armitage and Berry[12] or Kleinbaum et al,[14] or a more specialized text, eg, Draper and Smith.[15]) For example, Figure 7–4 shows the regression line that best fits the observed data shown in Figure 7–2. The notation traditionally used to represent the estimated linear regression line is as follows:

$$y = b_0 + b_1 x + e$$

That is, the symbols for the parameters denoted by the Greek letter beta (β) are replaced by the letter b to denote that these are *estimates*. The error term, e, represents the difference between each observed y

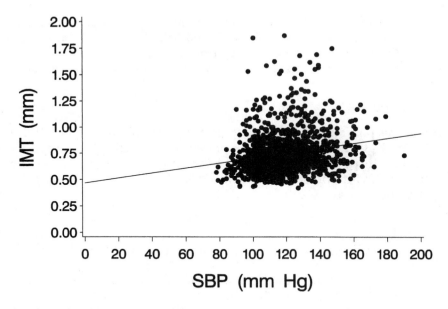

Figure 7–4 Regression line that best fits the data (least squares estimate) to the scatter points in Figure 7–2 (see text)

value and the corresponding predicted value (eg, the vertical distance between each point in the scatter in Figure 7–4 and the y value at the line). (For the sake of simplicity, the error term will be omitted from the remaining formulas in this chapter.) Returning to Figure 7–4, the mathematical formula for the estimated regression line shown in the figure is

[Equation 7.2]

   IMT (mm) = 0.4533 + 0.0025 × SBP (mm Hg)

The value of the intercept (0.4533 mm in this example) is purely theoretical; it does not have any real biological relevance in this case. It corresponds to the estimated IMT when SBP = 0: that is, when the above equation reduces to IMT (mm) = 0.4533. The fact that the intercept is biologically meaningless is frequent in many applications of linear regression in biomedical research because the value of 0 for many variables is not biologically viable or has no practical relevance. This is illustrated in Figure 7–4 and schematically in Figure 7–5, which shows how the intercept value is often a mere extrapolation of

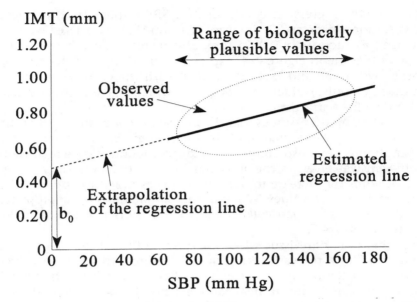

Figure 7-5 Observed data and extrapolation of regression line toward the axis (intercept)

the regression line to meet the ordinate (*y* axis), well beyond the range of biologically plausible values.*

More relevant in most circumstances when using linear regression is the value of the regression coefficient. In the above example, the es-

---

*The value of the intercept is useful if the investigator's intention is to use the regression results to *predict* the expected value of the dependent variable, given certain characteristics. To solve the equation, one needs to use the values of all the coefficients, including the intercept (see examples in the context of logistic regression in Section 7.4.3).

There are ways to improve the interpretability of the intercept by using transformations of the original continuous variables in the regression. For example, the mean systolic blood pressure could be subtracted from each individual's blood pressure value in the study population in Figure 7-4. This new variable (ie, the difference between each individual's blood pressure and the mean) could then be used in the regression, instead of the actual blood pressure value. In this case, even though the intercept is still defined as the estimated IMT for an individual with a value of 0 for the independent variables (*x*), it can be interpreted as the estimated IMT for an individual with the *average* blood pressure value in the study population.

timate of the regression coefficient for SBP implies that, in these cross-sectional data, an SBP increase of 1 mm Hg is associated with an average IMT increase of 0.0025 mm. This regression coefficient is the slope of the line in Figure 7–4, expressing the *strength* of the association between SBP and IMT, in contrast with the correlation coefficient, which only evaluates the degree to which a given set of quantitative data fits a straight line.

The above model assumes that the increase is *linear*: that is, that the increase in IMT as a function of the increase in SBP is constant. This assumption is obviously implicit in the fact that one single regression coefficient was given in the above equation (0.0025-mm increase in IMT per mm Hg increase in SBP), which is assumed to apply to the entire range of SBP values. Whether this simple model is appropriate will depend on each particular circumstance, as discussed in more detail in Section 7.4.7.

Another important issue when interpreting the "slope" (regression coefficient) of a regression function is the unit to which it corresponds. For example, it may be expressed as the increase in IMT per 5 mm Hg increase in SBP, rather than per 1 mm Hg, which would then be translated as a value of $5 \times 0.0025 = 0.0125$ mm in this example. The importance of specifying the units of variables x and y when reporting and interpreting the magnitude of the regression coefficient (slope) for all regression models (Table 7–14) cannot be sufficiently emphasized.

It is important to keep in mind, however, that comparison of the strength of the association between different variables (particularly continuous variables) based on the size of the regression coefficients should generally be avoided. This is related to the general problem of comparing the strength of the associations across different variables that was discussed in Chapter 3 (Section 3.5); further discussion of this issue is presented in Chapter 9, Section 9.3.4.

The regression coefficient (b_1) estimates the average increase in the dependent variable (eg, IMT) per unit increase in the independent variable (eg, SBP), and like any other statistical estimate, it is subject to uncertainty and random error. Thus, it is important to estimate the standard error of the regression coefficient to evaluate its statistical significance and to calculate the confidence limits around its point estimate (see Section 7.4.8 and Appendix A). The standard error estimate is readily provided by most statistical packages performing linear regression; for the regression coefficient $b_1 = 0.0025$ in the example above, it was estimated as $SE(b_1) = 0.00032$.

Both the line in Figure 7–4 and the corresponding mathematical formula (Equation 7.2) can be seen as a way to summarize data (a sort of "sketch") that tries to capture their "essence," while avoiding unnecessary and cumbersome details subject to random variability and measurement error (see Section 7.7). The attractiveness of the model proposed in the example—that the relationship between SBP and IMT is linear—lies in its simplicity and the fact that the regression coefficient has a very straightforward and easy interpretation: it is the slope of the regression function, or the average increase in IMT (in mm) per mm Hg increase in SBP. However, this model may not be either appropriate or the best to describe the data. It is, for example, possible that additional parameters describing more complex relationships (eg, a curve) may better describe the data. Adding new parameters to the model (eg, a square term) might add to its predictive capabilities—for example, by taking into account curvilinear relationships (see Section 7.4.7). However, this often results in a more complex interpretation of the regression coefficient(s). There is usually a trade-off between simplicity (interpretability) and completeness (predictive power, statistical fit) of any statistical model. In the last section of this chapter (Section 7.7), conceptual issues related to the art and science of statistical modeling are briefly discussed.

An additional example of the use of linear regression is based on the ecological analysis discussed in Chapter 1. Figure 1–10 displays the death rates for coronary heart disease in men from 16 cohorts included in the Seven Countries Study versus an estimate of the mean fat intake in each study site.[16] That figure also shows the value of the correlation coefficient ($r = 0.84$), which indicates to which extent the scatter of points fits a straight line; the corresponding regression equation is

$$y = -83 + (25.1 \times x)$$

where y is the 10-year rate of coronary mortality (per 10,000) and x is the percentage of calories from fat in the diet. The regression estimates can be interpreted as follows:

- The intercept (-83) has a basically meaningless "real-life" interpretation, since it represents the theoretical rate in a country where there is no consumption of fat whatsoever. Its negative value underscores its merely theoretical interpretation.
- The regression coefficient (25.1) represents the estimated average increase in the 10-year coronary mortality (per 10,000) associated

with a 1% increase in the proportion of calories from fat in the diet. In other words, according to this model, an increment of 1% in the proportion of calories from fat is related to an increase of 0.00251 (or 2.51 per thousand) in coronary mortality over 10 years. (Obviously, any causal inference from data such as these must take into consideration the possibility of ecologic fallacy.) As in the preceding example, the above model also assumes that the increase is *linear*: that the increase in mortality as a function of the increase in dietary fat is constant, so that it is as harmful for the level of fat in the diet to change from 10% to 11% as it is to change from 40% to 41%. On the other hand, careful inspection of the data in the figure suggests that the increase in mortality may be *nonlinear*: that the relationship may be curvilinear, with sharper increases in mortality at higher than at lower levels of dietary fat intake. To examine this alternative hypothesis, it would be necessary to test nonlinear models by including quadratic terms or dummy variables (see Section 7.4.7).

Finally, it is beyond the scope of this text to discuss statistical properties and assumptions related to the use of linear regression. Detailed discussions of these topics can be found in general statistics textbooks (eg, Armitage and Berry[12]) as well as more specialized textbooks (eg, Draper and Smith[15]).

7.4.2 Multiple Linear Regression

The extension of the simple linear regression model (see previous section) to a multivariate situation is based on the so-called multiple–linear regression models. Multiple–linear regression models are typically used for adjustment when the outcome (the y or dependent variable) is a continuous variable, although an application for a binary outcome is briefly discussed at the end of this section. The question is whether a given variable (x_1) is *linearly* associated with the outcome (y), after controlling for a number of other covariates (eg, x_2 and x_3). The corresponding linear regression model is written as follows:

$$y = \beta_0 + \beta_1 x_1 + \beta_2 x_2 + \beta_3 x_3$$

The postulated risk factors (x's or independent variables) can be either continuous or categorical (eg, dichotomous), as in the example below. Categorical variables can have multiple levels, which can be either treated as ordinal or transformed in a set of binary (indicator) variables (see Section 7.4.7).

As an example of the use of multiple linear regression, it may be of interest to know whether systolic blood pressure (SBP) is linearly associated with carotid IMT (as a proxy for atherosclerosis) and whether this association is independent of age, gender, and body weight. The results of a series of multiple regression analyses to answer this question, using the subset of individuals from the ARIC study that was used in the example in the preceding section[13] are shown in Table 7–15.

The first model is based on the same example discussed above and includes only SBP as the independent variable (Figure 7–4 and Equation 7.2). Model 2 adds the variable age and can be written as follows:

$$IMT(mm) = \beta_0 + \beta_1 \times SBP(mm\ Hg) + \beta_2 \times Age(years)$$

The estimated values of the regression coefficients, obtained by the least squares method (see above), are displayed in Table 7–15 (model 2). Using these values, the equation can be rewritten as a function of the estimates: that is, b_0, b_1, and b_2 (again omitting the error term, e, for simplicity):

[Equation 7.3]

$$IMT(mm) = -0.0080 + 0.0016 \times SBP(mm\ Hg) + 0.0104 \times Age(years)$$

To represent this model graphically, a three-dimensional plot is needed: one for SBP, one for age, and one for IMT. The scatter of

Table 7–15 Multiple–Linear Regression Analyses of the Cross-Sectional Association Between Systolic Blood Pressure and Carotid IMT (mm) in a Subset of Participants of the Washington County Cohort of the Atherosclerosis Risk in Communities (ARIC) Study, Ages 45 to 64 Years, 1987 to 1989

	Linear Regression Coefficient			
	Model 1	*Model 2*	*Model 3*	*Model 4*
Intercept	0.4533	−0.0080	0.0107	−0.0680
Systolic blood pressure (1 mm Hg)	0.0025	0.0016	0.0014	0.0012
Age (1 yr)	Not included	0.0104	0.0096	0.0099
Gender (1 = male, 0 = female)	Not included	Not included	0.0970	0.0981
Body mass index (1 kg/m²)	Not included	Not included	Not included	0.0033

Note: Intimal-medial thickness of the carotid arteries (measured in millimeters): average of B-mode ultrasound measurements taken at six sites of the carotid arteries in both sides of the neck.

points will be a three-dimensional *cloud* of points in this three-axis space. The model in Equation 7.3 expresses the formula of a *plane* that is supposed to provide a good representation of the three-dimensional scatter: that is, of the linear relations between the three variables. Each of the regression coefficients in model 2 can be interpreted as follows:

- The intercept ($b_0 = -0.008$) corresponds to the estimated IMT of a 0-year-old individual with SBP = 0 mm Hg; as in the preceding example, this represents an extrapolation with no practical use or meaningful interpretation (see Section 7.4.1).
- The regression coefficient for SBP ($b_1 = 0.0016$ mm) represents the estimated average increase in IMT per mm Hg increase in SBP *while controlling for age effects*: that is, after the associations of age with both SBP and IMT have been removed.
- Similarly, the regression coefficient for age ($b_2 = 0.0104$ mm) represents the estimated average increase in IMT per year increase in age *while controlling for SBP*: that is, after removing the associations of SBP with both age and IMT.

(For a succinct derivation and additional interpretation of the adjusted regression coefficients in multiple linear regression, the reader should consult Kahn and Sempos.[8] More detailed discussions of multiple regression can be found in the statistical textbooks referred to above.)

Note that the estimated coefficient for SBP ($b_1 = 0.0016$ mm) in model 2 is smaller than the corresponding coefficient in model 1 (0.0025 mm). This is because age is a confounder of the relationship between SBP and IMT. In other words, some of the apparent relation between SBP and IMT observed in the crude analysis (model 1) was due to the fact that people with higher SBP tend to be older, and older people tend to have a higher degree of atherosclerosis. In model 2, the strength of the association between SBP and IMT is reduced because the (positive) confounding effect of age is removed, at least partially (see Section 7.5).

An important assumption in the model represented in Equation 7.3 is that there is *no interaction between SBP and age*, the two variables included in the model. In other words, implicit in the formulation of this statistical model ($y = \beta_0 + \beta_1 x_1 + \beta_2 x_2$) is the fact that the change in y associated with a unit change in x_1 is assumed to be constant for the entire range of x_2, and vice versa. In the above example, the increase in IMT per unit increase in SBP, the estimate $b_1 = 0.0016$ mm, not only is adjusted for age but also should be applicable to individuals of all ages (and the converse is true for b_2). If interaction is present—that is, if the effect of SBP on IMT is, for example, deemed to be different between older and younger individuals—the above model (Equation 7.3) will not be appropriate. As discussed in Chapter 6, when a given factor (in this example, age) modifies the effect of the variable of interest (in this example, SBP), it is recommended that the association between the variable of interest and the outcome be assessed in strata formed by the effect modifier categories. Thus, rather than age adjustment, age-stratified models (ie, separate models for each age group) should be used, a situation that is analogous to the examples discussed in Section 7.2. An alternative analytical technique to deal with interaction in the context of multiple-regression analyses is to include *interaction terms* (also known as *product terms*) in the regression equation. For instance, in the present example, if an interaction between SBP and age is suspected, the following model can be used:

[Equation 7.4]

$$\text{IMT} = \beta_0 + (\beta_1 \times \text{SBP}) + (\beta_2 \times \text{age}) + [\beta_3 \times (\text{SBP} \times \text{age})]$$

where (SBP × age) represents a new variable that is obtained by multiplying the values of SBP and age in each individual. Note that if SBP and age were binary variables, the above model would be analogous to stratified models. In comparison with stratified analyses, the use of interaction terms increases the statistical efficiency and has the advantage of allowing the evaluation of interaction with or between continuous variables. The interaction term can be conceptualized as the excess change not explained by the sum of the individual independent effects of two independent (x) variables; it is schematically represented in Figure 6–3 of Chapter 6 (Interaction) by the excess, "I," on the joint-effect column (right-hand side). If interaction is present, the inclusion of the interaction term in the model is important for prediction, as it increases the amount of the variability in the outcome explained by the full model vis-à-vis the sum of the isolated effects of the individual predictors in the model.

Note that when two variables x_2 and x_3 interact, and the effect of another variable x_1 is of interest, it is important to adjust x_1 for x_2, x_3, *and* the interaction term ($x_2 \times x_3$). Adjusting for the interaction term is important because the distributions of x_2 or x_3 (when examined individually) may be the same for the different categories of x_1 (say, exposed vs unexposed), but the distributions of the *joint* presence of x_2 and x_3 ($x_2 \times x_3$) may be different, and thus the interaction term may act as a confounding variable. In addition, as interaction itself is amenable to confounding effects (see Chapter 6, Section 6.10.2), it is obviously important to adjust the interaction term for the other variables in the model. For more details, refer to biostatistics textbooks (eg, Armitage and Berry[12]).

Model 3 in Table 7–15 adds a new variable, gender. This is a dichotomous variable, arbitrarily assigned a value of 1 for males and 0 for females. As with any other variable, the coefficient $b_3 = 0.097$ is interpreted as the adjusted increase in IMT (mm) per "unit increase in gender," only that what this actually means in the case of gender is the average difference in IMT between males and females, adjusted for the other variables in the model (SBP and age) (Figure 7–6). (If the variable gender had been coded as 1 for females and 0 for males, the results would have been identical to those shown in Table 7–15, except that the sign of the coefficient would have been negative—ie, $b_3 = -0.097$, representing the difference, females minus males, in IMT.)

The interpretation of the coefficients in model 4, shown in Table 7–15, is consistent with that of models 2 and 3, except that there is additional adjustment for body mass index (BMI). As seen in the table, the magnitude of the coefficient for SBP decreased in models 3 and 4, thus implying that not only age but also gender and BMI were (positive) confounders of the observed relationship between SBP and IMT. The increase in IMT per mm Hg increase in SBP after simultaneously controlling for age, gender, and BMI (model 4; 0.0012 mm) is about one half of the estimated value when none of these variables was adjusted for (model 1; 0.0025 mm). For inferential purposes, it is important to consider the possibility that confounders not included in the model and residual confounding due, for example, to misclassification of covariates such as BMI may be responsible for at least part of the apparent residual "effect" of SBP, denoted by a regression coefficient of 0.0012 mm (see Section 7.5).

As indicated in Figure 7–4, a model with one independent variable (model 1) can be easily represented in a graph; so can model 2, although it would require a three-dimensional graph. In contrast, models 3 and 4 (ie, regression models with more than three dimensions—with one y variable and more than two x variables) cannot be represented graphically. However, the interpretation of the regression coefficients of models 3 and 4 remains analogous to that of models 1 and 2: these coefficients still represent the average estimated increase in the y variable per unit increase in the corresponding x variable, simultaneously adjusted for all other x variables in the model. Note that, as an extension of the discussion of model 2 above, the formulations for models 3 and 4 also imply *lack of interaction between the independent*

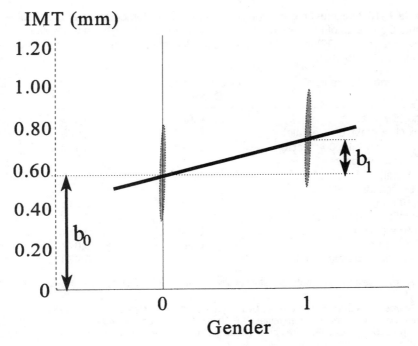

Figure 7–6 Graphical interpretation of the regression coefficient for a dichotomous variable, such as gender (as in models 3 and 4 in Table 7–15). For analogy with the regression situation with a continuous independent variable (eg, Figure 7–4), the regression line is plotted between the two clusters, even though no values are possible between $x = 0$ and $x = 1$. Note that intercept (b_0) corresponds to the mean IMT value in females ($x = 0$), while the regression coefficient (b_1) represents the average difference between males and females.

variables included in the model: in other words, the effect of each variable (each estimated b) is assumed to be constant across all levels of the other variables. Presence of interactions would require conducting stratified analysis or including "interaction terms" in the model (see above).

A further example of multiple–linear regression results taken from a study assessing correlates of leukocyte count in middle-aged adults[17] is shown in Table 7–16. In interpreting the findings in the table, the following points must be emphasized: (1) all coefficients refer to units of the dependent variable—that is, 1000 leukocytes/mm^3; and (2) each linear regression coefficient represents the expected change in

Table 7–16 Multiple–Linear Regression Analysis of Demographic and Constitutional Correlates of Leukocyte Count (in Thousands per mm^3) among Never-Smokers (n = 5,392) in the Atherosclerosis Risk in Communities (ARIC) Study Cohort, 1987 to 1989

Variable (Increment for b)	Linear Regression Coefficient*	Standard Error of b
Age (5 years)	−0.066	0.019
Sex (1 = male, 0 = female)	0.478	0.065
Race (1 = white, 0 = black)	0.495	0.122
Work activity score (1 unit)	−0.065	0.021
Subscapular skinfold (10 mm)	0.232	0.018
Systolic blood pressure (10 mm Hg)	0.040	0.011
FEV1 (1 L)	−0.208	0.047
Heart rate (10 beats/min)	0.206	0.020

*All regression coefficients are statistically significant (Wald statistic; see Section 7.4.8), $P < 0.01$.

Source: Data from FJ Nieto et al, Leukocyte Count Correlates in Middle-Aged Adults: The Atherosclerosis Risk in Communities (ARIC) Study, American Journal of Epidemiology, Vol 136, pp 525–537, © 1992, The Johns Hopkins University School of Hygiene & Public Health.

the mean leukocyte count for a given unit change of the independent variable, while simultaneously adjusting for all other variables included in the regression model. To be interpretable, the units of the regression coefficients must be specified (eg, for age, a 5-year increment) (see Section 7.4.1). The negative sign of a coefficient means that, on average, the leukocyte count *decreases* as the corresponding x variable increases.

Examples of how to interpret data from Table 7–16 are as follows:

- The mean leukocyte count decreases by (0.066 × 1000)/mm^3 (or 66 cells/mm^3) per unit increase in age (ie, 5 years), after controlling for the other variables in the table. This is equivalent to an average adjusted decrease of 13.2 cells/mm^3 per year of age (ie, 66/5 years), or 132 cells/mm^3 per 10 years of age, and so on.
- Because the variable sex is categorical, the "unit increase" actually represents the average difference between males and females. The regression coefficient estimate (b = 0.478) can thus be interpreted as males having on average 478 more leukocytes per cubic

millimeter than females, after adjusting for the other variables listed in the table.

Note that the value of the intercept was omitted from Table 7–16, as it has no practical value or meaningful interpretation in this example. (Its interpretation would be the expected leukocyte count value for a person with a 0 value in all the independent variables—ie, a newborn black woman, with zero systolic blood pressure, no heartbeats, etc.)

In this and the previous sections, linear regression methods have been described in the context of their usual application—that is, the assessment of predictors of a continuous outcome variable (eg, IMT). It is, however, possible to extend this method to the evaluation of binary (dichotomous) variables, such as the presence of carotid atherosclerosis defined as a categorical variable (present or absent), or the occurrence of an incident event (eg, disease, death), using the approach proposed by Feldstein.[18] In this situation, the regression coefficients are interpreted as the *predicted increase in the probability (prevalence or incidence) of the outcome* of interest in relation to a given increase or change in the value of the independent variable(s), while simultaneously adjusting for all the other variables in the model.[8(pp144–147)] One theoretical caveat of this method relates to the violation of some of the basic assumptions of linear regression (eg, that the errors e are normally distributed; see Armitage and Berry[12]). Another important problem is related to extrapolations to extreme values, which can result in absurd estimates of the predicted probability (eg, <0 or >1). As a consequence of these problems, Feldstein's binary linear regression model has fallen into disuse, particularly in the presence of alternatives resulting from the increasing availability and power of computational resources, such as the logistic regression model and related methods (see following sections). However, the approach appears to provide adjusted estimates in line with those obtained by other regression strategies.

7.4.3 Multiple Logistic Regression

For binary outcome variables such as the occurrence of death, disease, or recovery, the logistic regression model offers a more robust alternative to binary multiple linear regression. The logistic regression model assumes that the relationship between a given value of a variable x and the probability of a binary outcome follows the so-called logistic function:

[Equation 7.5]

$$P(y|x) = \frac{1}{1 + e^{-(b_0 + b_1 x)}}$$

where $P(y|x)$ denotes the probability (P) of the binary outcome (y) for a given value of x. The outcome of this equation, a probability, is constrained to values within the 0 to 1 range.

Figure 7–7A shows a graphical depiction of this function in the case of a continuous variable x. It is noteworthy to point out that this function's shape seems to be biologically plausible for the kinds of dose-response relationships observed in toxicology and risk assessment—that is, situations in which low doses of x induce a weak response up to a certain threshold, after which the response increases markedly and in which, beyond a certain level of x, a saturation effect then occurs (when the probability of the outcome becomes close to 1). Biological plausibility, however, is not the main reason for the popularity of the logistic regression for the multivariate analysis of predictors of a binary outcome. Rather, the reasons why this is one of the most popular methods for multivariate analysis of epidemiologic

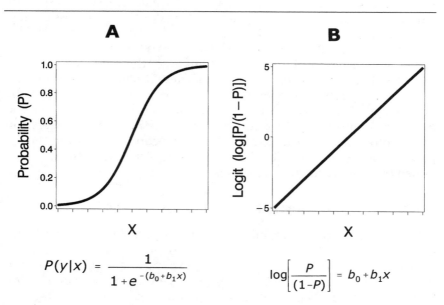

Figure 7–7 Two mathematically equivalent formulations of the logistic regression function

data are the convenience and interpretability of its regression estimates, which are easily translated into odds ratio estimates; this is
readily apparent when Equation 7.5 above is expressed in the following mathematically equivalent form:

[Equation 7.6]

$$\log \left(\frac{P}{1 - P}\right) = \log \text{ odds} = b_0 + b_1 x$$

where P is the short notation for $P(y|x)$ in Equation 7.5.

This expression is analogous to the simple linear regression function (Section 7.4.1), except that the ordinate is now the logarithm of
the odds (log odds, also known as *logit*), rather than the usual mean
value of a continuous variable. Thus, if the relationship between exposure (x) and the occurrence of the outcome is assumed to fit the logistic regression model, that implies that the log odds of the outcome
increases linearly with x (Figure 7–7B).

In the context of a *cohort study* (in which data on the incidence of
the outcome are obtained), the interpretation of the parameters from
the logistic regression equation is analogous to that of the parameters
of the linear regression model (Section 7.4.1), as follows:

- The intercept (b_0) is an estimate of the log odds of the outcome
  when $x = 0$. As in linear regression, this value may not have a
  useful interpretation in itself if $x = 0$ is a mere extrapolation of
  the realistic (possible) range of the exposure values.
- The logistic regression coefficient (b_1) is the estimated increase in
  the log odds of the outcome per unit increase in the value of x;
  or, in other words, $e^{(b_1)}$ is the odds ratio associated with a 1-unit
  increase in x.

As an illustration of the meaning of b_1 in a logistic function, consider a situation where x is the dichotomous variable, sex, for which
values of 1 and 0 are assigned to males and females, respectively.
Once the value of the regression coefficient is estimated, the predicted logistic regression equations can be formulated for each gender
as follows:

For males: $\log(\text{odds})_{\text{males}} = b_0 + b_1 \times 1 = b_0 + b_1$

For females: $\log(\text{odds})_{\text{females}} = b_0 + b_1 \times 0 = b_0$

Thus, b_1 is the difference in log odds between males and females,
which, as a result of the arithmetic properties of logarithms, is also
the log odds ratio comparing males and females:

$$b_1 = \log(\text{odds})_{\text{males}} - \log(\text{odds})_{\text{females}} = \log\left(\frac{(\text{odds})_{\text{males}}}{(\text{odds})_{\text{females}}}\right) = \log(\text{OR})$$

Similarly, if the variable x in Equation 7.6 is continuous, the regression coefficient, b_1, representing the increase in log odds per unit increase in x, can be translated into the log odds ratio when comparing any value of x with a value $(x - 1)$.

It follows that the odds ratio corresponding to a unit increase in the independent variable (eg, when comparing males to females in the example above) is the antilogarithm (ie, the exponential function) of the regression coefficient, b_1:

$$\text{OR} = e^{b_1}$$

For example, Table 7–17 shows the logistic regression coefficients corresponding to the associations between several risk factors and coronary heart disease (CHD) incidence in a subset of participants from the ARIC study.[19] These analyses are based on the cumulative incidence of CHD between the baseline examination (1987–1989) and December 1994, among 3597 Washington County participants who were free of clinical CHD at baseline. A total of 171 incident CHD events (myocardial infarction, CHD death, or coronary bypass surgery) was identified by the end of the follow-up. (For more details on methods and results from the follow-up study in the full ARIC cohort, see Chambless et al.[20]) The column labeled "Logistic Regression Coefficient" in Table 7–17 presents the intercept as well as the adjusted regression coefficients for each assessed independent variable. Each regression coefficient shown in Table 7–17 is adjusted for all the other variables in the model (listed in the table) and can be converted to an adjusted odds ratio (shown in the last column). For example, for gender, the adjusted odds ratio of incident CHD comparing males to females is

$$\text{OR}_{\text{males/females}} = e^{1.3075} = 3.70$$

Taking an example of a continuous variable, systolic blood pressure (SBP), the adjusted odds ratio for a 1-unit increase (1 mm Hg) is

$$\text{OR}_{1\text{ mm Hg SBP}} = e^{0.0167} = 1.017$$

Note that the odds ratio for SBP is very small because it is calculated for a very small increase in the independent variable (1 mm Hg). An odds ratio related to a more clinically meaningful SBP unit, such as a 10–mm Hg increase, can, however, be easily obtained by transforming the value of the coefficient into this SBP unit and then recalculating the corresponding odds ratio:

Table 7–17 Results from a Logistic Regression Analysis of Binary and Continuous Predictors of Coronary Heart Disease (CHD) Incidence in the Washington County Cohort of the Atherosclerosis Risk in Communities (ARIC) Study, Ages 45 to 64 Years at Baseline, 1987 to 1994

Variable	Logistic Regression Coefficient	Odds Ratio
Intercept	−8.9502	–
Gender (male = 1, female = 0)	1.3075	3.70
Smoking (yes = 1, no = 0)	0.7413	2.10
Age (1 yr)	0.0114	1.011
Systolic blood pressure (1 mm Hg)	0.0167	1.017
Serum cholesterol (1 mg/dL)	0.0074	1.007
Body mass index (1 kg/m²)	0.0240	1.024

$$OR_{10 \text{ mm Hg SBP}} = e^{10 \times 0.0167} = 1.18$$

The odds ratios for age, serum cholesterol, and body mass index in Table 7–17 also correspond to small changes (1 year, 1 mg/dL, and 1 kg/m², respectively) and can similarly be converted to more meaningful units. For serum cholesterol, for example, the odds ratio corresponding to a 20-mg/dL increase in serum cholesterol is

$$OR_{20 \text{ mg/dL chol}} = e^{20 \times 0.0074} = 1.16$$

For age, the odds ratio corresponding to a 5-year increase in age is

$$OR_{5 \text{ years age}} = e^{5 \times 0.0114} = 1.06$$

The validity of these calculations depends on one of the main assumptions underlying the use of continuous variables in multiple-regression methods (see also Sections 7.4.1 and 7.4.7): that the relationships are linear (in the log odds scale, in this particular case) across the entire range of the data (eg, for age, that the increase in the log odds of CHD incidence associated with an age unit increase is the same throughout the age range of study participants). This assumption, however, may be relaxed if continuous variables are categorized into binary exposure variables, such as, "older" versus "younger" age categories, or "hypertension present" versus "hypertension absent," as illustrated in Table 7–18.

Note the changes in the values of the estimates shown in Table 7–18, compared with those in Table 7–17. The definitions of gender and smoking did not change, but because those of the adjusting covariates (all the other variables) did, the "adjusted" regression coeffi-

Table 7–18 Results from a Logistic Regression Analysis of Binary Predictors of Coronary Heart Disease (CHD) Incidence in the Washington County Cohort of the Atherosclerosis Risk in Communities (ARIC) Study, Ages 45 to 64 Years at Baseline, 1987 to 1994

Variable	Logistic Regression Coefficient	Odds Ratio
Intercept	−4.5670	−
Gender (male = 1, female = 0)	1.3106	3.71
Smoking (yes = 1, no = 0)	0.7030	2.02
Older age* (yes = 1, no = 0)	0.1444	1.16
Hypertension† (yes = 1, no = 0)	0.5103	1.67
Hypercholesterolemia‡ (yes = 1, no = 0)	0.4916	1.63
Obesity§ (yes = 1, no = 0)	0.1916	1.21

* Age ≥ 55 yr.

† Blood pressure ≥ 140 mm Hg systolic or ≥ 90 mm Hg diastolic or antihypertensive therapy.

‡ Total serum cholesterol ≥ 240 mg/dL or lipid-lowering treatment.

§ Body mass index ≥ 27.8 kg/m² in males and ≥ 27.3 kg/m² in females.

cients and corresponding odds ratios for gender and smoking are slightly different. However, the estimates for the other predictors obviously changed more markedly, as a result of their transformation from continuous (Table 7–17) to categorical (Table 7–18) variables. For example, the adjusted odds ratio for hypertension (1.67) in Table 7–18 is interpreted as the ratio of the CHD incidence odds for individuals meeting the criteria used to define hypertension (blood pressure ≥140 mm Hg systolic or ≥90 mm Hg diastolic or antihypertensive therapy) to the odds of those not meeting any of these hypertension criteria. This is very different from the estimate for SBP in Table 7–17, both in value and in interpretation. Note that the dichotomous definition of hypertension (or that of any other intrinsically continuous variable), while avoiding the assumption of linearity inherent to the continuous definition, is not assumption-free, as it implies that the risk of CHD is homogeneous *within* categories of hypertension. If there is a gradient of risk within the hypertension categories, this information is lost in the model. Note that this loss of information may result in residual confounding (Section 7.5). Consider, for example, the assessment of the association between smoking and CHD odds, with adjustment for hypertension (and other variables), as depicted in Table 7–18: given the fact that the relationship between blood pressure and CHD follows a dose-response (graded) pattern, residual confounding may have occurred if hypertensives among smokers had higher blood pressure values than hypertensives among nonsmokers. Notwithstanding the possible loss of information, unlike some of the examples discussed previously, the use of dichotomous variables as shown in Table 7–18 allows an interpretation of the *intercept* in logistic regression that may be useful in a couple of ways.

First, in the context of data from a prospective study, and on the basis of Equation 7.6, the intercept can be interpreted as the log(odds) for individuals with values of 0 for all the independent variables. For example, according to the results presented in Table 7–18, the intercept represents the log(odds) of incident CHD for nonsmoking females who are aged 45 to 54 years, nonhypertensive, nonhypercholesterolemic, and nonobese. This value is calculated as $-4.567 + 0$, or, transformed to the corresponding value in an arithmetic scale, Odds $= e^{-4.567} = 0.0104$.

For predictive purposes, this result can be translated into the more readily interpretable cumulative incidence (probability, P) estimate (see Chapter 2, Section 2.4) as follows:

$$P = \frac{\text{Odds}}{1 + \text{Odds}} = \frac{0.0104}{1 + 0.0104} = 0.0103, \text{ or } 1.03\%$$

This example underscores the utility of the intercept when the assigned values of 0 fall within biologically plausible ranges of values of the independent variables. In contrast, interpretation of the intercept per se is meaningless when using results such as those from Table 7–17.

Second, as for regression models in general, the intercept is needed in logistic regression for obtaining the predicted probability (cumulative incidence) of the outcome for an individual with a given set of characteristics. For example, based on the results in Table 7–18, the probability of CHD for a male smoker who is younger than 55 years, hypertensive, nonhypercholesterolemic, and obese can be estimated simply by substituting the values of each x variable in an equation of the form shown in Equation 7.5, as follows:

$$P = \frac{1}{1 + e^{-[-4.567 + (1.3106 \times 1) + (0.703 \times 1) + (0.1444 \times 0) + (0.5103 \times 1) + (0.4916 \times 0) + (0.1916 \times 1)]}} =$$

$$\frac{1}{1 + e^{-(-4.567 + 1.3106 + 0.703 + 0.5103 + 0.1916)}} = 0.1357 = 13.57\%$$

Similarly, the results from Table 7–17 can be used to estimate the probability of CHD in an individual with specific values of each of the physiologic parameters measured. This could be done for an individual with average values for all the covariates. For example, the average values of the covariates presented in Table 7–17 for the individuals in this ARIC cohort were as follows (note that the average value of dichotomous covariates is the *proportion* of individuals with the value that was coded as 1): male gender = 0.469; smoking = 0.229; age = 54.7 years; SBP = 119.1 mm Hg; cholesterol = 217.7 mg/dL; BMI = 27.8 kg/m^2. Thus, using the results from Table 7–17, the predicted probability of incident CHD for an "average individual" in the cohort will be

$$P = \frac{1}{1 + e^{-[-8.9502 + (1.3075 \times .469) + (.7413 \times .229) + (.0114 \times 54.7) + (.0167 \times 119.1) + (.0074 \times 217.7) + (.024 \times 27.8)]}}$$

$$= \frac{1}{1 + e^{-(-3.27649948)}} = 0.0364 = 3.64\%$$

(The concept of an "average individual" is an abstract one, particularly with respect to the average of binary variables. For example, in this case, it means an individual who is "0.469 male" and "0.229 smoker" and who has the mean value of all the other continuous covariates.)

As another example of the application of the logistic model for prediction, Framingham study investigators produced the so-called Framingham multiple–logistic risk equation, which can be used to estimate the risk of cardiovascular disease over time for a person with a given set of values for a number of relevant variables (gender, age, serum cholesterol, systolic blood pressure, cigarette smoking, left ventricular hypertrophy by ECG, and glucose intolerance).[11]

The use of these models for prediction purposes assumes, of course, that the model fits the data reasonably well. Furthermore, the above discussion about the interpretation of the intercept and the calculation of predicted probabilities of the event is relevant when the data are prospective. The use of the logistic regression model for the analyses of cohort data, however, is limited in that the model uses cumulative incidence data and therefore has to rely on two important assumptions: that follow-up of study participants is complete and that time to event is not important. That these assumptions are usually not met is underscored by staggered entries in many cohort studies in which recruitment is carried out over a more or less extended time period; by subsequent losses of follow-up; and by the variability of latency periods for most outcomes of interest, thus making time to event important (see Chapter 2, Section 2.2). For the analysis of cohort data with incomplete follow-up for some observations, more appropriate multivariate analysis tools are available, as discussed in the following two sections.

The most frequent application of the logistic regression model is in the context of case-control studies, where it constitutes the primary analytical tool for multivariate analyses.[21,22] In a *case-control study*, the interpretation of regression coefficients is identical to that of the cohort study (ie, the log of the odds ratio), as shown in the examples below. On the other hand, when the data come from a case-control study, the intercept is not readily interpretable, as the sampling fractions for cases and controls are arbitrarily selected by the investigator (for a more technical discussion of this issue, see Schlesselman[22]). An example of the use of multiple regression in a case-control study is based on a study of the seroprevalence of hepatitis B virus in health care workers in Boston in the late 1970s and early 1980s—that is, before the introduction of the hepatitis B virus vaccine.[23] Some findings of this study are presented in Table 7–19, which shows the results of a multiple–logistic regression analysis aimed at identifying variables associated with the odds of positivity for hepatitis B serum antibodies. The table shows both the logistic regression coefficients and the corresponding odds ratios (as well as their 95% confidence interval; see Section 7.4.8 and Appendix A, Section A.9). The intercept was omitted because of its irrelevance (see above). Note that the first three variables are dichotomous; thus, the regression coefficient for each of these variables represents the difference in the log odds between the two corresponding categories (in other words, the antilog of the regression coefficient represents the odds ratio comparing the "exposure" category—coded as 1—with the reference category—coded as 0). For example, for the variable "recent needlestick," the value 0.8459 is the estimated difference in the log odds of positive antibodies between those with and those without a history of a recent needlestick, after adjusting for all the other variables in the table. Consequently, the odds ratio associated with recent needlestick is estimated as $e^{0.8459} = 2.33$. The two bottom variables in Table 7–19 (age and years in occupation) were entered in the model as continuous, and the regression coefficients and corresponding odds ratios are given for increments of 1 year. For example, for "Years in Occupation," the value 0.0198 represents the adjusted estimated increase in log odds of positive antibodies per year increase in length of employment as a health worker. In other words, the adjusted odds ratio corresponding to an increase in 1 year of occupation is estimated as $e^{0.0198} = 1.02$.

Table 7–19 Multivariate Logistic Regression Analysis of Risk Factors for the Presence of Hepatitis B Virus Serum Antibodies in Health Workers, Boston, Massachusetts, 1977 to 1982

Characteristic	Logistic Regression Coefficient	Odds Ratio (95% Confidence Interval)
Occupational/blood exposure (yes/no)	0.7747	2.17 (1.31–3.58)
Recent needlestick (yes/no)	0.8459	2.33 (1.19–4.57)
Hepatitis A virus positive serology (yes/no)	0.6931	2.00 (1.13–3.54)
Age (1 yr)	0.0296	1.03 (0.99–1.06)
Years in occupation (1 yr)	0.0198	1.02 (0.97–1.08)

Source: Data from A Gibas et al, Prevalence and Incidence of Viral Hepatitis in Health Workers in the Prehepatitis B Vaccination Era, *American Journal of Epidemiology*, Vol 136, pp 603–610, © 1992, The Johns Hopkins University School of Hygiene & Public Health.

It should be reemphasized that the logistic regression model is a *linear model in the log odds scale*, as was seen in Equation 7.6. What this means in practical terms is that when a continuous variable is entered as such, the resulting coefficient (and corresponding odds ratio) is assumed to represent the linear increase in log odds (or the exponential increase in odds) per unit increase in the independent variable *across the entire range* of x values. For example, the estimated increase in the odds of positive hepatitis B antibodies per year of occupation (ie, OR = 1.02) shown in Table 7–19 is assumed to be the same when comparing 3 with 2 years as it is when comparing 40 with 39 years of occupation. Again, as discussed in Sections 7.4.1 and 7.4.7, if this assumption is incorrect (eg, if the increase in the risk of infection associated with a 1-year change in the occupation is higher in more recently hired, less experienced workers), the above model will be incorrect, and alternative models using categorical definitions of the variable (dummy variables) or other forms of parametrization (eg, quadratic terms) must be used.

7.4.4   Cox Proportional Hazards Model

When the analysis is based on time-to-event (or survival) data, one of the options is to model the data using the hazard (or instantaneous force of morbidity or mortality) scale (see Chapter 2, Section 2.2.4).

The assumption underlying the use of this approach is that exposure to a certain risk factor (or the presence of a certain characteristic) is associated with a fixed relative increase in the instantaneous risk of the outcome of interest, compared to a baseline or reference hazard (eg, the hazard in the unexposed). In other words, it is assumed that at any given time (t), the hazard in those exposed to a certain risk factor $[h_1(t)]$ is a multiple of some underlying hazard $[h_0(t)]$. Figure 7–8 illustrates this model, which can be mathematically formulated as follows:

[Equation 7.7]

$$h_1(t) = h_0(t) \times B$$

That is, at any given point in time, the hazard among those exposed to the risk factor x_1 is the hazard among those not exposed to it, multiplied by a constant factor (B). The hazards in both the exposed and the reference groups may be approximately constant or may increase over time (see Figure 7–8A—eg, the instantaneous risk of mortality as individuals age) or fluctuate over time (see the hypothetical example in Figure 7–8B, eg, the risk of an accident as the driving speed changes). In both examples in Figure 7–8, it is assumed that at any given point in time, the hazard among those exposed (eg, car wearing old tires) is multiplied by 2 regardless of the baseline hazard (eg, wear-

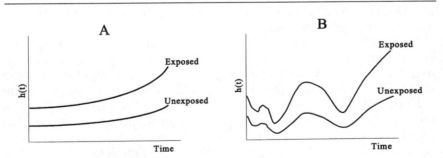

Figure 7–8 Hazard over time in two hypothetical situations in which exposed individuals have twice the hazard of those unexposed. **A** represents a situation with a relatively stable hazard that slowly increases over time, such as hazard of death as adult individuals age; **B** represents a situation in which the hazard fluctuates with time, such as the hazard of a car accident that increases or decreases as a function of the car's velocity at any given point in time, with the presence of the exposure (eg, having worn-out tires) doubling the risk of having an accident, compared with its absence (having new tires).

ing new tires): in other words, that the hazard ratio (or relative hazard) comparing exposed and unexposed is constant.

For estimating B—that is, the constant multiplication factor in Equation 7.7—it is convenient to define it in terms of an exponential function: $B = e^b$, obtained by reformulating Equation 7.7 as

[Equation 7.8]

$$h_1(t) = h_0(t) \times e^b$$

If $h_0(t)$ represents the hazard in the unexposed group at any given point in time, then the hazard ratio (HR) comparing the exposed and the unexposed is

$$HR = \frac{h_1(t)}{h_0(t)} = e^b$$

Or, taking logarithms:

$$\log(HR) = b$$

Note that because both the hazard ratio and the odds ratio are multiplicative measures of association (ie, linear in a log scale), many issues related to the interpretation of the regression coefficient in the proportional hazards model (which estimates log hazard ratio) are similar to the interpretation of the regression coefficient in the logistic regression model (which estimates log odds ratio). Thus, the interpretation issues related to the type of independent variable included in the model (continuous, ordinal, categorical) are similar in the Cox and logistic regression models.

Table 7–20 shows the results of two alternative analyses using Cox proportional regression (models 1 and 2) to assess predictors of incident CHD in the Washington County cohort of the ARIC study. Note that in this table, the independent variables included as predictors are the same as those used previously to illustrate the logistic regression model (Tables 7–17 and 7–18). Here, the outcome of interest is also incident CHD, but in contrast with the logistic regression analysis (which assumes that all participants had complete follow-up and the cumulative incidence odds were obtained), the regression coefficients in Table 7–20 take into account the *time of occurrence* of each event, as well as the time of censoring for the participants who were not observed for the entire follow-up (see Chapter 2, Section 2.2). Thus, also in contrast with the logistic regression, where the regression coefficients antilogs were interpreted as odds ratios, exponentiation of the regression (beta) coefficients in Table 7–20 results in hazards ratios (analogous to relative risks).

Table 7–20 Results of Cox Proportional Regression Analyses of Binary and Continuous Predictors of Coronary Heart Disease (CHD) Incidence in the Washington County Cohort of the Atherosclerosis Risk in Communities (ARIC) Study, Ages 45 to 64 Years at Baseline, 1987 to 1994

Model	Variable	Cox Regression Coefficient	Hazard Ratio
1	Gender		
	(male = 1, female = 0)	1.2569	3.52
	Smoking (yes = 1, no = 0)	0.7045	2.02
	Age (1 yr)	0.0120	1.012
	Systolic blood pressure		
	(1 mm Hg)	0.0152	1.015
	Serum cholesterol (1 mg/dL)	0.0067	1.007
	Body mass index (1 kg/m^2)	0.0237	1.024
2	Gender (male = 1,		
	female = 0)	1.2669	3.55
	Smoking (yes = 1, no = 0)	0.6803	1.97
	Older age* (yes = 1, no = 0)	0.1391	1.15
	Hypertension[†] (yes = 1, no = 0)	0.5030	1.65
	Hypercholesterolemia[‡]		
	(yes = 1, no = 0)	0.4552	1.58
	Obesity[§] (yes = 1, no = 0)	0.1876	1.21

* Age ≥ 55 yr.

[†] Blood pressure ≥ 140 mm Hg systolic or ≥ 90 mm Hg diastolic or antihypertensive therapy.

[‡] Total serum cholesterol ≥ 240 mg/dL or lipid-lowering treatment.

[§] Body mass index ≥ 27.8 kg/m^2 in males and ≥ 27.3 kg/m^2 in females.

There is a remarkable similarity between the estimates obtained from logistic regression in Tables 7–17 and 7–18 (cumulative incidence odds ratio; time to event and censoring not considered) and the Cox estimates in Table 7–20 (hazard ratio; time to event and censoring taken into account). This similarity is probably due to the following facts: (1) CHD is relatively rare, and thus the odds ratio estimated from logistic regression approximates the hazard ratio (which is akin to a relative risk) estimated by Cox's regression; and (2) losses to follow-up and time to events are likely to be nondifferential between the exposure groups, and thus the biases resulting from time-related factors tend to cancel out, which represents a phenomenon comparable to "compensating bias," described in Section 4.2.

It should be underscored that, unlike the output obtained from logistic regression, there is no intercept in the Cox model. Cox's important contribution was to devise a method for estimating the regression parameters in the proportional hazards model without the need to specify the value or the shape of the baseline hazard (h_0), which is the equivalent of the intercept.[24] Methods have been devised that permit the estimation of the underlying survival function based on the results of a multivariate Cox regression analysis; details on this and other applications of the Cox model can be found in the growing literature and textbooks on survival analysis.[25,26]

The Cox model is also called the *proportional hazards model*. This term emphasizes the "proportionality assumption"; that is, the assumption that the exposure of interest multiplies the baseline hazards (the hazards in those unexposed) by a constant factor, e^b (see Equation 7.8 above) at any given point during follow-up. As illustrated in Figure 7–8, this implies that regardless of the value of the baseline hazard at any given point in time, those exposed have a hazard equal to the baseline hazard multiplied by e^b. The need for this assumption is implicit in the fact that *one* hazard ratio is estimated for the entire follow-up. If the hazards are not proportional over time—that is, if the hazard ratio changes during the follow-up—the model needs to account for this by stratifying according to follow-up time. This situation could be properly described as a case of "time × exposure" interaction—that is, effect modification (see Chapter 6)—in which time modifies the relationship between exposure and outcome. For a more detailed description of methods to assess the proportionality assumption when applying the Cox model as well as approaches to account for time × exposure interactions, the reader is referred to a more specialized text (eg, Collet[25] or Parmar and Machin[26]).

7.4.5 Poisson Regression

The Poisson regression model is another method for multiple-regression analysis of cohort data with a dichotomous outcome and one or more categorically defined predictors. It is mostly used in situations in which the outcomes of interest are rates (and rate ratios); it is especially suitable for studying rare diseases in large populations. The model specifies that the magnitude of the rate is an exponential function of a linear combination of covariates and unknown parameters:

$$\text{Rate} = e^{(b_0 + b_1 x_1 + b_2 x_2 + \ldots + b_k x_k)}$$

This equation can be rewritten as the log of the rate being the dependent variable of a linear function:

[Equation 7.9]

$$\log(\text{rate}) = b_0 + b_1 x_1 + b_2 x_2 + \ldots + b_k x_k$$

Equation 7.9 is also called a *log-linear model*, reflecting the fact that it is simply a log transformation of an outcome variable (a rate in this case) related to a linear equation of predictors. If the "rate" is decomposed into its two components (number of events in the numerator and person-time in the denominator), Equation 7.9 can be rewritten in the following ways:

$$\log(\text{events/person-time}) = b_0 + b_1x_1 + b_2x_2 + \ldots + b_kx_k$$

$$\log(\text{events}) - \log(\text{person-time}) = b_0 + b_1x_1 + b_2x_2 + \ldots + b_kx_k$$

$$\log(\text{events}) = [\log(\text{person-time})] + b_0 + b_1x_1 + b_2x_2 + \ldots + b_kx_k$$

$$\log(\text{events}) = b_0{}^* + b_1x_1 + b_2x_2 + \ldots + b_kx_k$$

Note that in the above equation, the log person-time is incorporated ("offset" in statistical terms) into the intercept (now noted as $b_0{}^*$) of the multiple linear predictor, and the outcome variable is now a count, the number of events (log transformed). For this type of outcome variable (a count), and for reasonably rare events, as are assessed in most epidemiologic studies, it is assumed that the most appropriate basis for the statistical procedure of estimation of the parameters in the model above is the Poisson distribution. (Several statistical textbooks provide more details regarding the statistical properties and uses of the Poisson distribution. See, eg, Armitage and Berry.[12])

Again, the interpretation of the Poisson regression coefficients is analogous to those in logistic regression and Cox models, except that where in the latter models the odds ratio and the hazard ratio were, respectively, obtained, in the Poisson regression is the *rate ratio*. For example, when comparing exposed (eg, $x_1 = 1$) and unexposed ($x_1 = 0$) groups, Equation 7.9 will reduce to the following:

$$\text{For the exposed: } \log(\text{rate}_{\text{exp}}) = b_0 + b_1 \times 1 + b_2x_2 + \ldots + b_kx_k$$

$$\text{For the unexposed: } \log(\text{rate}_{\text{unexp}}) = b_0 + b_1 \times 0 + b_2x_2 + \ldots + b_kx_k$$

Subtracting the above equations:

$$\log(\text{rate}_{\text{exp}}) - \log(\text{rate}_{\text{unexp}}) = b_1$$

And thus,

$$\log\left(\frac{\text{rate}_{\text{exp}}}{\text{rate}_{\text{unexp}}}\right) = \log(\text{rate ratio}) = b_1$$

Consequently, the antilog of the regression coefficient estimate (e^{b_1}) corresponds to the rate ratio comparing exposed and unexposed, adjusted for all the other variables included in the model ($x_2, \ldots x_k$).

As pointed out previously, for using the Poisson regression, all independent (x) variables need to be categorical, as the method is set to use the total amount of person-time and the total number of events per category or cell (representing each unique combination of the predictors). For example, the application of the Poisson regression method to the analysis of CHD incidence in the ARIC study and including the same variables as in model 2 of the Cox regression example (Table 7–20) results in the data shown in Table 7–21. The exponentiation of the Poisson regression coefficients provides estimates of the adjusted rate ratios comparing exposed (or those with the characteristic coded as 1) and unexposed individuals.

To carry out the Poisson regression analyses in Table 7–21, each unique combination of the six independent variables had to be identified (total $2^6 = 64$ cells), the total person-time contributed to by all individuals in each cell had to be added up, and the total number of events among these individuals had to be identified. The cell-specific data look as shown in Table 7–22, in which 8 of the 64 cells are shown, with PY denoting the total person-years in each cell (LogPY is

Table 7–21 Results from a Poisson Regression Analysis of Binary Predictors of Coronary Heart Disease (CHD) Incidence in the Washington County Cohort of the Atherosclerosis Risk in Communities (ARIC) Study, Ages 45 to 64 Years at Baseline, 1987 to 1994

Variable	Poisson Regression Coefficient	Rate Ratio
Intercept	−6.3473	−
Gender (male = 1, female = 0)	1.1852	3.27
Smoking (yes = 1, no = 0)	0.6384	1.89
Older age* (yes = 1, no = 0)	0.2947	1.34
Hypertension† (yes = 1, no = 0)	0.5137	1.67
Hypercholesterolemia‡ (yes = 1, no = 0)	0.6795	1.97
Obesity§ (yes = 1, no = 0)	0.2656	1.30

* Age ≥ 55 yr.

† Blood pressure ≥ 140 mm Hg systolic or ≥ 90 mm Hg diastolic or antihypertensive treatment.

‡ Total serum cholesterol ≥ 240 mg/dL or lipid-lowering therapy.

§ Body mass index ≥ 27.8 kg/m² in males and ≥ 27.3 kg/m² in females.

Table 7–22 Data Used for Calculating the Results Shown in Table 7–21

Cell	Male	Smok	Old Age	Hyperten	Hypercho	Obese	PY	CHD	LogPY
1	0	0	0	0	0	0	1740.85	1	7.46213
2	0	0	0	0	0	1	1181.40	2	7.07446
3	0	0	0	0	1	0	539.97	0	6.29152
4	0	0	0	0	1	1	521.93	1	6.25754
... /									
61	1	1	1	1	0	0	24.485	1	3.19804
62	1	1	1	1	0	1	37.415	0	3.62208
63	1	1	1	1	1	0	171.409	1	5.14405
64	1	1	1	1	1	1	85.372	5	4.44701

the logarithm of that value), and CHD the number of corresponding coronary heart disease events. The calculation of the regression (beta) coefficients shown in Table 7–21 was based on these data.

7.4.6   A Note on Models for the Multivariate Analyses of Data from Matched and Nested Case-Control Studies

In *matched case-control studies* (see Section 1.4.5), the multivariate analysis technique most frequently used is *conditional logistic regression*. This model is analogous to the logistic regression model presented above (Section 7.4.3), except that the parameters (the intercept and regression coefficients) are estimated taking into account ("conditioned on") the pairing or matching of cases and controls with respect to the variables that determined the matching. The interpretation of the coefficients in conditional logistic regression is the same as in ordinary logistic regression, except that these coefficients are to be considered "adjusted" not only for the variables included in the model but also for the matching variables. Details on the statistical properties and applications of the conditional logistic regression model can be found elsewhere (eg, Hosmer and Lemeshow,[21] Breslow and Day[27]). This model is particularly useful for the analyses of studies in which cases and controls are *individually matched (paired)*. An example is given by the cross-sectional examination of variables associated with carotid atherosclerosis in the ARIC study.[28] For this analysis, cases ($n = 386$) were defined as individuals with elevated carotid artery intimal-medial thickness (IMT, see above) based on B-mode ultrasound imaging measurements. Controls in this study were selected among individuals with low IMT and were individually matched to each case on sex, race, age group (45–54 or 55–64 years), study center, and date of examination. Selected results from this study are presented in Table 7–23. Each of the odds ratios in this table was obtained by exponentiating the regression coefficient estimate (e^b) obtained from a logistic regression model conditioned on the matching variables; thus, by definition, the estimates shown on the table are adjusted not only for all variables shown in the table but also for the matching factors. Note that to avoid potential residual confounding resulting from the use of broad age-matching categories, the study investigators also adjusted for age as a continuous variable (see Section 1.4.5, Figure 1.24, and Section 7.5).

In studies in which cases and controls are frequency matched (see Section 1.4.5), a more efficient strategy is simply to use ordinary logistic regression and include the matching variables in the model. An

Table 7–23 Adjusted Odds Ratios* for Carotid Atherosclerosis in Relation to Selected Cardiovascular Risk Factors in 386 Matched Pairs† from the Atherosclerosis Risk in Communities (ARIC) Study Cohort Examined Between 1987 and 1989

Variable and Reference Category	Age-Adjusted Odds Ratio (95% Confidence Interval)	Multivariate-Adjusted‡ Odds Ratio (95% Confidence Interval)
Current smoker vs ex- and never-smoker	3.3 (2.3–4.7)	3.9 (2.6–5.9)
Ever smoker vs never-smoker	2.8 (2.0–4.0)	3.1 (2.1–4.6)
Hypertensive vs normotensive	2.7 (1.9–3.8)	2.9 (1.9–4.3)
LDL cholesterol		
≥160 vs <100 mg/dL	2.6 (1.6–4.4)	2.0 (1.1–3.7)
100–159 vs <100 mg/dL	1.6 (1.0–2.6)	1.4 (0.8–2.4)

* Obtained by conditional logistic regression.

† Matched on sex, race, age group (45–54 or 55–64 yr), study center, and date of examination.

‡ Adjusted for age (as a continuous variable) and all the other variables listed in the table, in addition to matching variables.

Source: Data from G Heiss et al, Carotid Atherosclerosis Measured by B-Mode Ultrasound in Populations: Associations with Cardiovascular Risk Factors in the ARIC Study, *American Journal of Epidemiology,* Vol 134, pp 250–256, © 1991, The Johns Hopkins University School of Hygiene & Public Health.

example of a frequency-matched study, cited in Chapter 1, is the examination of the relationship between cytomegalovirus (CMV) antibodies and atherosclerosis.[29] Table 7–24 shows the association between CMV antibody levels in serum samples collected in 1974 and the presence of carotid atherosclerosis in the ARIC study's first two examinations (1987–1992).[29] These odds ratios were obtained from the estimated coefficients in logistic regression models that contained the matching variables (*matched odds ratio*) and additional variables adjusted for (*adjusted odds ratio*).

Nested case-control studies, in which the controls are selected among the members of the "risk set," that is, among the cohort members at risk at the time when the case occurs (see Chapter 1, Section 1.4.2), can be considered and analyzed as "matched case-control studies" in which cases and controls are matched by length of follow-up (Figure 1–21). Thus, as in other matched case-control studies, the multivariate analysis technique most frequently indicated is the conditional

Table 7–24 Intimal-Medial Thickness Case-Control Status in the Atherosclerosis Risk in Communities (ARIC) Study (1987–1992) in Relation to High or Moderate Versus Low Positive/Negative Values for Cytomegalovirus (CMV) Antibodies in Serum Samples Collected in 1974

CMV Antibody Levels*	Cases	Controls	Matched OR[†] (95% Confidence Interval)	Adjusted OR[‡] (95% Confidence Interval)
Low	31	51	1.0[§]	1.0[§]
Moderate	104	94	1.9 (1.1–3.2)	1.5 (0.8–2.9)
High	15	5	5.2 (1.7–16.0)	5.3 (1.5–18.0)

* Low: positive/negative ratio < 4; moderate: positive/negative ratio 4 to 19; high: positive/negative ratio ≥ 20.

[†] Odds ratios obtained by multiple–logistic regression analysis including the frequency-matching variables age (10-year categories) and gender.

[‡] Odds ratios obtained by multiple–logistic regression analysis including the frequency-matching variables age (10-year categories and gender) plus continuous age, cigarette smoking (current/former vs never), years of education (> 12 vs ≤ 12), hypercholesterolemia, hypertension, diabetes, and overweight.

[§] Reference category.

Source: Data from FJ Nieto et al, Cohort Study of Cytomegalovirus Infection as a Risk Factor for Carotid Intimal-Medial Thickening, a Measure of Subclinical Atherosclerosis, *Circulation*, Vol 94, pp 922–927, © 1996.

logistic regression, in which the conditional variable is length of follow-up. This type of conditional logistic regression model is analogous to the Cox proportional hazards regression model.[30] In addition to its inherent logistical advantages (see Chapter 1, Section 1.4.2), the nested case-control study has become a popular study design as a result of the wide availability in recent years of statistical packages that can carry out this type of conditional analysis. Its increasing popularity is attested by the increasing number of studies that use it.

In the alternative design for case-control studies within a well-defined cohort, the so-called *case-cohort study*, cases occurring in the cohort during follow-up are compared with a random sample of the baseline cohort (*subcohort*) (see Chapter 1, Section 1.4.2). Because a sample of the baseline cohort and the cases occurring during follow-up are identified (see Figure 1–20), the Cox proportional hazards regression can be used for the multivariate analyses in this type of study. It should be emphasized that sampling heterogeneity may occur when using this design, as the case group may include both cases who are and cases who are not in the cohort sample. This heterogeneity has to be taken into consideration; otherwise, biases may be introduced. Fortunately, as described elsewhere,[31,32] the Cox model can be adapted to this situation by allowing for staggered entries (for the cases outside the subcohort).

As an example of this approach, Table 7–25 shows results for a study described at the end of Section 1.4.2. This is a case-cohort study conducted within the ARIC cohort looking at the association between serum antibodies against *C. pneumoniae* and incident CHD over a follow-up of 3 to 5 years.[33] The 246 incident CHD cases were compared to a stratified sample of 550 participants from the original cohort using a Cox regression analysis, which takes into consideration time to event and allows for staggered entries to handle the case-cohort sampling design. As in the previous examples, each of the hazard ratios shown in the table was obtained by exponentiating the corresponding regression coefficient from the Cox regression model. The results shown in Table 7–25 suggest that the apparent increased hazard of coronary heart disease in those with high levels of *C. pneumoniae* antibodies at baseline can be largely explained by a positive confounding effect by other risk factors.

7.4.7 Modeling Nonlinear Relationships with Linear Regression Models

Epidemiologic studies often use continuous scales to measure physiologic parameters or other characteristics, such as those in the exam-

---

Table 7–25 Estimated Crude and Adjusted Hazard Ratios of Incident Coronary Heart Disease (and 95% Confidence Intervals) by Level of *C. Pneumoniae* Antibody Titers at Baseline, 1987 to 1991*

	C. Pneumoniae *IgG Antibody Titers*		
	Negative	*1:8–1:32*	*≥1:64*
Adjusted for demographics†	1.0	1.2 (0.7–2.1)	1.6 (1.0–2.5)
Adjusted for demographics† and risk factors‡	1.0	1.1 (0.6–2.3)	1.2 (0.7–2.1)

* Estimated using weighted proportional hazards regression models with staggered entries for cases outside the subcohort and Barlow's robust variance estimates.[31]

† Age (continuous), gender, race, and center.

‡ Smoking, hypercholesterolemia, hypertension, diabetes, and educational level.

Source: Data from FJ Nieto et al, *Chlamydia Pneumoniae* Infection and Incident Coronary Heart Disease: The Atherosclerosis Risk in Communities (ARIC) Study, *American Journal of Epidemiology,* Vol 150, pp 149–156, © 1999, The Johns Hopkins University School of Hygiene & Public Health.

ples discussed in previous sections. Two different definitions of such variables were used to illustrate the application of a number of adjustment models: continuous (eg, systolic blood pressure levels—Tables 7–15; 7–17; and 7–20, model 1) or dichotomous (eg, hypertension—Tables 7–18; 7–20, model 2; and 7–21). In this section, the possible limitations of these models and some alternative approaches are briefly discussed.

To illustrate the problems related to the selection of the modeling approach, Figure 7–9A shows a hypothetical observed (assumed to be true) "J-shape" relationship between a given continuous predictor (x) and an outcome variable (y). Note that y here could be any of the dependent variables in the models summarized in Table 7–14—for example, a continuous variable such as the carotid intimal-medial thickness when using linear regression, or the log(odds) of carotid atherosclerosis (defined as a binary variable) when using logistic regression. This type of relationship has been found, for example, in epidemiologic studies of body weight and mortality,[34,35] in which a higher risk of mortality has been observed in low-weight individuals (possibly because of underlying chronic morbidity), the lowest risk in individuals of "normal" weight, and a steady increase in mortality in overweight and obese individuals. (Other examples of such J- or U-type relationships are those between serum cholesterol and mortality,[36] and between alcohol intake and coronary heart disease.[37])

Figure 7–9B illustrates the problems of using a linear regression model to explain the observed relationship between x and y. In Figure 7–9B, an estimate of the regression coefficient, b, would represent the average linear increase of y (eg, mortality) per unit increase in the continuous variable x (eg, body weight): that is, the slope of the straight line in Figure 7–9B. Obviously, the estimation of an overall linear regression coefficient, as shown in Figure 7–9B, ignores the fact that there is actually a *decrease* in y in the lower x range, a slow increase in y in the mid x range, and a pronounced increase in y in the upper x range. Because the latter is more pronounced than the former, the average value of b will come out positive; however, as readily inferred from Figure 7–9B, this estimate misrepresents the true relationship of x to y, to the extent that it falsely "reverses" the observed negative association for lower values of x and underestimates the strong positive association seen for higher x values.

For the model shown in Figure 7–9C, x is defined as a dichotomous variable, with the categories 0 and 1 represented in the abscissa of the graph. By so modeling x, the model assumes that there is a "threshold" phenomenon: that is, that the relationship between x

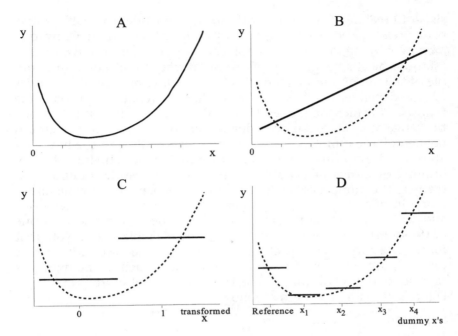

Figure 7–9 Hypothetical example of an observed (true) J-shape relationship between X and an outcome variable Y (**A**); **B** through **D** illustrate the observed relationship (broken line) with alternative models superimposed: continuous x (**B**), dichotomous x (**C**), and dummy variables for x quintiles (**D**).

and y is flat for the lower range of x values and that there is a sudden increase in y at a certain x threshold (which is the cutoff point used to define x as a categorical variable), after which there is no further increase in y as x increases. The estimated regression coefficient in this case represents the difference in the average y value between the higher and the lower x-range categories (see Figure 7–6)—that is, the vertical distance (in y units) between the two horizontal bars depicted in Figure 7–9C. As for the model shown in Figure 7–9B, it also neglects an important feature of the relationship between x and y, namely that y decreases as x increases for low values of x, while the opposite is true for higher values.

Use of Indicator ("Dummy") Variables

To take into account these patterns, more elaborate and complex models are necessary. One option, often used in epidemiology, consists of breaking down the continuous independent variable x into categories (based, eg, on quartiles or quintiles), then using one *dummy* variable as indicator for each category and allowing the "slope" (the change in y) to vary from category to category. An example of the use of dummy variables for modeling multilevel categories of an independent variable that is not linearly related to the outcome follows. Consider the model illustrated in Figure 7–9D. In this panel, the range of x values has been divided in fifths: that is, in five groups defined by the quintiles, each containing about 20% of the individuals ordered according to the value of x from lowest to highest. A set of dummy or indicator variables (categories) can be then defined, as many as the number of categories for the independent variable minus 1 or 4 in this case. One of the categories is chosen as the "reference," and each of the remaining categories is assigned a value of 1 for one of the dummy variables and 0 for the others (Table 7–26). Note that for the category arbitrarily chosen as reference (the lowest fifth in this case), all four dummy variables have 0 values. Each of the dummies represents the remaining fifths. Thus, the model corresponding to Figure 7–9D can be written as follows:

[Equation 7.10]

$$y = b_0 + b_1x_1 + b_2x_2 + b_3x_3 + b_4x_4$$

It should be noted that these four dummy variables correspond to different categories of a single variable, x. In fact, because of the complete lack of overlap between these "variables" (no one individual can have a value of 1 for more than one such "variable," simply because no individual can belong to more than one of these mutually exclusive fifths), the model in Equation 7.10 can be reduced to the following equations for each of the fifths:

Table 7–26 Definitions of Dummy Variables for the Model in Figure 7–9D

Fifth of x	Dummy Variables			
	x_1	x_2	x_3	x_4
1 (reference)	0	0	0	0
2	1	0	0	0
3	0	1	0	0
4	0	0	1	0
5	0	0	0	1

- For the individuals in the bottom fifth, all dummies have a value of 0, and thus $y = b_0$
- For individuals in the second fifth, where only x_1 is equal to 1, $y = b_0 + b_1 x_1$
- For individuals in the third fifth, $y = b_0 + b_2 x_2$
- For individuals in the fourth fifth, $y = b_0 + b_3 x_3$
- For individuals in the top fifth, $y = b_0 + b_4 x_4$

Thus, the regression coefficients have the following interpretation:

- b_0 = the average value of y among individuals in the reference category (bottom fifth).
- b_1 = the average difference in the value of y between individuals in the second fifth and those in the bottom fifth.
- b_2 = the average difference in the value of y between individuals in the third fifth and those in the bottom fifth.
- b_3 = the average difference in the value of y between individuals in the fourth fifth and those in the bottom fifth.
- b_4 = the average difference in the value of y between individuals in the top fifth and those in the bottom fifth.

The difference between each fifth and a different fifth other than the reference is easily obtained by subtraction of the regression coefficients. For example, the difference between the top fifth and the second fifth can be calculated as $b_4 - b_1$.

In Figure 7–9D, b_0 represents the y value corresponding to the horizontal bar for the "reference" category, and each of the other b's represents the vertical distance (in y units) between the horizontal bars for each of the fifths and the reference fifth. In the hypothetical example shown in this figure, the values of b_1 and b_2 will be negative (because the average y values in subjects in the second and third fifth are lower than the average y value in the bottom fifth), whereas the values of b_3 and of b_4 will be positive. Note that the choice of the reference category is purely arbitrary and largely inconsequential. For example, because the second fifth is the category with the lowest y value, which thus might be considered the "normal" range for x, it could have been chosen as the reference category in the above example. If this had happened, b_0 would have represented the average value of the individuals in this new reference category, and the remaining b's (all positive in this situation) would have been the average differences between each of the other fifths and the second fifth. Note, in addition, that if the model in Equation 7.10 had included other variables, each of the estimates for the difference between each category and the reference category would have been adjusted for these other variables.

An example of breaking down continuous independent variables into several categories when using the multiple–logistic regression model is presented in Table 7–27. This table shows results pertaining to the examination of the cross-sectional associations between sociodemographic characteristics and the prevalence of depressive symptoms among Mexican Americans participating in the US Hispanic Health and Nutrition Examination Survey.[38] In this table, logistic regression coefficients and corresponding odds ratios (and the attached P values—see Wald statistic, Appendix A, Section A.9) are presented side by side. Note that all variables were entered in the model as categorical variables, including variables that could have been entered as continuous (eg, age, income). With the exception of sex and employment status, all variables in the table have more than two categories. For each of these variables, one of the categories is used as the reference (ie, it has no regression coefficient), with the value of its odds ratio being, by definition, 1.0. All other categories have been modeled as dummy variables. For each of these categories, a logistic regression coefficient is estimated; exponentiation of this coefficient results in an estimate of the odds ratio that compares this category with the reference. For example, for age, the younger age group (20–24 years) was chosen as reference. The coefficient for "25 to 34 years" is 0.1866, corresponding to an odds ratio of $e^{0.1866}$, or 1.2; for the next age group ("35–44 years"), the coefficient is negative (-0.1112), thus indicating that the log odds in this category is lower than that in the reference, which translates into an odds ratio below 1 (OR $= e^{-0.1112} = 0.89$); and so forth. For years of education and income, the highest categories were chosen as reference; had the authors chosen the lowest instead, the results would have been the reciprocals of those shown in the table. Very importantly, note that, as discussed previously in this section, by breaking down the continuous variables into dummy variables (categories), it is possible to adequately model nonlinear relationships observed in these data by using a linear model. For example, the use of five dummy variables (plus a reference category) for age in Table 7–27 suggests the presence of an inverse "J-shape" pattern, as the odds ratio is higher for the category 25 to 34 years than for the reference category (20–24 years), but consistently and increasingly lower for the older age categories.

Use of dummy variables is sometimes mandatory, as when modeling *nonordinal* polychotomous categorical variables such as "marital status" and "place of birth/acculturation" in Table 7–27. For example,

Table 7–27 Logistic Regression Analysis of the Association Between Various Sociodemographic Characteristics and Prevalence of Depressive State, Hispanic Health and Nutrition Examination Survey, Mexican Americans Aged 20 to 74 Years, 1982 to 1984

Characteristic	Logistic Regression Coefficient	Odds Ratio	P Value
Intercept	−3.1187		
Sex (female vs male)	0.8263	2.28	0.0001
Age (years)			
20–24	−	1.00	
25–34	0.1866	1.20	0.11
35–44	−0.1112	0.89	0.60
45–54	−0.1264	0.88	0.52
55–64	−0.1581	0.85	0.32
65–74	−0.3555	0.70	0.19
Marital status			
Married	−	1.00	
Disrupted marriage	0.2999	1.35	0.18
Never married	0.7599	2.14	0.004
Years of education			
0–6	0.8408	2.32	0.002
7–11	0.4470	1.56	0.014
12	0.2443	1.28	0.21
≥13	−	1.00	
Annual household income (US$)			
0–4,999	0.7055	2.02	0.019
5,000–9,999	0.7395	2.09	0.009
10,000–19,999	0.4192	1.52	0.08
≥20,000	−	1.00	
Employment			
(unemployed vs employed)	0.2668	1.31	0.20
Place of birth/acculturation			
US-born/Anglo oriented	−	1.00	−
US-born/bicultural	−0.3667	0.69	0.004
Foreign-born/bicultural	−0.6356	0.53	0.026
Foreign-born/Mexican oriented	−0.8729	0.42	0.0003

Source: Data from EK Mościcki et al, Depressive Symptoms among Mexican-Americans: The Hispanic Health and Nutrition Examination Survey, *American Journal of Epidemiology,* Vol 130, pp 348–360, © 1989, The Johns Hopkins University School of Hygiene & Public Health.

one potentially important finding of this analysis is that, compared with US-born/Anglo-oriented Mexican Americans, the prevalence of depressive state seems to be significantly lower among the foreign born, particularly those who are Mexican oriented. Again, it is important to bear in mind that the estimate for each variable is adjusted for all other variables shown in the table. Variables not included in the model, however, could still confound these associations (see Section 7.5); furthermore, causal inferences based on the data shown in Table 7–27 may be affected by their cross-sectional nature and its related biases (see Chapter 4, Section 4.4.2).

With respect to continuous or ordinal categorical variables, dummy variables can serve as an intermediary or exploratory step to evaluate whether a straight linear model is appropriate or whether several categories have to be redefined or regrouped. For example, after seeing the results shown in Table 7–27, one could simplify the definition for the variable "income" by grouping the two categories of <US$10,000 into one, in view of their seemingly homogeneous odds of depression. Furthermore, because of the appearance of an approximately linear increase in the odds of depression according to decreasing levels of education, the authors could have further simplified the model by replacing the three dummy variables for education with a single ordinal variable (1 to 4—or 0 to 3); the value of the coefficient in the later case would be interpreted as the increase in the log odds per unit increase (or decrease in this case) in the level of education. In other words, the antilog of this coefficient would be the estimate of the odds ratio comparing any one pair of adjacent ordinal categories of education (ie, comparing those with ≥13 years versus those with 12 years, or those with 12 years vs those with 7–11 years, or those with 7–11 years vs those with 0–6 years).

The latter approach, frequently used in epidemiology (as when redefining the levels of certain serum parameters, nutrients, etc, according to quartiles, quintiles, etc) is essentially equivalent to using a continuous variable, except that the possible values of x are now restricted to the integer values from 1 to 4, or 1 to 5, and so on. The advantages of this approach as compared to a more complex model including a number of dummy variables are that (1) the resulting model is more parsimonious and simpler to explain (see Section 7.7) and (2) the statistical testing of the corresponding regression coefficient (see next section and Appendix A, Section A.9) is the multivariate adjusted analogue of the test for dose response described in Appendix B. It is important to bear in mind, however, the risks of using these ordinal definitions of the independent variables without consideration of the possible presence of patterns such as those schematically represented in Figure 7–9A.

Alternative Modeling Techniques for Nonlinear Associations

The use of more complex mathematical functions constitutes another approach to modeling associations for which a simple linear function (eg, a straight line) does not seem to represent a proper fit. Examples of these alternative models include the use of quadratic terms (which can model simple curve relationships) or more complex polynomial or other types of functions to model U- or J-shape relationships (eg, Figure 7–9A). Although a discussion of these models is outside the purview of this book (see, eg, Armitage and Berry[12]), two examples are displayed in Figures 7–10 and 7–11.

Figure 7–10 is based on a study that examined the relationship between BMI and percent body fat in several populations of African descent.[39] Figure 7–10A shows the scatter diagram for the combined male and female subjects from the Nigeria subset in that study; whereas Figures 7–10B and C show the estimated regression lines separately for males and females. Note that after evaluating different modeling options, the authors concluded that the relationship between BMI and body fat was well described by a simple linear model in men.

$$\%body\ fat = -21.37 + 1.51(BMI)$$

whereas a curvilinear model (quadratic term) was needed for women:

$$\%body\ fat = -44.24 + 4.01(BMI) - 0.043(BMI)^2$$

Figure 7–11 is from a simulation study of the spread of two sexually transmitted diseases (gonorrhea and *Chlamydia trachomatis*) based on different assumptions regarding transmission patterns.[40] Specifically, Figure 7–11 shows the prevalence of these diseases according to the effective contact rate (a function of the mean and variance of the number of sexual partners); shown in the figure are the estimated (observed) prevalence in each of the simulations (the dots), as well as the estimated statistical models that best fit the observed data for either disease. These complex hyperbolic functions are useful for prediction (see above). On the other hand, none of the parameters from these models (eg, $b_1 = 1.89$) has a clear interpretation in terms of summarizing the association between the variables of interest (eg, effective contact rate and prevalence of gonorrhea). The trade-off between simplicity and interpretability on the one hand and proper fit on the

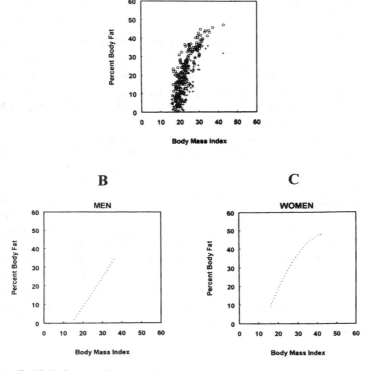

Figure 7–10 Relations between body mass index and percentage of body fat among men and women in Nigeria, 1994–1995. **A,** scatter diagram of raw data (men, + ; women, O). **B** and **C,** estimated regression lines for males and females, respectively. *Source:* Reprinted with permission from A Luke et al, Relation Between Body Mass Index and Body Fat in Black Population Samples from Nigeria, Jamaica, and the United States, *American Journal of Epidemiology,* Vol 145, pp 620–628, © 1997, The Johns Hopkins University School of Hygiene & Public Health.

---

other is at the core of the art and science of statistical modeling, as briefly discussed in the summary section of this chapter (Section 7.7).

7.4.8 Statistical Testing and Confidence Intervals of Regression Estimates

The values of the regression parameters in linear regression, whether simple (Section 7.4.1) or multiple (Section 7.4.2) linear re-

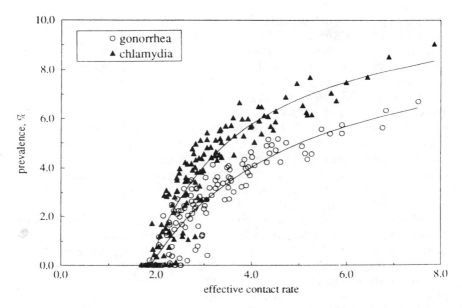

Figure 7–11 Simulation models for the spread of gonorrhea and *Chlamydia trachomatis:* the prevalence rates of gonorrhea and chlamydia (as percentages of the model population) as a function of the effective contact rates. Each data point represents one simulation run. The solid lines represent hyperbolic functions of the form $y = [b_0(x - b_1)]/[b_2 + (x - b_1)]$, which were fitted to the data points with a nonlinear curve–fitting program. In this equation, y is prevalence and x is the effective contact rate; the resulting parameter value estimates were for gonorrhea, $b_0 = 10.08$, $b_1 = 1.89$, $b_2 = 3.18$, and for chlamydia, $b_0 = 11.12$, $b_1 = 1.85$, $b_2 = 2.0$. *Source:* Reprinted with permission from M Kretzschmar, YTHP van Duynhoven, and AJ Severijnen, Modeling Prevention Strategies for Gonorrhea and Chlamydia Using Stochastic Network Simulations, *American Journal of Epidemiology,* Vol 144, pp 306–317, © 1996, The Johns Hopkins University School of Hygiene & Public Health.

gression, are estimated using the *ordinary least squares* (OLS) method. This method of estimation is fairly simple and, in the case of simple linear regression, can be done with a simple pocket calculator; for multivariate linear regression, however, matrix algebra is required. On the other hand, the simple least squares method cannot be applied to the other three regression methods described in the previous sections. Logistic regression, Cox regression, and Poisson regression methods require an iterative estimation process based on the *maximum likelihood method* (MLE), a task that is greatly facilitated by using modern computers and statistical software. (For a general introduction to the principles of likelihood and MLE, see Clayton and Hills.[41])

As with any other statistical estimate, the regression parameters obtained using OLS or MLE for the regression methods presented in the previous sections are subject to uncertainty due to sampling variability. Thus, in addition to the regression coefficient, the estimation algorithm provides the standard error associated with that parameter estimate (see, eg, Table 7–16). With the point estimate of the regression coefficient and its standard error (in any of the regression methods described in the preceding sections), a test of hypothesis can be performed to assess whether the regression coefficient in question is statistically significant: that is, whether the null hypothesis (H_o: $b = 0$) can be rejected at a certain significance (alpha error) level. This test, called the Wald statistic, is briefly described with some examples in Appendix A, Section A.9. Similarly, a confidence interval for the value of the regression coefficients can be estimated using the point estimate and the standard error of the regression coefficient (see Appendix A). As shown in the examples in the appendix, for multiplicative models (eg, logistic, Cox, Poisson), the exponentiation of the lower and upper confidence interval for the regression coefficients provides the corresponding confidence limits for the multiplicative measures of effect (eg, odds ratio, hazards ratio, rate ratio).

In addition to the Wald statistic and confidence limits to evaluate the statistical relevance of each regression parameter estimated, other statistical parameters or tests are useful for the comparison of different models; these include the value of the R^2 in the context of linear regression, which gives an estimate of the proportion of the variance of the dependent variable explained by the independent variables, and the *likelihood ratio test (LRT)*, a significance test comparing models based on MLE-based regression methods. In addition, a number of numerical and graphical techniques can be used to evaluate the statistical assumptions and fit of the data to a particular model or set of independent variables. For more details on these methods, the reader is referred to more advanced textbooks, such as Armitage and Berry,[12] Kleinbaum et al,[14] or Clayton and Hills.[41]

7.5   INCOMPLETE ADJUSTMENT: RESIDUAL CONFOUNDING

The issue of residual confounding, which occurs when adjustment does not remove completely the confounding effect due to a given variable or set of variables, has been introduced in Chapter 5, Section 5.4.3. The sources for incomplete adjustment and/or residual confounding are diverse, and some of the most important ones are discussed below.

1. *Improper definition of the categories of the confounding variable.* This occurs, for example, when attempting to adjust for a continuous variable using categories that are too broad. For example, Table 7–28 shows the results of different alternatives for age adjusting when exploring the cross-sectional relationship between menopausal status and prevalent CHD using unpublished data from the ARIC study. The decrease in odds ratio when adjusting for age as a continuous variable indicates that the "age-adjusted" estimates using categorical definitions of age did not completely remove its confounding effect. The inference that the best alternative for the age adjustment in Table 7–28 is the model using age as a continuous variable obviously requires assuming that CHD prevalence increases linearly with age throughout the entire age range of study participants. This is an approximately correct assumption in this particular example, given the relatively narrow age range of the study population (middle-aged women). However, this may not be the case in other situations. For example, if the age range of individuals in the study covered the whole life span, a linear model would not be reasonable, as the rate at which the increase in CHD risk varies by age is different between younger and older individuals. In this situation, a model similar to model 3 in Table 7–28 (defining age categorically) might have been the most appropriate. Another example

Table 7–28 Cross-Sectional Relationship Between Natural Menopause and Prevalent Coronary Heart Disease (CHD), Atherosclerosis Risk in Communities (ARIC) Study, Ages 45 to 64, 1987 to 1989

Model		OR	95% Confidence Interval
1	Crude	4.54	2.67–7.85
2	Adjusted for age using two categories: 45–54 and 55–64 years (Mantel-Haenszel)	3.35	1.60–6.01
3	Adjusted for age using four categories: 45–49, 50–54, 55–59, and 60–64 years (Mantel-Haenszel)	3.04	1.37–6.11
4	Adjusted for age as a continuous variable (logistic regression)	2.47	1.31–4.63

of potential residual confounding relates to the adjustment for smoking using categorical definitions such as "current," "former," or "never." The variability in cumulative dose *within* the first two categories (ie, in average number of cigarettes per day, pack-years, time since quitting, etc) may be large, thus resulting in important residual confounding when evaluating relationships between variables confounded by smoking.

2. *The variable used for adjustment is an imperfect surrogate of the condition or characteristic the investigator wishes to adjust for.* When using a given variable in an epidemiologic study, it is important to consider the issue of its *construct validity*: that is, the extent to which it represents the exposure or the outcome it purports to represent.[42] A typical example leading to residual confounding is the use of education to adjust for social class when evaluating ethnic differences (eg, black-white differences) in a given outcome, as residual differences in access to goods and income level may exist between ethnic/racial groups, even *within* each educational level category.[43]

3. *Other important confounders are not included in the model.* If some of the confounding variables are left out of the model, the adjusted estimates will obviously still be confounded. The results in the first row of Table 7–25, for example, are adjusted for demographic variables; if these had been the only results provided (either because of missing data on the additional possible confounders considered in the second model or because these data, although available, had been deemed unimportant by the investigators), their interpretation would have been that a high level of *C. pneumoniae* antibodies was associated with a 60% increase in the "adjusted" hazard ratio of coronary heart disease. Note that even the second model, which implies that the association is either weak or nonexistent, may be subject to residual confounding, due to the failure to include additional (unmeasured or unknown) confounders. Another example is the study showing an association between frequent sexual activity and lower mortality[44] that was discussed in Chapter 5, Section 5.4.3. As mentioned in that section, the lower mortality of study participants with a higher frequency of sexual intercourse persisted when a number of putative confounding variables were adjusted for using multiple logistic regression. In their discussion, the authors of that study speculated that unknown confounders may account for the results. Although they did not discuss which specific variables might account for residual confounding, at least

two possibilities can be suggested: first, social class, an important determinant of both disease and mortality, has been taken into consideration in only a very crude manner by a dichotomous occupational variable ("manual" and "nonmanual" occupations); thus, substantial residual confounding may have remained. In addition, the only prevalent disease adjusted for was coronary heart disease; other diseases affecting both sexual activity and mortality (eg, diabetes, perhaps psychiatric conditions) apparently were not considered and could result in residual confounding of the reported results.

4. *Misclassification of confounding variables.* Another source of residual confounding is misclassification of confounders, which results in imperfect adjustment.[45] Thus, for example, if there is no causal association between exposure and outcome, but the confounded association is reflected by a risk ratio or odds ratio greater than 1.0, adjustment for misclassified confounders may not result in an adjusted risk ratio or odds ratio of 1.0. An example of this phenomenon, based on hypothetical data, is presented in Table 7–29. This table shows the same data from Table 7–1 (left-hand side); in this example, although the crude odds ratio suggested that, compared to females, males were at a 71% higher risk of malaria, in occupation-stratified analyses this association all but vanished, and the occupation-adjusted OR_{MH} was 1.01 (see Sections 7.2 and 7.3.3). When misclassification of the confounder occurs (right-hand side of the table), the resulting "adjusted" OR_{MH} (1.30) is affected by residual confounding and fails to completely remove the confounding effect of occupation. Note that the example in Table 7–29 is one of the simplest cases of misclassification: nondifferential and only in one direction. More complex patterns of misclassification (eg, bidirectional and/or differential) may lead to unpredictable consequences in terms of the magnitude of the "adjusted" estimates.

7.6 OVERADJUSTMENT

As mentioned in Chapter 5 (Section 5.2.3), adjustment for a given variable implies an adjustment, at least partially, for variables related to it. Thus, when adjusting for educational level, adjustment for income is to a certain extent also carried out. As mentioned previously, depending on the specific characteristics of the study population, adjustment for residence may result in adjustment for related variables, such as socioeconomic status or ethnic background. *Overadjustment*

Table 7–29 Hypothetical Data Showing Residual Confounding Resulting from Nondifferential Misclassification of a Confounder (Occupational Status)

All Cases and Controls

	Cases	Controls	Total	
Males	88	68	156	OR = 1.71
Females	62	82	144	
Total	150	150	300	

CORRECTLY CLASSIFIED
Occupational Status*

MISCLASSIFIED
Occupational Status†

Mostly Outdoor Occupations

	Cases	Controls	Total		Cases	Controls	Total	
Males	53	15	68	OR = 1.06	35†	10	45	OR = 1.00
Females	10	3	13		7	2	9	
Total	63	18	81		42	12	54	

Mostly Indoor Occupations

	Cases	Controls	Total		Cases	Controls	Total	
Males	35	53	88	OR = 1.00	53†	58	111	OR = 1.33
Females	52	79	131		55	80	135	
Total	87	132	219		108	138	246	

"Correct" OR_{MH} = 1.01   "Misclassified" OR_{MH} = 1.30

* See Table 7–1.

† Nondifferential misclassification: one third of all individuals with mostly outdoor occupation (regardless of case-control or gender status) are misclassified to mostly indoor occupation. (All the misclassified numbers are rounded to the nearest integer.) For example, of the 53 male cases in outdoor occupations, 18 ($\approx$ 53 × 0.333) are misclassified to mostly indoor, which leaves 35 subjects in that cell; in turn, as many as 53 male cases (35 correctly classified + 18 misclassified) are now included in the corresponding indoor occupation stratum.

(or *overmatching*, for a variable adjusted for by matching) is said to occur when adjustment is inadvertently carried out for a variable which is either in the causal pathway between the exposure and the outcome (thus being an "intermediate" cause) or so strongly related to either the exposure or the outcome that their true relationship is distorted.[46] Overadjustment can, therefore, obscure a true effect or create an apparent effect when none exists.[47]

An example is given by the adjustment for hypertension when examining the association between overweight and hemorrhagic stroke. As hypertension is likely to be the most common mechanism explaining this association, adjustment for it may lead to obscuring the obesity-stroke relationship. As discussed in Chapter 5, it would nevertheless be appropriate to adjust for an intermediate cause or a mechanistic link when assessing the presence of residual effects due to alternative mechanisms.

Overadjustment may also occur when adjusting for a variable closely related to the exposure of interest. An example that epitomizes gross overadjustment is the adjustment for residence when studying the relationship of air pollution to respiratory disease. Other examples include situations when different variables representing overlapping constructs are simultaneously adjusted, as when including education, income, occupation, and aggregate (ecologic) measures of income or other socioeconomic indicators in the same regression model. Because all these variables are markers of "social class," their collinearity would render the corresponding regression coefficients hard to interpret, or even meaningless.

The issue of overadjustment underscores the need to consider the biologic underpinnings of the postulated relationship, as well as to carry out a thorough assessment of the relationships between the postulated confounding variable on the one hand and the exposure and outcome variables on the other, as discussed in Chapter 5.

7.7 CONCLUSION

Our aim is to discover and ascertain the nature and substance of the soul, and, in the next place, all the accidents belonging to it.

Aristotle (quoted in Durrant[48(p15)])

Statistical models are conceptual and mathematical summaries that establish the presence of a certain pattern or association between the elements of a system (eg, suspected risk factors and disease outcome). The epidemiologist uses statistical models "to concisely summarize broad patterns in data and to interpret the degree of evidence in a data set relevant to a particular hypothesis."[49(p1064)] When trying to identify patterns of associations between exposures and outcomes in epidemiology, the goal of the modeling process is usually to find the most *parsimonious* statistical model—that is, the simplest model that satisfactorily describes the data. One simple way to understand this idea is to conceive the statistical model as a *sketch* or a *caricature* of the association under investigation. Thus, statistical modeling could be seen as a process analogous to that of a cartoonist trying to find the few lines that capture the essence of the character being portrayed, as illustrated in Figure 7–12. The four panels in this figure can be conceived as four "models" of US president William J. Clinton. The model in Figure 7–12A is the simplest but fails to effectively represent the person that it is trying to portray (most people would not recognize President Clinton if shown only this picture). Some, but not all people, would recognize Clinton if shown Figure 7–12B, and probably almost everyone would recognize him in the sketch in Figure 7–12C. Thus, when looking for a succinct, parsimonious model to describe the essence of that portrait, those shown in Figures 7–12B or C would be the best choices. The "model" in Figure 7–12D fits "the data" better, but at the expense of making each of the elements in the sketch less useful in portraying the *essence* of the character.

This process is similar when using statistical modeling in epidemiologic analysis. As discussed by Zeger,[49] statistical models should be considered as "tools for science" rather than "laws of nature": "Statistical models for data are *never true*. The question of whether a model is true is irrelevant. A more appropriate question is whether we obtain the correct scientific conclusion if we pretend that that process under study behaves according to a particular statistical model."[49(p1064)]

Thus, the key question is whether the model fits the data reasonably well in order to help the investigator to derive appropriate inferences. This means that whether the estimated value of the parameter (eg, $b_1 = 0.0025$ mm in Table 7–15, model 1) is a *perfect* estimate of the "true" relation between systolic blood pressure and carotid IMT or whether the true relationship between these two variables is *exactly* linear (eg, Figure 7–4) is not that important. Often, the relevant questions are whether there is a more or less linear increment and what the approximate average increment is on y per unit of x after controlling for certain covariates. However, it should be again emphasized that, as in the example in Figure 7–9, a model should never be adopted just because it is simple if it does not describe the association of interest properly (eg, Figures 7–9B or C).

The attractiveness of simple linear models is precisely their simplicity and the interpretability of the parameters, such as the straight line that expresses the expected increase in carotid IMT for a given increase in systolic blood pressure (Figure 7–4). Assuming that the model is appropriate (ie, that the association is linear), it is possible to calculate the parameters (intercept and linear regression coefficient of the line—the model) that would best fit the data (Equation 7.2). Thus, the assumption is that the line in Figure 7–4 reflects the true *essence* of the relation between systolic blood pressure and IMT and that the scatter around the line (the observed data) is just *noise*: that is, within-individual variability or random error.

A

B

C

D

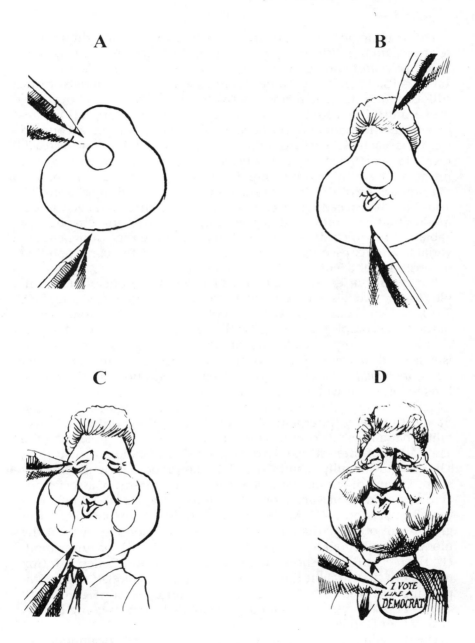

Figure 7–12 Building a "model" of President Clinton. *Source:* Copyright ©
Kevin "KAL" Kallaugher, 1986, *Baltimore Sun,* Cartoonists and Writers Syndicate.

The same logic applies to situations that incorporate the mutual relations among different correlates of both "exposure" (eg, systolic blood pressure) and "outcome" (eg, IMT), such as models 2 to 4 in Table 7–15. These *multivariate* or multiple-regression models, while still assuming that the relation between these variables is linear, define a multidimensional space where the mutual correlations between the independent and dependent variables can be accounted for. Thus, each estimate from these multiple-regression models (each regression coefficient) is said to be *adjusted* for all the other variables in the model, although it is important to always consider the potential limitations of this kind of inference, as discussed in Sections 7.5 and 7.6. The preceding discussion applies to all generalized linear models that were presented in preceding sections in this chapter (see Table 7–14), which differ only with regard to the type of dependent variable and, consequently, the interpretation of the corresponding regression coefficient.

It may, of course, be found that the data do not fit one of these simple "linear" models. For example, if the type of scatter in Figures 7–9, 7–10, or 7–11 is observed, it would probably be necessary to use some of the more complex modeling approaches that were discussed in Section 7.4.7 (dummy variables, quadratic terms, etc). Furthermore, if it is suspected that two or more of the covariates in the model interact (ie, if one *modifies the effect* of the other), stratification or inclusion of interaction terms will be needed to account for such interactions.

Again, the investigator has to take a stand in the trade-off between fit and simplicity (interpretability) of the model. Ignoring the possibility that a linear association may not be a good way to describe the association of interest may lead to seriously misleading conclusions. The need to carefully examine the data cannot be sufficiently emphasized. The use of dummy variables to examine patterns of associations across the range of values of continuous variables was briefly discussed in Section 7.4.7. More advanced statistical textbooks cover in great detail other statistical tools to assess the goodness of fit of the models described above (see, eg, Draper and Smith[15] for linear models, Hosmer and Lemeshow[21] for logistic models, and Collet[25] for Cox regression). If a straight line is not an appropriate model, more complex models need to be adopted, such as those seen in Figures 7–10 and 7–11, a process that could be seen as analogous to going from A or B to C or D in Figure 7–9.

The preceding discussion pertains to the use of statistical models in identifying and describing associations between exposures and outcomes in epidemiology. However, statistical models can also be used for *prediction*, as discussed with examples in the logistic regression section in this chapter (Section 7.4.3). In this case, obtaining a model as parsimonious as possible is no longer that important. In fact, for obtaining an accurate prediction of the *expected* value of a dependent variable, the more complex the model, the better. Because the interpretation of the parameters in themselves is not the goal, complex models (eg, Figures 7–10 and 7–11) are perfectly suitable for prediction. Again, using the analogy of the cartoonist (Figure 7–12), if the goal was to accurately identify the subject (eg, if the cartoonist was working for the police in creating—predicting—a suspect's portrait!), the most complex "model" of the type shown in Figure 7–9D would be chosen.

7.7.1   Selecting the Right Statistical Model

So far, this discussion has focused mainly on modeling issues with respect to the *shape* of the relationship between a certain independent variable and a dependent variable. Obviously, however, this is not the only issue in statistical modeling. Other fundamental decisions in any multivariate or multiple-regression analysis are (1) the choice of the specific regression/stratification-based technique and (2) the choice of the variables to be included in the multivariate equation or stratification scheme.

The choice of the adjustment technique (stratification or regression based) is often a matter of convenience and personal preference. The choice of a particular adjustment technique over all others described in the preceding sections of this chapter (and others not covered here) is often based on the type of study design, the type of variables (dependent and independent) under investigation, and the type of measure of association that one wishes to obtain. Table 7–30 summarizes how the adjustment techniques described in this chapter relate to the main study designs, variable types, and measures of association.

Analysis-of-variance methods and linear regression models are indicated when the outcome variable is continuous. When the outcome is a binary variable (as is often the case in epidemiology), the adjustment techniques based on the popular multiplicative models described above (eg, Mantel-Haenszel summary odds ratio or rate ratio, logistic regression, Cox regression, Poisson regression) tend to provide similar results. This is illustrated by the similarity of results obtained in Tables 7–15, 7–17, 7–18, 7–20, and 7–21. A similar example can be found in Kahn and Sempos,[8] where different stratification-based and multiple-regression–based adjustment methods were used

Table 7–30 Commonly Used Analytic Techniques Available to the Epidemiologist for the Assessment of Relationships Between Exposures and Outcomes

Type of Study	Type of Dependent Variable (Outcome)	Multivariate Technique	Adjusted Measure of Association
Any	Continuous biological parameter	ANOVA	Difference in means
		Linear regression	Linear regression coefficient
Cross-sectional	Diseased/ nondiseased	Direct adjustment	Prevalence rate ratio
		Indirect adjustment	Standardized prevalence ratio
		Mantel-Haenszel	Odds ratio
		Logistic regression	Odds ratio
Case-control	Diseased/ nondiseased	Mantel-Haenszel	Odds ratio
		Logistic regression	Odds ratio
Cohort	Cumulative incidence (by the end of follow-up)	Direct adjustment	Relative risk
		Indirect adjustment	Standardized incidence ratio
		Mantel-Haenszel	Odds ratio
		Logistic regression	Odds ratio
	Cumulative incidence (Time-to-event data)	Cox model	Hazard ratio
	Incidence rate (per person-time)	Mantel-Haenszel	Rate ratio
		Poisson regression	Rate ratio
Nested case-control nested case-cohort	Time-dependent disease status (Time-to-event data)	Conditional logistic regression	Hazard ratio
		Cox model with staggered entries	

to obtain the adjusted estimates of the associations of three risk factors (hypertension, age, and male sex) with CHD in a subset of participants from the Framingham Heart Study. All methods resulted in comparable estimates leading to similar conclusions. As discussed by Greenland,[50] many of these methods often used in epidemiology (eg, Mantel-Haenszel, logistic, Poisson, Cox) are based on similar assumptions (multiplicative relationships between risk factors and disease) and have similar epidemiologic meanings. Thus, it is not surprising that, with the exception of unusually extreme circumstances (eg, gross violations of the basic assumptions of the model, extreme outliers), these methods often will produce similar results.

The issue of *which independent variables (confounders) ought to be included* in the model is at the core of the discussion on the topic of confounding in general (Chapter 5) and of residual confounding in particular (Section 7.5). A detailed discussion of the statistical techniques that could be helpful in choosing a particular set of variables for a model is outside of the scope of this textbook. A useful overview was provided by Greenland.[50]

An important recommendation when choosing a particular statistical model is to conduct a *sensitivity analysis*: that is, to check whether similar results are obtained when different models or assumptions are used for the analysis.[50,51]

Due to the increased ease and availability of computers and computer software, the last few years have seen a flourishing of the options for and frequency of use of multivariate analysis in the biomedical literature. These highly sophisticated mathematical models, however, rarely eliminate the need to carefully examine the raw data by means of scatter diagrams, simple $n \times k$ tables, and stratified analyses.

REFERENCES

1. Miettinen OS, Cook EF. Confounding: essence and detection. *Am J Epidemiol.* 1981;114:593–603.

2. Greenland S. Absence of confounding does not correspond to collapsibility of the rate ratio or rate difference. *Epidemiology.* 1996;7:498–501.

3. Reif JS, Dunn K, Ogilvie GK, et al. Passive smoking and canine lung cancer risk. *Am J Epidemiol.* 1992;135:234–239.

4. Shapiro S, Slone D, Rosenberg L, et al. Oral-contraceptive use in relation to myocardial infarction. *Lancet.* 1979;1:743–747.

5. Gordis L. *Epidemiology.* Philadelphia, Pa: WB Saunders; 1996.

6. Armstrong BG. Comparing standardized mortality ratios. *Ann Epidemiol.* 1995;5:60–64.

7. Mantel N, Haenszel W. Statistical aspects of the analysis of data from retrospective studies of disease. *J Natl Cancer Inst.* 1959;22:719–748.

8. Kahn HA, Sempos CT. *Statistical Methods in Epidemiology.* New York, NY: Oxford University Press; 1989.

9. Pandey DK, Shekelle R, Selwyn BJ, et al. Dietary vitamin C and β-carotene and risk of death in middle-aged men: the Western Electric study. *Am J Epidemiol.* 1995;142:1269–1278.

10. Sorlie PD, Adam E, Melnick SL, et al. Cytomegalovirus/herpesvirus and carotid atherosclerosis: the ARIC Study. *J Med Virol.* 1994;42:33–37.

11. Kannel WB, McGee D, Gordon T. A general cardiovascular risk profile: the Framingham study. *Am J Cardiol.* 1976;38:46–51.

12. Armitage P, Berry G. *Statistical Methods in Medical Research.* 3rd ed. London, England: Blackwell, 1994.

13. Nieto FJ, Diez-Roux A, Sharrett AR, et al. Short and long term prediction of atherosclerosis by traditional risk factors. *J Clin Epidemiol.* 1999;52:559–567.

14. Kleinbaum DG, Kupper LL, Morgenstern H. *Epidemiologic Research: Principles and Quantitative Methods.* Belmont, Calif: Lifetime Learning Publications; 1982.

15. Draper NR, Smith H. *Applied Regression Analysis*. 3rd ed. New York, NY: John Wiley; 1998.
16. Keys A. *Seven Countries: A Multivariate Analysis of Death and Coronary Heart Disease*. Cambridge, Mass: Harvard University Press; 1980.
17. Nieto FJ, Szklo M, Folsom A, et al. Leukocyte count correlates in middle-aged adults: the Atherosclerosis Risk in Communities (ARIC) study. *Am J Epidemiol*. 1992;136:525–537.
18. Feldstein MS. A binary multiple regression method for analyzing factors affecting perinatal mortality and other outcomes of pregnancy. *J Roy Stat Soc [A]*. 1966;129: 61–73.
19. ARIC investigators. The Atherosclerosis Risk in Communities (ARIC) study: design and objectives. *Am J Epidemiol*. 1989;129:687–702.
20. Chambless LC, Heiss G, Folsom AR, et al. Association of coronary heart disease incidence with carotid arterial wall thickness and major risk factors: the Atherosclerosis Risk in Communities (ARIC) study. *Am J Epidemiol*. 1997;146:483–494.
21. Hosmer DW, Lemeshow S. *Applied Logistic Regression*. New York: John Wiley; 1988.
22. Schlesselman JJ. *Case-Control Studies: Design, Conduct, Analysis*. New York, NY: Oxford University Press; 1982.
23. Gibas A, Blewet DR, Schoenfeld DA, Dienstag JL. Prevalence and incidence of viral hepatitis in health workers in the prehepatitis B vaccination era. *Am J Epidemiol*. 1992;136:603–610.
24. Cox DR. Regression models and life table (with discussion). *J Roy Stat Soc [B]*. 1972; 34:187–220.
25. Collet D. *Modelling Survival Data in Medical Research*. London, England: Chapman & Hall; 1994.
26. Parmar MKB, Machin D. *Survival Analysis: A Practical Approach*. Chichester, England: John Wiley; 1995.
27. Breslow NE, Day NE. *Statistical Methods in Cancer Research: Vol 1. The Analysis of Case Control Studies*. Lyon, France: International Agency for Research on Cancer Scientific Publications; 1980.
28. Heiss G, Sharrett AR, Barnes R, et al. Carotid atherosclerosis measured by B-mode ultrasound in populations: associations with cardiovascular risk factors in the ARIC study. *Am J Epidemiol*. 1991;134:250–256.
29. Nieto FJ, Adam E, Sorlie P, et al. Cohort study of cytomegalovirus infection as a risk factor for carotid intimal-medial thickening, a measure of subclinical atherosclerosis. *Circulation*. 1996;94:922–927.
30. Pearce N. Incidence density matching with a simple SAS computer program. *Int J Epidemiol*. 1989;18:981–994.
31. Barlow WE. Robust variance estimation for the case-cohort design. *Biometrics*. 1994;50:1064–1072.
32. Thomas D. New techniques for the analysis of cohort studies. *Epidemiol Rev*. 1998; 20:122–136.
33. Nieto FJ, Folsom AR, Sorlie P, et al. *Chlamydia pneumoniae* infection and incident coronary heart disease: the Atherosclerosis Risk in Communities (ARIC) study. *Am J Epidemiol*. 1999;150:149–156.
34. Waaler HT. Height, weight and mortality: the Norwegian experience. *Acta Med Scan Suppl*. 1984;679:1–56.

35. Allison DB, Faith MS, Heo M, Kotler DP. Hypothesis concerning the U-shaped relation between body mass index and mortality. *Am J Epidemiol.* 1997;146:339–349.
36. Fagot-Campagna A, Hanson RL, Narayan V, et al. Serum cholesterol and mortality rates in a Native American population with low cholesterol concentrations: a U-shaped association. *Circulation.* 1997;96:1408–1415.
37. Thun MJ, Peto R, Lopez AD, et al. Alcohol consumption and mortality among middle-aged and elderly U.S. adults. *N Engl J Med.* 1997;337:1705–1714.
38. Mościcki EK, Locke BZ, Rae DS, Boyd JH. Depressive symptoms among Mexican Americans: the Hispanic Health and Nutrition Examination Survey. *Am J Epidemiol.* 1989;130:348–360.
39. Luke A, Durazo-Arvizu R, Rotimi C, et al. Relation between body mass index and body fat in black population samples from Nigeria, Jamaica, and the United States. *Am J Epidemiol.* 1997;145:620–628.
40. Kretzschmar M, van Duynhoven YTHP, Severijnen AJ. Modeling prevention strategies for gonorrhea and chlamydia using stochastic network simulations. *Am J Epidemiol.* 1996;144:306–317.
41. Clayton D, Hills M. *Statistical Models in Epidemiology.* Oxford, England: Oxford University Press; 1993.
42. Krieger N, Williams DR, Moss NE. Measuring social class in US public health research: concepts, methodologies, and guidelines. *Annu Rev Public Health.* 1997;18: 341–378.
43. Kaufman JS, Cooper RS, McGee DL. Socioeconomic status and health in blacks and whites: the problem of residual confounding and the resiliency of race. *Epidemiology.* 1997;8:621–628.
44. Davey Smith G, Frankel S, Yarnèll J. Sex and death: are they related? Findings from the Caerphilly Cohort Study. *Br Med J.* 1997;315:1641–1644.
45. Greenland S. The effect of misclassification in the presence of covariates. *Am J Epidemiol.* 1980;112:564–569.
46. Last JM. *A Dictionary of Epidemiology.* New York: Oxford University Press; 1995.
47. Breslow N. Design and analysis of case-control studies. *Annu Rev Public Health.* 1982;3:29–54.
48. Durrant M. *Aristotle's De Anima in Focus.* London, England: Routledge; 1993.
49. Zeger SL. Statistical reasoning in epidemiology. *Am J Epidemiol.* 1991;134: 1062–1066.
50. Greenland S. Modeling and variable selection in epidemiologic analysis. *Am J Public Health.* 1989;79:340–349.
51. Robins JM, Greenland S. The role of model selection in causal inference from nonexperimental data. *Am J Epidemiol.* 1986;123:392–402.

CHAPTER 8

Quality Assurance and Control

8.1 INTRODUCTION

As with other types of empirical research, the *validity* of the inferences made from results of epidemiologic research depends on the accuracy of its methods and procedures. In epidemiologic jargon, the term *validity* (or *accuracy*) refers to absence of bias. The most common biases and some approaches to prevent their occurrence so as to maximize the validity of the study's results and inferences were discussed in Chapter 4. This chapter extends the discussion of issues related to the accuracy of data collection and data processing that should be considered when designing and conducting epidemiologic studies. In addition to validity or lack of bias, the present chapter also addresses issues related to assessing and ensuring *reliability* (precision, reproducibility) of the data collected.

Although the terms *quality assurance* and *quality control* are sometimes used interchangeably or, even more often, lumped together under a common term, *quality control*, for systematization purposes in this chapter, the activities to ensure quality of the data before data collection are regarded as quality assurance, and the efforts to monitor and maintain the quality of the data during the conduct of the study are regarded as quality control.

Quality control and quality assurance activities are key components of epidemiologic research and are best understood in the context of the key features of an epidemiologic study design. The important features of a study design, aptly described in Kahn and Sempos's textbook,[1] provide the background for further elaboration in the context of this chapter (Table 8–1). Most components of a study can be said to relate to quality assurance or quality control in one way or another in the broad context of validity and reliability of epidemiologic research. This chapter, however, will focus on the activities more traditionally regarded as belonging to the realm of quality assurance or control— that is, items 7 and 8 in Table 8–1. For an additional systematic review on this topic, see Whitney et al.[2]

To illustrate some of the issues covered in the discussion that follows, Appendix D includes a verbatim transcription of the quality assurance and control protocol for two procedures carried out in a multicenter cohort study of atherosclerosis, the Atherosclerosis Risk in Communities (ARIC) study[3]: blood pressure and venipuncture.[4]

8.2   QUALITY ASSURANCE

Quality assurance activities before data collection relate to standardizing procedures and thus preventing or at least minimizing systematic or random errors in collecting and analyzing data. Traditionally, these activities have comprised detailed protocol preparation, development of data collection instruments and procedures and their manuals of operation, and training and certification of staff. (The development of manuals specifying quality control activities can be also regarded as a quality assurance activity.)

The design of quality assurance activities should be followed by pretesting and pilot-studying these activities. Results of pretests and pilot studies, in turn, assist in modifying and/or making adjustments to these procedures so as to make them more efficient, valid, and reliable.

8.2.1   Study Protocol and Manuals of Operation

The *study protocol* consists of a description of the general components of the investigation, including those shown in Table 8–1. It provides a global picture of the strategies leading to the development of more detailed manuals of operation. The protocol describes the general design and procedures used in the study (including those related to sampling and recruiting study participants) and assists the staff in understanding the context in which their specific activities are carried out.

Table 8–1 Key Features of the Design of an Epidemiologic Study

Activity *(Quality Assurance, QA,* *or Quality Control, QC)*	*Comments*
1. Formulation of study's main hypothesis/hypotheses (QA)	The hypothesis should specify the independent (eg, risk factor) and the dependent (eg, disease outcome) variables. If the investigators plan to analyze interaction, the study's hypothesis should specify the potential effect modifier(s).
2. A priori specification of potential confounding variables (QA)	A review of the pertinent literature may assist the investigators in identifying the main confounding variables, and thus help in choosing the most appropriate study design (eg, matched vs unmatched case-control) and in selecting the data that need to be collected.
3. Definition of the characteristics of the study population for external validity (generalizability) purposes (QA)	The ability to generalize results to other populations is conditional on several circumstances, including differences in the distribution of effect modifiers and the characteristics of the study population. A detailed characterization of the study participants allows data "consumers" to decide whether findings are applicable to their target population.
4. Definition of the design strategy (eg, cohort, case-control, case-cohort) and of the groups to be compared, and specification of selection procedures for internal validity (comparability) purposes (QA)	Selection of groups to be compared relates to prevention of selection bias and the level of confounding to be expected. The strategy for the search of confounders in addition to those suggested by previous studies should be specified.
5. Definition of the design strategy and samples for studies of reliability and validity (QA/QC)	The approach for selection of samples for studies of repeat measurements (reliability) or comparison with "gold standards" (validity) should be specified.

continues

Table 8–1 continued

Activity (Quality Assurance, QA, or Quality Control, QC)	Comments
6. Specification of the study power necessary to detect the hypothesized association(s) at a given level of significance (QA)	The estimation of sample size is an important guidepost to decide whether the study has sufficient power at a given alpha error level, and it should take into account the potential interaction(s), if specified in the study hypothesis.
7. Standardization of procedures (QA)	This includes preparation of written manuals that contain a detailed description of the procedures for selection of the study population and data collection, as well as training and certification of staff.
8. Activities during data collection, including analysis of quality control data and remedial actions (QC)	These include ongoing monitoring of data collection procedures, as well as conducting studies on samples to assess validity and reliability of measurements, which may result in retraining and recertification of study staff.
9. Data analysis	Data analysis should be done according to a preestablished plan. Efforts should be made to establish analytic strategies in advance (eg, the choice of "cutoff" points when using continuous or ordinal data to create discrete categories). Analysis should proceed from the more parsimonious strategies (description of data, calculation of unadjusted measures of association, simple adjustment approaches) to the more complex models (eg, Cox, logistic regression). Investigators should also specify analytic strategies to evaluate validity and reliability of procedures.

continues

Table 8–1 continued

Activity (Quality Assurance, QA, or Quality Control, QC)	Comments
10. Reporting of data	Findings should be reported as soon as possible after data collection activities are finished so as to preserve the timeliness of the study. To avoid publication bias, data should be reported regardless of the direction of findings (see Chapter 4, Section 4.5). The study instruments and quality control data should be available to the scientific community on request.

Source: Data from HA Kahn and CT Sempos, *Statistical Methods in Epidemiology,* © 1989, Oxford University Press.

Manuals of operation should contain detailed descriptions of exactly how the procedures specific to each data collection instrument are to be carried out so as to maximize the likelihood that tasks will be performed as uniformly as possible. For example, the description of the procedures for blood pressure measurements should include the calibration of the sphygmomanometer, the position of the participant, the amount of resting time before and between measurements, the size of the cuff, and the position of the cuff on the arm. With regard to interviews, the manual of operations should contain instructions as to exactly how each question should be asked during the course of the interview ("question-by-question" instructions or, to use epidemiologic jargon, "q by q's"). Standardization of procedures is particularly critical in multicenter studies in which several technicians carry out the same exams or administer the same questionnaires to study participants recruited and examined at different clinics or locations. A detailed manual of operations is important to achieve the highest possible level of uniformity and standardization of data collection procedures in the entire study population.

In large studies involving different measurements, the manuals of operation may be activity specific: that is, separate manuals of operations may be prepared for different data-related activities, such as interviews, collection and processing of blood samples, and pulmonary function testing. Manuals of operation must be also developed for reading and classifying data, as when coding electrocardiographic findings using the Minnesota Code[4] or assigning a disease to different diagnostic categories, such as "definite," "probable," or "absent" myocardial infarction.[5] A manual may also have to be developed specifying how "derived" variables are created for the purposes of the study, that is, analytical variables based on combinations of "raw" variables obtained during data collection. An example is the definition of *hypertension* (present or absent) based on sphygmomanometer-measured blood pressure levels *or* a participant's report of physician-diagnosed hypertension *or* use of antihypertensive medications.

8.2.2 Data Collection Instruments

Development (or choice) of data collection instruments and their corresponding operation manuals is a key step in the study design and should be carried out according to well-established rules, as in the case of designing a questionnaire.[6,7]

Whenever possible, it is advisable to choose data collection instruments and procedures that have been effectively used in previous studies to measure both suspected risk factors and disease outcomes. Examples include the questionnaire to identify angina pectoris developed by Rose[8] (the so-called "Rose questionnaire"), the American Thoracic Society questionnaire to assess respiratory symptoms,[9] the blood pressure measurement procedures followed by the National Health Examination Surveys,[10] and the food frequency questionnaires designed by Block et al[11] or Willett et al[12] to assess dietary habits. Validity and reliability of such previously tested instruments and procedures are sometimes known,[12] allowing to some extent the assessment of possible bias and misclassification (see below). In addition, use of established instruments and procedures permits comparing findings of the study with those of previous studies, thus facilitating the preparation of overviews and meta-analyses.[13]

On occasion, a well-established instrument is modified to suit a study's purposes. For example, modification of a questionnaire may be done either to include or exclude variables or to reduce interview time. The extent to which the modified version maintains the reliability and validity of the original instrument can be assessed by comparing results using the two instruments in the same sample. Such assessment, however, may be affected by the lack of independence between the two instruments when they are applied to the same individuals (ie, responses to the questionnaire administered last may be influenced by the study participants' recall of the responses to the first questionnaire).

When instruments effectively used in the past are not available, making it necessary to create special instruments to suit the purposes of the study, pilot studies of the validity and reliability of the instruments and related measurement procedures should be carried out, preferably before data collection activities begin (see below).

8.2.3 Training of Staff

Training of each staff person should aim at making him or her thoroughly familiar with the procedures under his or her responsibility. These procedures include not only data collection and processing procedures but also setting up appointments for interviews or visits to study clinics, preparing materials for the interviewers and other data collectors, calibrating instruments, and assigning interviewers to study participants. Training should also involve laboratory technicians and those in charge of reading and classifying data obtained from exams such as electrocardiograms and magnetic resonance or B-mode imaging studies. In multicenter studies, training of technicians from all field centers is usually done at a central location. Training culminates with the certification of the staff member to perform the specific procedure. Particularly in studies with a relatively long duration (such as concurrent prospective studies; see Gordis[14]), periodic recertification is carried out, with retraining of any staff member whose performance in conducting recertification tasks is deemed to be inadequate. But because retraining and recertification are done when data collection activities are already ongoing, they are usually classified as quality control rather than quality assurance activities.

Careful training of all study personnel involved in data collection is required for standardization of data collection and classification procedures and should emphasize adherence to the procedures specified in the manual of operations (see above). A thorough training of data collectors is key to prevent misclassification (Chapter 4, Section 4.3.3), which may occur if data collection procedures are not used in a standardized manner.

8.2.4 Pretesting and Pilot Studies

Verification of the feasibility and efficiency of the study procedures is carried out through pretests and pilot studies. Often, the terms *pretesting* and *pilot testing* are used interchangeably; however, a useful distinction is that the pretest involves assessing specific procedures on a "grab" or convenience sample (eg, on staff persons themselves or their friends or relatives) in order to detect major flaws, whereas the pilot study is a formal "rehearsal" of study procedures that attempts to reproduce the whole flow of operations in a sample as similar as possible to study participants. Results of pretesting and pilot studies are used to assess participant recruitment and data collection procedures and, if necessary, to correct these procedures before fieldwork begins. For example, after pretesting and carrying out a pilot study of a questionnaire, the following elements can be assessed: flow of questions, presence of sensitive questions, appropriateness of categorization of variables, clarity of wording to the respondent and the interviewer, and clarity of the "question-by-question" instructions to the interviewer.

Pilot studies also allow evaluating alternative strategies for participant recruitment and data collection. For example, a pilot study can be carried out to assess whether telephone interviews are a good alternative to the more expensive and time-consuming in-person interviews.

A summary of some of the key quality assurance steps is shown in Exhibit 8–1.

8.3 QUALITY CONTROL

Quality control activities begin after data collection and processing start. Monitoring of quality control data is the basis for possible remedial actions aiming at minimizing bias and reliability problems. Quality control strategies include observation of procedures and perfor-

---

Exhibit 8–1 Steps in Quality Assurance

1. Specify study hypothesis.
2. Specify general design to test study hypothesis → Develop an overall study protocol.
3. Choose or prepare specific instruments, and develop procedures for data collection and processing → Develop operation manuals.
4. Train staff → Certify staff.
5. Using certified staff, pretest and pilot-study data collection and processing instruments and procedures; pilot-study alternative strategies for data collection (eg, telephone vs mail interviews).
6. If necessary, modify 2 and 3, and retrain staff on the basis of results of 5.

mance of staff members—which allows the identification of obvious protocol deviations—and special studies of validity and reliability usually carried out in samples of study subjects at specified intervals throughout data collection and processing (see Appendix D). What follows is a summary of the most common quality control strategies and indices. The in-depth statistical discussion of reliability and validity indices is beyond the scope of this textbook; instead, the focus of the following sections is on their applicability, interpretation, and limitations.

8.3.1 Observation Monitoring and Monitoring of Trends

To identify problems in the implementation of study procedures by interviewers, technicians, and data processors, supervisors can monitor the quality of these procedures by "over-the-shoulder" observation of staff. For example, observation monitoring of the quality of blood pressure measurements is often done by "double stethoscoping": that is, using a stethoscope that allows two observers to measure blood pressure levels simultaneously. Observation monitoring of interviews can be done by taping all interviews and reviewing a random sample of these so as to assess interviewers' adherence to protocol and accuracy of recorded responses.

Another monitoring technique routinely performed in epidemiologic studies, particularly in multicenter studies in which participants are recruited and data collected over prolonged periods, is the statistical assessment of trends over time in the performance of each observer (interviewer and clinic or laboratory technician).[2] In the ARIC study, for example, the coordinating center routinely (quarterly) performs calculation of statistics on blood pressure and other variables measured by each technician for all study participants. After adjustment for age, sex, and other relevant characteristics, the temporal trends in these statistics are analyzed for each technician (see Appendix D). If drifts are detected that cannot be explained by changes in the demographic composition of the participant pools, the corresponding clinic coordinator is notified, and a review of the protocol adherence for the affected technician is conducted.

Each type of measurement may require a special quality monitoring approach. For blood pressure and anthropometric measurements, for example, the routine assessment of digit preference is carried out in a straightforward manner. For studies using specialized reading centers for the reading and scoring of measurements performed at different field centers (eg, ultrasound, magnetic resonance imaging, X-rays), monitoring data quality over time is more complicated because both field center data collection and centralized reading/scoring procedures can be sources of errors and variability.[2] Monitoring of laboratory data quality may require using external or internal standards (pools), as discussed below.

8.3.2 Validity Studies

In epidemiologic studies, particularly those conducted on large numbers of individuals, a compromise between accuracy on the one hand and costs and participants' burden on the other is often necessary. Highly accurate diagnostic procedures are usually too invasive and/or expensive for use in large-scale studies in healthy individuals; accurate information on complex lifestyle characteristics or habits often requires the use of lengthy (and therefore time-consuming) questionnaires. Thus, epidemiologists must frequently settle for less invasive or less time-consuming instruments or procedures that, although cheaper and more acceptable to study participants, may result in relatively important errors in the assessment of the variables of interest. Validity studies in subsamples of participants who undergo both the studywide procedure and a more accurate procedure serving as a "gold standard" allow assessing the impact of these errors on the study estimates.

Some of the approaches applicable to the evaluation of validity in the context of epidemiologic studies are described next. In Section 8.4, the most commonly used indices of validity are described.

Standardized Pools for Laboratory Measurements

When using blood or other biological specimens, a possible approach for conducting a validity study is to take advantage of a well-established external quality control program. This approach consists of using the same biological (eg, serum) pool to compare measurements obtained from applying study procedures with those resulting from the application of the "gold standard" procedures. The reference values serving as the "gold standard" may be measured either in a pool *external* to the study (such as a pool provided by the Centers for Disease Control and Prevention [CDC] serum cholesterol standardization program).[15] Alternatively, an internal pool can be created by combining specimens obtained from study participants and tested by a "standard" laboratory outside the study. (Each sample unit in the pool is formed by biologic specimens contributed to by several participants so as to use as small an amount of specimen of each study individual as possible.) Ideally, deviations, if any, of the study measurements from the "true" (standard) results should be random during data collection and measurement activities; importantly, these deviations should not vary according to the presence and level of key variables, such as the main exposure and outcome of interest and participant accrual or follow-up time, lest differential misclassification occur (Chapter 4, Section 4.3.3).

An example of the use of an "internal" pool is a validity study based on a mass serum cholesterol screening program involving 1880 Washington County, Maryland, residents. Screening measurements were done on blood obtained by the fingerstick method in a nonfasting state. In a subset of 49 screenees who also participated in a major cardiovascular study, serum cholesterol could also be assayed in a nationally recognized standard laboratory (Comstock, personal communication, 1991). The standard measurements were done in the fasting state under carefully controlled conditions. The validity (ie, sensitivity and specificity; see Section 8.4.1) of the screening measurements could thus be evaluated by using the standard laboratory values as the "gold standard."

An example of a study that participated in the CDC serum cholesterol standardization program is the study by Burke et al[16] of the time trends in mean cholesterol levels in participants in the Minnesota Heart Survey (MHS). In this study, values obtained from applying MHS procedures were compared with those obtained from applying "gold standard" (CDC) procedures. MHS values were found to be lower than CDC values, and the difference was found to be greater at the beginning than at the end of the study. This phenomenon of differential bias over time, generically referred to as a temporal "drift," is schematically shown in Figure 8–1. Once the magnitude of the "drift" is estimated using the standard, statistical techniques can be used to estimate "corrected" values. Thus, with correction for the temporal drift, the temporal decrease in serum cholesterol over time in the MHS was estimated to be even larger than that observed without the correction.[16]

Other Approaches To Examine Validity

The approach of comparing studywide data with "gold standard" results in samples of study participants is not limited to laboratory measurements; it applies to questionnaire data as well. For example, in a case-control study assessing the relation of hormone replacement therapy to breast cancer, information given by study participants was verified by contacting the physicians who had presumably written

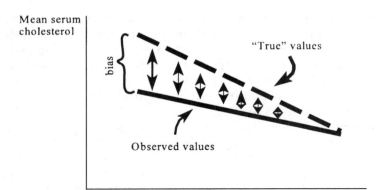

Figure 8-1 Difference between "true" and observed values in an epidemiologic study with follow-up over time. True values are those determined by the standard laboratory, and observed values are those determined by the study laboratory.

these prescriptions.[17] Another example is given by a study that assessed the validity of Willett's food frequency questionnaire in a sample of 173 women selected from among the over 90,000 participants in the Nurses' Health Study.[12] All study participants responded to the 61-item food frequency questionnaire, which is relatively simple and easy to administer and which measures the approximate average frequency of intake of selected food items. In addition, the women in the sample filled a 1-week diet diary, which was then used as the "gold standard" to assess the validity of the food frequency questionnaire applied to the whole cohort. (This sample was also given the same food frequency questionnaire twice over a 1-year period to assess its reliability; see Section 8.3.3.)

In some studies, "validation" is sought only for "positive" responses given by study participants. However, assessing samples of both "positive" and "negative" answers is important because it allows estimation of both sensitivity and specificity of the study's basic data collection strategy (see Section 8.4.1)—as, for example, when confirming interview data given by both participants who report and those who do not report oral contraceptive pill use. In addition, information should be collected separately for the groups being compared (eg, cases and controls, or exposed and unexposed) so as to permit establishing whether misclassification, if present, is nondifferential or differential (see Chapter 4, Section 4.3.3).

Availability of Validity Data from Previous Studies

On occasion, data on the validity of a given procedure are available from previous studies. For example, data have been published on self-reported hypertension ever diagnosed by a health professional in approximately 8400 participants of the National Health and Nutrition Examination Survey III (NHANES III), a nationwide inquiry conducted in the United States between 1988 and 1991.[18] Availability of "gold standard" data comprising the actual blood pressure levels measured in these participants and reports of antihypertensive medication use makes it possible to estimate the sensitivity and specificity of the participants' self-reports both for the total sample and according to sociodemographic characteristics (see Section 8.4.1).

Similarly, a study of the validity of self-reported anthropometric variables was conducted in participants of the Lipid Research Clinics (LRC) Family Study, whose weights and heights were both self-reported and measured.[19] As in the previous example, the authors of this study examined the validity of self-reported weight and height information according to the participant's age and gender and identified important differences (see Section 8.4.1).

Studies that rely on self-reported information, such as that on hypertension or weight/height, may use the estimates of validity of previous studies to evaluate the possible misclassification resulting from the use of such information in their own study population. In this case, it will be necessary to judge whether the estimates of validity obtained in these previous studies (eg, NHANES III or the LRC Family Study) are relevant and applicable to the study population in question, as briefly discussed in the following paragraphs.

Importance and Limitations of Validity Studies

As extensively illustrated in Chapter 4, the presence and strength of associations observed in epidemiologic studies are a function of the validity (and reliability) of key study variables, which in turn determines the presence and degree of misclassification (see Chapter 4, Section 4.3.3). Thus, an important element in the causal inferential process is the knowledge of the validity of exposure, outcome, and main confounding variables. That many variables, even those considered as fairly "objective," have a relatively poor validity has been clearly shown (Table 8–2).[20] Consider, for example, a case-control study in which information on smoking is obtained from next of kin, rather than directly from cases and controls. In this study, assume that the prevalence of smoking in controls is 10%. Assume, in addition, that the "true" odds ratio associated with smoking (2.25) can be

Table 8–2 Examples of Reported Sensitivities and Specificities of Tests Used in Epidemiologic Studies

Test	Validation Approach*	Sensitivity (%)	Specificity (%)
	Cohort		
Glucose tolerance by University Group Diabetes Project criteria	World Health Organization criteria	91	94
Pap smear	Biopsy	86	91
Peptic ulcer by questionnaire	Radiologic diagnosis	50	98
Protoporphyrin assay-microhematocrit	Blood lead concentration	95	73
Rose questionnaire	Clinical interview	44	93
	Case-Control		
Circumcision status by questionnaire	Physician's examination	83	44
Smoking status by next of kin	Personal questionnaire	94	88

*For bibliographic sources of original validation studies, see Copeland et al.[20]

Source: Data from KT Copeland et al, Bias Due to Misclassification in the Estimation of Relative Risk, *American Journal of Epidemiology,* Vol 105, pp 488–495, © 1977, The Johns Hopkins University School of Hygiene & Public Health.

obtained by direct personal interviews. Using the sensitivity and specificity figures for smoking shown in Table 8–2 (bottom row), if misclassification were nondifferential, the study's observed (biased) relative odds would be almost 30% closer to the null hypothesis (ie, 1.63) than would the true value. (For the calculation of biased estimates based on sensitivity and specificity figures, see Chapter 4, Section 4.3.3.) A weaker association might have been missed altogether with these same levels of sensitivity and specificity. Obviously, as also mentioned in Chapter 4, Section 4.3.3, knowledge of the sensitivity and specificity levels of misclassified variables (as shown in the table) allows the correction of a biased estimate. In addition, assessment of validity levels is crucial to the continuous efforts to develop ever more accurate data collection procedures without sacrificing their efficiency.

Notwithstanding the importance of carrying out validity studies, it should be emphasized that these studies, especially (but not exclusively) those dealing with questionnaire data, may have important limitations, and their results should be interpreted with caution. First, the "gold standard" itself may not be entirely valid. In validation studies of dietary information, for example, diary data, often used as gold standard, may have its own limitations with regard to measuring food intake.[21] Similarly, the use of medical charts, which are not primarily used for research purposes, to "validate" information collected by interview may be problematic; as these records are not tightly standardized, they often lack relevant information. As a consequence, even important data regarding the patients' medical history may have limited accuracy (and reliability). For information on habits or behaviors (eg, past history of smoking) not routinely collected and recorded in medical records, information relayed by participants may well be more accurate.

Another problem related to validity studies is that although these studies are usually attempted on a random sample of participants, the study sample frequently constitutes a selected group of especially willing individuals. Because, by definition, the "gold standard" procedure tends to be more invasive and burdensome (which, in addition to its cost, may be precisely why it has not been used as the primary means of studywide data collection in the first place), often validity studies primarily include compliant volunteers. As a result, validity levels estimated in these participants may not be representative of the true validity levels in the entire study population, particularly for questionnaire data. For example, in the validation study of Willett's dietary questionnaire described above, 224 female nurses randomly selected among the Boston participants were invited to participate (participants from other locations were excluded for logistical reasons); of these 224, 51 declined, dropped out, or had missing information on key items for the validation study. Thus, the 173 women on whom the validity and reproducibility were eventually assessed (73% of those originally invited from the Boston subset) may be unrepresentative of all study participants.

An additional concern is that the usually small sample size and resulting statistical imprecision of validity studies limit the applicability of their findings. This is especially problematic if the derived estimates of sensitivity and specificity are used to "correct" the study's observed relative risk or odds ratio estimates. A correction based on validation estimates that are markedly affected by random error may do more harm than good: in other words, the "corrected" estimate may be even less "correct" than the original one.

Finally, it is important to realize that caution should be used when extrapolating the results of a validation study from one population to another, particularly if the data collection instrument is a question-naire. For example, the validity of Willett's food frequency question-naire, even if estimated accurately and precisely in a cohort of nurses, may not be generalizable to other study populations with different so-ciodemographic characteristics, educational level, and health-related attitudes and awareness. Particularly problematic is the generalizabil-ity of validity figures for interview instruments to study populations from different cultures. Often, culture-specific instruments need to be specifically developed: an example is the food frequency questionnaire developed by Martin-Moreno and colleagues[22] for use in the Spanish population.

8.3.3 Reliability Studies

In contrast with validity studies, reliability studies assess the extent to which results agree when obtained by different approaches—that is, different observers, study instruments, or procedures—or by the same approach at different points in time. To assess reliability, it is important to consider all sources of variability in an epidemiological study. Ideally, the only source of variability in a study should be that *between study participants.* Unfortunately, other sources of variability also influence any given measurement in most real-life situations; these include

- *Variability due to the imprecision of the observer or the method,* which can be classified in two types:
  1. *Within- (or intra-) observer or method variability,* such as the vari-ability of a laboratory determination conducted twice on the same sample by the same technician using the same technique or the variability of a response to a question by the same study participants when the interview is conducted at different points in time (assuming that the response is not time depen-dent)
  2. *Between- (or inter-) observer or method variability,* such as the variability of a laboratory determination conducted on the same sample by two (or more) different technicians using the same assay or the variability of a laboratory determination done on the same individuals by the same technician using different assays
- *Variability within study participants,* such as variability in habits and behaviors (eg, day-to-day dietary intake variability) or physi-ological variability in hormone levels or blood pressure. For ex-

ample, Figure 8–2 shows systolic blood pressure values of two individuals over time. In this hypothetical example, one of the individuals is hypertensive, and the other is not (ie, their average blood pressure levels are respectively above and below the cutoff level for the definition of systolic hypertension, 160 mm Hg). However, because of the physiological within-individual blood pressure variability, participant A's blood pressure occasionally dips below the hypertension cutoff level. If the measurement turns out to be at one of those moments, that participant will be erroneously classified as "normotensive." In this example, the within-individual variability masks the between-individual variability (the difference in "true" average values that distinguish

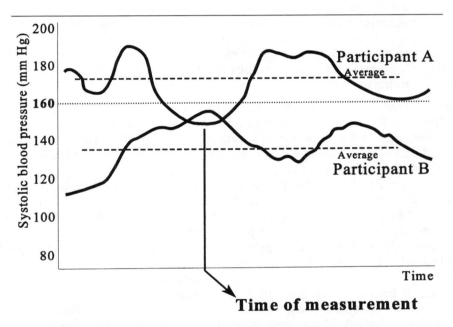

Figure 8–2 Hypothetical systolic blood pressure values of two individuals over time. Participant A is "hypertensive" (average or usual systolic blood pressure, 174 mm Hg); participant B is "normotensive" (average systolic blood pressure, 135 mm Hg). If they are measured at the time indicated by the arrow, misclassification will result due to within-individual variability: participant A will be misclassified as "normotensive" (systolic blood pressure < 160 mm Hg); moreover, participant B's blood pressure will be considered higher than participant A's blood pressure.

participants A and B as hyper- and normotensive, respectively). Unlike observer method variability, within-individual variability is real; however, it has consequences similar to those resulting from variability due to measurement errors in that it also introduces "noise" in detecting differences between study participants, the usual goal in epidemiologic research. Like errors due to the measurement method (originating from the observer, the instrument, or the procedure), intraindividual variability masks the true between-individual variability and by doing so also produces misclassification. Obviously, whereas quality assurance procedures attempt to prevent or minimize within- and between-observer or method variability, physiological within-individual variability is not amenable to prevention. However, its influence can be minimized by standardizing the timing of data collection for measures with known temporal fluctuations, such as levels of steroid hormones or physical activity, or standardizing measurement conditions for variables affected by stress or activity (eg, blood pressure should be measured after a resting time in a quiet environment).

All these sources of variability, if present, tend to decrease the reliability of the measured value of a given variable; for any given measurement, they will add to the variability of the "true value" for the individual in question when compared with the rest of the individuals in the study population.

Reliability studies during data collection and processing activities usually consist of making random repeat measurements, often referred to as "phantom" measurements. Figure 8–3 schematically illustrates an approach to reliability studies in the case of a biologic specimen.[23] Reliability studies may include repeated measures in the same individual to assess within-individual variability. Measurements of within-laboratory (or technician) reliability can be done by splitting a sample into two aliquots, which are then measured by the same laboratory (or technician) on separate occasions (Figure 8–3, aliquots 1.1 and 1.2). An additional split aliquot (aliquot 1.3) can be sent to another laboratory (or technician) to assess between-laboratory reliability. It is important that all these repeat determinations in phantom samples be conducted in a masked fashion. Typically, phantoms are interspaced in the general pool of samples that are sent to a given laboratory or technician so that masking can be achieved.

As for laboratory determinations, reliability studies of other types of measurements (eg, X-rays) can be conducted by repeat exams or repeat readings. Within-individual variability for many of these exams

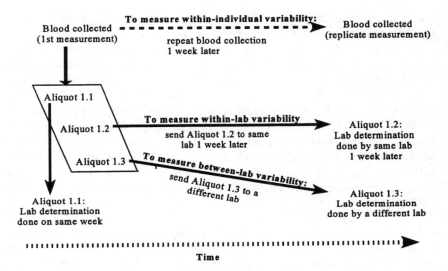

Figure 8–3 Design of a study to evaluate within-individual and within- and between-laboratory variability. *Source:* Data from LE Chambless et al, Short-Term Intraindividual Variability in Lipoprotein Measurements: The Atherosclerosis Risk in Communities (ARIC) Study, *American Journal of Epidemiology,* Vol 136, pp 1069–1081, © 1992, The Johns Hopkins University School of Hygiene & Public Health.

is limited or null (eg, the short-term variability of an X-ray image of a tumor). Sources of variability that should be assessed include the conduct of the exam (eg, the participant's positioning in the machine) and the reading (or interpretation). (See examples in Section 8.4.2 that illustrate the assessment of reliability of readers of polysomnographic studies to determine the presence of sleep-related breathing disorders.)

Assessing the reliability of each type of measurement has its own singularities and challenges. Anthropometric determinations, such as adult height, have little (if any) within-individual variability (at least in the short term); assessment of between-observer variability is fairly straightforward. On the other hand, assessment of within-observer reliability of such measurements may be challenging because it is difficult to "blind" the reader, as he or she may recognize the study participant as a "repeat" measurement (and thus remember the previous reading and/or make an effort to be more "precise" than usual). Similarly, studying the reliability of answers to questionnaires is difficult, as the participant's recall of his or her previous answers will influence the responses to the repeat questionnaire (whether it is administered by the same or by a different interviewer).

As with validity studies, it is important to assess whether reliability estimates obtained for a sample of study participants differ according to relevant characteristics, which may result in differential rates of misclassification. For example, the reliability of Willett's food frequency questionnaire was compared across subgroups of participants in the Nurses' Health Study, defined according to age, smoking and alcohol intake status, and tertiles of relative body weight.[24] In this study, no important differences in reproducibility of nutrient intake estimates among these different categories were observed, suggesting that the measurement errors resulting from the imperfect reliability of nutrient intake information were probably nondifferential (see Chapter 4, Section 4.3.3).

Finally, as with results of validity studies, it is important to be cautious when generalizing results from a reliability study of a given instrument to another study population: like validity, reliability may be a function of the characteristics of the study population. Even though it is appropriate to use published reliability and validity estimates in the planning stages of the study, it is recommended that, whenever possible, reliability and validity of key instruments, particularly questionnaires, be assessed in study participants. It is in addition important to evaluate within-individual variability, as it may also differ according to certain population characteristics, thus further affecting the generalizability of reliability results. For example, the daily variability in levels of serum gonadal hormones (eg, estrogens) is much larger in pre- than in postmenopausal women; thus, regardless of the measurement assays, reliability of levels of gonadal hormones for younger women is not applicable to older women.

8.4   INDICES OF VALIDITY AND RELIABILITY

In this section, some of the most frequently used indices of validity and reliability are briefly described, along with examples from published studies. Some of these indices, such as sensitivity and specificity, relate to the assessment of validity, whereas others, such as kappa or intraclass correlation, are usually applied in the evaluation of reliability (Table 8–3). However, some of these indices are used interchangeably to evaluate validity and reliability. For example, indices that are typically used as reliability indices, such as percent agreement or intraclass correlation coefficient, are sometimes used to report validity results. In real life, a true "gold standard" may not be available, thus sometimes making it difficult to distinguish between validity

Table 8–3 Summary of Indices or Graphic Approaches Most Frequently Used for the Assessment of Validity and Reliability

Type of Variable	Index or Technique	Mostly Used to Assess . . .	
		Validity	Reliability
Categorical	Sensitivity/specificity	+ +	
	Youden's *J* statistic	+ +	+
	Percent agreement	+	+ +
	Percent positive agreement	+	+ +
	Kappa statistic	+	+ +
Continuous	Scatter plot (correlation graph)	+	+ +
	Linear correlation coefficient (Pearson)	+	+
	Ordinal correlation coefficient (Spearman)	+	+
	Intraclass correlation coefficient	+	+ +
	Mean within-pair difference	+	+ +
	Coefficient of variation		+ +
	Bland-Altman plot	+ +	+ +

Note: + +, the index is indicated and used to measure the magnitude of validity or reliability; +, although the index is used to measure the magnitude of either validity or reliability, its indication is somewhat questionable.

and reliability measures. When a "gold standard" is not clearly identified, "validity" results are often referred to as *inter-method reliability estimates.*

8.4.1   Indices of Validity/Reliability for Categorical Data

Sensitivity and Specificity

Sensitivity and specificity are the two traditional indices of validity when the definitions of exposure and outcome variables are categorical. The study exposure or outcome categorization is contrasted with that of a more accurate method (the "gold standard," which is assumed to represent the "true" value and thus to be free of error). Sensitivity and specificity are measures also frequently used in the context of the evaluation of diagnostic and screening tools; in that context, basic epidemiology textbooks usually describe them in relation to the assessment of disease status (the "outcome"). As quality control measures in an analytic epidemiologic study, however, these indices apply to the evaluation of both exposure and outcome variables.

The definitions of the terms *sensitivity* and *specificity* were presented in Chapter 4, Exhibit 4–1. The calculation of sensitivity and specificity for a binary variable is again schematically shown in Table 8–4. (Appendix A, Section A.10 shows the method for the calculation of the confidence interval for estimates of sensitivity and specificity.)

An example is shown in Table 8–5, based on a study done in Washington County, Maryland, and previously discussed in Section 8.3.2, in which fingerstick tests were compared with standard laboratory ("gold standard") measurements of serum cholesterol. For Table 8–5, abnormal values are arbitrarily defined as those corresponding to 200 mg/dL. Sensitivity and specificity for these data were found to be $18/19 = 0.95$ and $11/30 = 0.37$, respectively. Although the screening test's ability to identify truly hypercholesterolemic individuals was quite acceptable, its ability to identify "normals" was poor (63% of normals were false positives).

In the study of the validity of self-reported weight and height information among participants in the LRC Family Study mentioned previously,[19] participants were classified in four categories according to their body mass index (BMI, measured as kg/m^2): "underweight" (BMI $<$ 20), "normal" (BMI $=$ 20–24.9), "overweight" (BMI $=$ 25–29.9), and "obese" (BMI $\geq$ 30). BMI was calculated on the basis of either "self-reported" or measured weight and height. The cross-tabulation between self-reported and measured BMI categories is presented in Table 8–6. Based on these data, the validity of binary definitions of overweight and obesity based on self-reported information can be evaluated by constructing the two-by-two tables shown in Table 8–7. Note that the validity estimates differ according to the cutoff adopted. For example, for definition A, *overweight* was defined as BMI ≥ 25 kg/m^2, resulting in a sensitivity of $3234/3741 = 0.86$ and a specificity of $3580/3714 = 0.96$. For definition B (right-hand side of

---

Table 8–4 Schematic Representation of the Calculation of Sensitivity and Specificity for a Binary Variable

	Gold Standard's Result		
Study's Result	Positive	Negative	Total
Positive	a	b	a + b
Negative	c	d	c + d
Total	a + c	b + d	N

Sensitivity $= a/(a + c)$
Specificity $= d/(b + d)$

Table 8–5 Comparison of Screening Values of Serum Cholesterol under Field Conditions and Values Done in a Standard Laboratory

	Standard Laboratory Values		
Screening Values	Abnormal*	Normal	Total
Abnormal	18	19	37
Normal	1	11	12
Total	19	30	49

*Abnormal: serum cholesterol ≥ 200 mg/dL for screening and standard laboratory, respectively.

Source: Unpublished data from GW Comstock, 1991.

Table 8–7), "obesity" was defined as BMI $\geq$ 30 kg/m^2, with corresponding sensitivity and specificity estimates of 0.74 and 0.99, respectively. Note that in this example, sensitivity is lower than specificity: that is, there is a lower proportion of "false positives" than of "false negatives," probably as a consequence of the stigma associated with obesity in our society, resulting in a higher proportion of individuals underestimating than of those overestimating their weight.

Other issues related to sensitivity and specificity that should be underscored include the following. First, the dependence of sensitivity and specificity estimates on the cutoff level used shows that there is a

Table 8–6 Cross-Tabulation of Self-Reported and Measured Four Body Mass Index (BMI) Categories: 7455 Adult Participants of the Lipid Research Clinics Family Study, 1975–1978

	Measured BMI Category				
BMI Based on Self-Reports	Underweight	Normal	Overweight	Obese	Total
Underweight	462	178	0	0	640
Normal	72	2868	505	2	3447
Overweight	0	134	2086	280	2500
Obese	0	0	59	809	868
Total	534	3180	2650	1091	7455

Note: Underweight, BMI < 20 kg/m^2; Normal, BMI = 20–24.9 kg/m^2; Overweight, BMI = 25–29.9 kg/m^2; Obese, BMI $\geq$ 30 kg/m^2.

Source: Data from FJ Nieto-Garcia, TL Bush, and PM Keyl, Body Mass Definitions of Obesity: Sensitivity and Specificity Using Self-Reported Weight and Height, *Epidemiology*, Vol 1, pp 146–152, © 1990.

Table 8–7 Cross-Tabulation of Self-Reported and Measured Binary Body Mass Index (BMI) Categories: 7455 Adult Participants of the Lipid Research Clinics Family Study, 1975–1978 (see Table 8–6)

	Definition A: Overweight*			Definition B: Obese†		
	Measured BMI Category				Measured BMI Category	
BMI Based on Self-Report	Overweight	Nonoverweight		BMI Based on Self-Report	Obese	Nonobese
Overweight	3234	134		Obese	809	59
Nonoverweight	507	3580		Nonobese	282	6305
Total	3741	3714		Total	1091	6364

*Overweight: BMI $\geq$ 25 kg/m^2.

†Obese: BMI $\geq$ 30 kg/m^2.

Source: Data from FJ Nieto-Garcia, TL Bush, and PM Keyl, Body Mass Definitions of Obesity: Sensitivity and Specificity Using Self-Reported Weight and Height, *Epidemiology,* Vol 1, pp 146–152, © 1990.

certain arbitrariness in assessing and reporting the validity of binary definitions of continuous exposure and outcome variables. This problem should not be confused, however, with the dependence of "predictive values" on the prevalence of the condition.* Unlike positive

---

*Positive and negative predictive values are measures used in the context of the evaluation of screening and diagnostic procedures, in addition to sensitivity and specificity. *Positive predictive value* (PPV) is the proportion of true positives among individuals who test positive (eg, in Table 8–7, definition A, 3234/(3234 + 134) = 0.96). *Negative predictive value* (NPV) is the proportion of true negatives out of the total who test negative. An important feature of these indices is that, in addition to their dependence on the sensitivity/specificity of the test in question, they are a function of the prevalence of the condition. For example, in Table 8–7, the prevalence of overweight (definition A) is 50.2% (3741/7455); if the prevalence had been 10% instead, even at the same self-reported weight and height sensitivity and specificity levels as those from the LRC Family Study, the PPV would have been only 0.71. (This can be shown as follows: using the notation from Table 8–4, and assuming the same total N = 7455, the expected value of cell *a* would be 641.1 (7455 × 0.10 × 0.86) and that of cell *b* would be 268.4 [7455 × (1 − 0.10) × (1 − 0.96)]; thus PPV = 641.1/(641.1 + 268.4) = 0.70.)

These indices have limited relevance in the context of evaluating the influence of validity on estimates of measures of association and are thus not discussed here. A detailed discussion of their interpretation and use, as well as a discussion of the likelihood ratio and other validity issues more relevant to screening and clinical decision making, can be found in basic clinical epidemiology textbooks.[25,26]

and negative predictive values, sensitivity and specificity are conditioned on the table's bottom totals (the "true" numbers of positives and negatives) and thus are theoretically independent of the prevalence of the condition. However, the common belief that sensitivity and specificity are inherent (fixed) properties of the test (or diagnostic criteria or procedure) itself, regardless of the characteristics of the study population, may be an oversimplification. This is particularly true for conditions based on a continuous scale that is more or less arbitrarily changed into a binary one (eg, obesity, hypertension).[27,28] For a continuous trait, the probability of misclassifying a true positive as a negative (ie, 1 − sensitivity, or cell *c* in Table 8–4) tends to be higher for individuals whose true values are near the chosen cutoff value, such as hypertensives with systolic blood pressure values close to a value traditionally defined as a cutoff point to define "high" values (eg, 140 mm Hg). Thus, even for the same test (or diagnostic procedure) and the same cutoff point, the degree of misclassification will be larger if the distribution of values (ie, the "spectrum of severity" of the condition) is closer to that of the truly negative, as illustrated in Figure 8–4.

Thus, the sensitivity and specificity of a given definition of a condition (ie, based on a cutoff in a continuous distribution) does depend on the distribution of the severity of the condition. The validity of a test can also vary from population to population when the test is not a direct marker of the condition. For example, the specificity of positive occult blood in the stool *for the diagnosis of colon cancer* varies according to the prevalence of other conditions that also cause gastrointestinal bleeding, such as peptic ulcer or parasitic disorders. Similarly, the ability of the purified protein derivative (PPD) test to accurately diagnose human tuberculosis is a function of the prevalence of atypical mycobacterial infections in the study population.

As discussed previously, another limitation to the generalizability of sensitivity and specificity estimates obtained in validation studies, especially when the information is obtained by questionnaire, is that these measures can vary according to the characteristics of individuals in question. Examples are shown in Table 8–8. In Nieto-García et al's study,[19] the validity of the definition of *obesity* (BMI $\geq$ 30 kg/m^2) based on self-reported weight and height information varied substantially according to age and gender. Sensitivity estimates using "measured" BMI as the gold standard (74% overall) ranged from more than 80% in young adults of either sex to less than 40% in older males.

Table 8–8 also shows the marked differences in the sensitivity of self-reported information depending on ethnicity and health care uti-

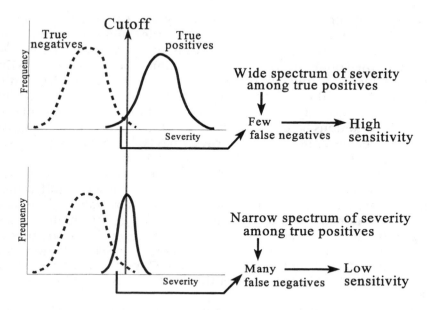

Figure 8–4 Two hypothetical situations leading to different estimates of sensitivity depending on the spectrum of severity of a given condition (eg, systolic blood pressure in the abscissa) even though the same test and cutoff (eg, systolic blood pressure ≥ 140 mm Hg for the definition of hypertension) is used in both situations.

lization (indicated by a doctor's visit in the previous year) in the NHANES III survey. On the basis of these data, the authors concluded that "use of self-reported hypertension as a proxy for hypertension prevalence . . . is appropriate among non-Hispanic whites and non-Hispanic black women and persons who had a medical contact in the past 12 months. However, self-reported hypertension is not appropriate . . . among Mexican-Americans and individuals without access to regular medical care."[18(p684)] These examples illustrate the influence of key sociodemographic variables on estimates of validity and serve as an empirical demonstration of the problems related to the extrapolation of validity estimates to populations with characteristics different from those in which validity was assessed. In addition, the large variability of validity estimates according to demographic variables, such as those shown in Table 8–8, suggests that if these variables represent the exposures of interest (or are correlated with them), differential misclassification may arise (see Chapter 4, Section 4.3.3).

Table 8–8 Examples of Results from Subgroup Analyses of Sensitivity of Information Obtained by Self-Reports in Two Epidemiologic Studies

			Males	Females
Study		*Category*	*Sensitivity (%)*	
Nieto-García et al[19]	Age (yr)	20–29	81	82
"Obesity" based on		30–39	73	85
self-reported		40–49	69	82
weight and height*		50–59	65	81
		60–69	46	75
		70–79	38	68
Vargas et al[18]	White			
"Hypertension"	Doctor visit last year	Yes	71	73
based on self-report[†]		No	43	57
	Black			
	Doctor visit last year	Yes	80	74
		No	36	73
	Mexican American			
	Doctor visit last year	Yes	61	65
		No	21	65

*Based on data from the Lipid Research Clinics Family Study (see text); true "obesity" defined as measured body mass index $\geq$ 30 kg/m^2.

[†]Based on data from NHANES III (see text); true "hypertension" defined as measured systolic blood pressure $\geq$ 140 mm Hg, diastolic blood pressure $\geq$ 90 mm Hg, or use of antihypertensive medication.

Finally, it is important to emphasize that, as discussed previously in Section 8.3.2, the validity of some information items that are widely used in clinical settings or epidemiologic studies cannot be taken for granted. Table 8–2 shows some examples of results from validation studies of diverse clinical or medical history data, as summarized in a review by Copeland et al.[20] Note that some of the tests included in Table 8–2 suffer from poor sensitivity but have acceptable specificity, such as self-reported peptic ulcer and Rose's questionnaire definition of angina. These miss 50% or more of the cases identified by X-rays or clinical interview, respectively, while correctly identifying almost all "noncases." On the other hand, other tests suffer from the opposite problem, such as the self-report of circumcision status, which tends to identify more than 80% of truly positive cases (according to a physician's examination), while at the same time labeling a large proportion of true negatives as (false) positives (1 − specificity = 56%). The poor specificity of self-reported circumcision status underscores the fact that even items of information that would be considered highly valid because of their "objective" nature are subject to error. Further illustration is given by findings from a study by Fikree et al[29] on the validity of husbands' report of their wives' pregnancy outcomes. In this study, carried out on a sample of 857 couples selected from a working population in Burlington, Vermont, the wives' reports were used as the standard against which the husbands' reports were evaluated. The sensitivity of men's report of low birth weight pregnancies was 74%, that of spontaneous abortions was 71.2%, and that of induced abortions was 35.1%. The validity was poorer among the younger and lower educated individuals. The authors of this study concluded that it "would be prudent to avoid the use of husbands as proxy informants of their wives' reproductive histories."[29(p237)]

Youden's J Statistic

Described by Youden[30] in 1950, the J statistic is a summary index of validity that combines sensitivity and specificity. It is calculated as

J = Sensitivity + Specificity − 1.0

For example, for the data shown in Table 8–5,

$J = (18/19) + (11/30) - 1.0 = 0.947 + 0.367 - 1.0 = 0.314$ (or 31.4%)

The value 1.0 is subtracted from the sum of sensitivity and specificity so that the maximum value of the index becomes 1 when there is perfect agreement. Although theoretically the value of J can be negative, down to −1 (ie, in the presence of perfect disagreement, when the test always disagrees with the "gold standard"), a more realistic minimum for the range of J in real life is $J = 0$, obtained when the test performs no better than chance alone (ie, sensitivity and specificity = 0.5). Note that this index gives equal weight to sensitivity and specificity, thus assuming that both are equally important components of validity. For example, for the data shown in Table 8–7, the values of J for the self-reported information are 82% and 73% for "overweight" and "obese," respectively. (Note that the latter is almost identical to the estimated sensitivity of obesity based on self-report [74%] because of the almost perfect specificity [99%]—in this case, a value that is essentially canceled out by subtracting 1.0 in the calculation.)

The formulas for the calculation of the confidence interval for a J statistic estimate are provided in Appendix A, Section A.11.

Because the *J* statistic assigns equal weight to sensitivity and specificity, alternative indices need to be used when these validity components are deemed not to be equally important in a given situation.

Percent Agreement

Percent agreement between two sets of observations is obtained by dividing the number of paired observations in the agreement cells by the total number of paired observations (Figure 8–5). As an example of calculation of percent agreement, Table 8–9 shows results of repeat readings of B-mode ultrasound images of the left carotid bifurcation, conducted to examine reliability of atherosclerotic plaque identification in the ARIC study.[31] When using a binary definition of the variable (plaque or normal), as in the example shown in the table, the percent agreement can be calculated simply as

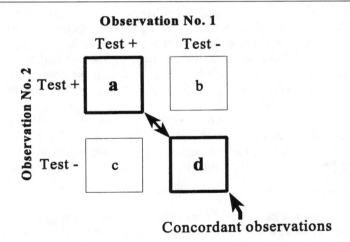

$$Percent\ agreement: \frac{(a+d)}{(a+b+c+d)} \times 100$$

Figure 8–5 Percent agreement for paired binary test results (positive vs negative) (eg, those obtained by two different observers or methods or by the same observer at two different points in time): proportion of concordant results among all tested

$$\text{Percent agreement} = \frac{140 + 725}{986} \times 100 = 87.7\%$$

Not only is the percent agreement the simplest method of summarizing agreement for categorical variables, but it has the added advantage that it can be calculated for any number of categories, not just two, as in the preceding example. Thus, in the carotid ultrasound reading reliability study,[31] readers who detected a carotid plaque were also asked to assess the presence of acoustic shadowing (an attenuation of echoes behind the plaque often reflecting the presence of plaque calcification: ie, an advanced atherosclerotic plaque). The results of the reproducibility readings of the left carotid bifurcation in this study when the finer definition of the plaque is used are shown in Table 8–10; the percent agreement in this case can be calculated as

$$\text{Percent agreement} = \frac{17 + 104 + 725}{986} \times 100 = 85.8\%$$

Results from another reliability evaluation, based on data from a study of the relationship between p53 protein overexpression and breast cancer risk factor profile, are shown in Table 8–11.[32] As part of the quality control procedures in this study, 49 breast tumor sections were stained twice, and the resulting cross-tabulation of the results after the first and second staining shows the percent agreement to be $100 \times (14 + 7 + 21)/49 = 85.7\%$.

Although the percent agreement is the epitome of reliability indices for categorical variables, it can be also used to assess validity: that is, it can be used to examine the agreement between the test results and a presumed "gold standard"; when this is done, the calculation is obvi-

---

Table 8–9 Agreement Between the First and the Second Readings To Identify Atherosclerosis Plaque in the Left Carotid Bifurcation by B-Mode Ultrasound Examination in the Atherosclerosis Risk in Communities (ARIC) Study

		First Reading		
		Plaque	Normal	Total
Second reading	Plaque	140	52	192
	Normal	69	725	794
	Total	209	777	986

Source: Data from R Li et al, Reproducibility of Extracranial Carotid Atherosclerosis Lesions Assessed by B-Mode Ultrasound: The Atherosclerosis Risk in Communities Study, *Ultrasound Med Biol*, Vol 22, pp 791–799, © 1996.

Table 8–10 Agreement Between the First and the Second Readings To Identify Atherosclerosis Plaque with or Without Acoustic Shadowing in the Left Carotid Bifurcation by B-Mode Ultrasound Examination in the Atherosclerosis Risk in Communities (ARIC) Study

		First Reading			
		P + S*	Plaque Only	Normal	Total
Second reading	P + S*	17	14	6	37
	Plaque only	5	104	46	155
	Normal	5	64	725	794
	Total	27	182	777	986

*Plaque plus (acoustic) shadowing.

Source: Data from R Li et al, Reproducibility of Extracranial Carotid Atherosclerosis Lesions Assessed by B-Mode Ultrasound: The Atherosclerosis Risk in Communities Study, *Ultrasound Med Biol,* Vol 22, pp 791–799, © 1996.

ously done without conditioning on the latter (as is the case with sensitivity/specificity calculations). For example, in Table 8–5 percent agreement is merely the percentage of the observations falling in the agreement cells over the total, or $100 \times (18 + 11)/49 = 59.2\%$. Likewise, in the validity study results shown in Table 8–6, the percent agreement between the weight categories based on self-report and measured weight and height is $100 \times (462 + 2868 + 2086 + 809)/7455 = 83.5\%$.

A limitation of the percent agreement approach is that its values tend to be high whenever the proportion of negative-negative results is high (resulting from a low prevalence of positivity in the study population), particularly when the specificity is high. For example, in Table 8–7, the percent agreement is higher for definition B (95.4%) than for definition A (91.4%), even though sensitivity was 12 points lower in B than in A (74% and 86%, respectively); this can be explained partly by the fact that the prevalence of the condition is lower in B than in A, thus inflating the negative-negative cell, and partly by the fact that the specificity is higher in B than in A (it is close to 100% for the former). As further illustration, Table 8–12 shows the hypothetical situation of a population in which the prevalence of obesity was 20 times lower than that observed in the LRC population but the sensitivity and specificity levels were *the same* as those observed in Table 8–7, definition B (except for rounding). In this situation, the percent agreement will increase from 95.4% to

Table 8–11 Reproducibility of the Staining Procedure for p53 Overexpression in 49 Breast Cancer Sections: Netherlands OC Study

		First Staining			
		p53+	p53±	p53−	Total
Second staining	p53+	14	1		15
	p53±		7	2	9
	p53−		4	21	25
	Total	14	12	23	49

Note: p53+, p53 overexpression; p53±, weak overexpression; p53−, no p53 overexpression.

Source: Data from K van der Kooy et al, p53 Protein Overexpression in Relation to Risk Factors for Breast Cancer, *American Journal of Epidemiology,* Vol 144, pp 924–933, © 1996, The Johns Hopkins University School of Hygiene & Public Health.

---

about 99%; that is, it will be almost perfect solely as a result of the decreased prevalence. Note that, in an analogous fashion, the percent agreement also tends to be high when the prevalence of the condition is very high (resulting in a high proportion of positive-positive observations), particularly when the sensitivity is high.

Table 8–12 Hypothetical Results Based on the Example Shown in Table 8–7 (Definition B), Assuming the Same Validity Figures But a Prevalence of Obesity Approximately 20 Times Lower Than That Found in the Lipid Research Clinics Population

	Measured BMI Category		
BMI Based on Self-Report	*Obese*	*Nonobese*	*Total*
Obese	41	69	110
Nonobese	14	7331	7345
Total	55	7400	7455

$$\text{Percent agreement} = \frac{(41 + 7331)}{7455} \times 100 = 98.9\%$$

$$\text{PPA}^* = \frac{2 \times 41}{(55 + 110)} \times 100 = 49.7\%$$

$$\text{Chamberlain's PPA}^* = \frac{41}{(41 + 69 + 14)} \times 100 = 33.1\%$$

*Percent positive agreement.

As for sensitivity and specificity, standard errors and confidence limits for percent agreement are calculated as for any observed proportion (see Appendix A, Section A.10).

Percent Positive Agreement

In part to overcome the limitations of the percent agreement as a reliability index when the prevalence of the condition is very low (or very high), at least two measures of *positive agreement* (PPA) have been proposed:[33]

1. *Percent positive agreement:* the number of occurrences for which both observers report a positive result, out of the average number of positives by either observer. Using the notation in Table 8–4, this is formulated as follows:

$$PPA = \frac{a}{\left(\frac{(a + c) + (a + b)}{2}\right)} \times 100 = \frac{2a}{[(a + c) + (a + b)]} \times 100 =$$

$$\frac{2a}{(2a + b + c)} \times 100$$

2. *Chamberlain's percent positive agreement:* the number of occurrences for which both observers report positive results out of the total number of observations for which at least one observer does so.[34]

$$\text{Chamberlain's PPA} = \frac{a}{(a + b + c)} \times 100$$

The calculation of these two indices is illustrated in the example shown in Table 8–12. Note that the two indices are closely related algebraically:

$$\text{Chamberlain's PPA} = \frac{PPA}{(2 - PPA)}$$

Kappa Statistic

The preceding measures of agreement have an important limitation. They do not take into account the agreement that may occur by chance alone: that is, they do not take into consideration the fact that even if both readings were completely unrelated (eg, both observers scoring at random), they would occasionally agree just by chance. A measure that corrects for this chance agreement is the kappa statistic (κ), defined as the fraction of the observed agreement not due to chance in relation to the maximum nonchance agreement when using a categorical classification of a variable.[35–37] This definition is readily grasped by consideration of the formula for the calculation of κ:

$$\kappa = \frac{P_o - P_e}{1.0 - P_e}$$

where P_o is the proportion of *observed* agreement and P_e is the chance agreement, that is, the proportion of agreement *expected* to occur by chance alone.

The κ is calculated from the cells shown in the diagonal of a cross-tabulation table, representing complete concordance between the two sets of observations. The chance agreement is the agreement that would be expected if both observers rated the responses at random. The total chance agreement is the sum of the chance agreement for each cell on the diagonal. The number expected in each cell by chance alone is the product of the corresponding marginal totals divided by the grand total. (Note that this is the same method as that used for calculating the expected values under the null hypothesis for a chi-square test in a contingency table.) For example, the chance agreement for the "plaque-plaque" cell in Table 8–9 is (209 × 192)/986, or 40.7, and that for the "normal-normal" cell is (777 × 794)/986, or 625.7. The total expected chance agreement is thus (40.7 + 625.7)/986 = 0.676. (A shortcut for the calculation of the proportion chance agreement for each cell is to divide the products of the marginals by the square of the total: that is, to combine both steps— calculation of the expected *number* and that of the expected *proportion*—into one. For example, for the data in Table 8–9, the expected proportion for the "plaque-plaque" cell is $[209 \times 192]/986^2$, and that for the "normal-normal" cell is $[777 \times 794]/986^2$. The total chance agreement is therefore $[209 \times 192 + 777 \times 794]/986^2 = 0.676$.) As the observed agreement for this table was 0.877 (see above),

$$\kappa = \frac{0.877 - 0.676}{1.0 - 0.676} = 0.62$$

Formulas for the standard error and confidence interval of kappa are given in Appendix A, Section A.12.

Possible values of kappa range from −1 to 1, although values below 0 are not very realistic in practice (the observed agreement would be worse than by chance alone). For the interpretation of a given value of kappa, different classifications have been proposed[36,38–40] (Figure 8–6). Of these, probably the most widely used is that proposed by Landis and Koch.[38] It is important to realize, however, that these clas-

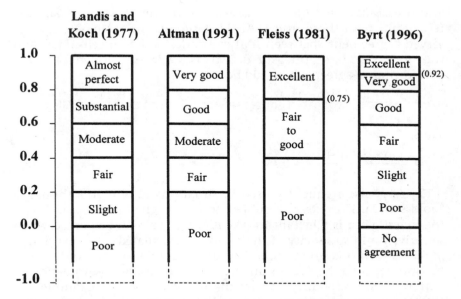

Figure 8–6 Proposed classifications for the interpretation of a kappa value

sifications are arbitrary;[41] for any given value of kappa, the degree of misclassification/bias that would result from using the corresponding instrument/reader will depend on other circumstances, such as the prevalence of the condition and the distribution of the marginals (see below).

Like the percent agreement, the kappa can be estimated from 3×3, 4×4, or $k \times k$ tables. For example, the value of kappa for the repeat readings of the ultrasound examinations of the carotid bifurcation in the ARIC study shown in Table 8–10 can be calculated as follows:

Observed agreement (see above) = 0.858

$$\text{Chance agreement} = \frac{[(27 \times 37) + (182 \times 155) + (777 \times 794)]}{(986)^2} = 0.665$$

$$\kappa = \frac{(0.858 - 0.665)}{(1 - 0.665)} = 0.576$$

Also like percent agreement, κ is primarily used for the assessment of reliability: that is, when there is no clear-cut standard and it is appropriate to give equal weight to both sets of readings. However, it is also occasionally used for the assessment of validity, to compare the test results with those from a "gold standard." In Table 8–6, the observed "agreement" between BMI categories based on self-report and the "gold standard" (measured BMI) is 0.835 (see above). The expected chance agreement would be

$$\frac{[(534 \times 640) + (3180 \times 3447) + (2650 \times 2500) + (1091 \times 868)]}{7455^2} = 0.340$$

Thus,

$$\kappa = \frac{(0.835 - 0.340)}{(1 - 0.340)} = 0.75$$

Kappa is also frequently used in situations in which, although a "gold standard" exists, it is subject to non-negligible error, and thus the investigator is reluctant to take it at face value (as assumed when sensitivity and specificity of the "test" are calculated). (As mentioned previously, in this situation, it may be preferable to refer to the comparison between the "gold standard" and the test as an evaluation of "intermethod reliability" rather than of validity). An example is a study using serum cotinine levels as the "gold standard" to assess the "validity" of reported current smoking among pregnant women; kappa between these two measures was estimated to be 0.83.[42] In this example, the "gold standard" is also subject to errors stemming from both laboratory and within-individual variability. In addition, to indirectly assess which method (self-report or serum cotinine) had better predictive validity (and reliability), the authors compared the magnitude of their correlation with an outcome known to be strongly related to maternal smoking: infant birth weight. The correlation between serum cotinine and birthweight ($r = 0.246$) was only slightly higher than that observed between smoking self-report and birthweight ($r = 0.20$), suggesting that, in this study population, serum cotinine and self-report are similarly adequate as markers of current smoking exposure. (The limitations of inferences based on the value of the correlation coefficient are discussed below; see Section 8.4.2.)

Another example of the application of kappa to evaluate intermethod reliability is a study comparing performance-based and self-rated functional capacity in an elderly population of Barcelona, Spain.[43] Selected results from this study are shown in Table 8–13. Note that the authors reported measures of both validity (sensitivity and specificity) and reliability (percent agreement and kappa), thus leaving to the reader the judgment as to whether performance evaluation at one point in time was an appropriate gold standard.

Table 8–13 Agreement Between Reported Disability and Observed Performance in a Sample of 626 Individuals Aged 72 Years and Older in Barcelona, Spain

Reported "need of help" to walk

		Performance: 4-Meter Walk			
	Unable	Able	Sensitivity*	Specificity*	% Agreement	Kappa
---	---	---	---	---	---	---
Yes	15	12	0.58	0.98	96	0.55
No	11	571				

Reported "difficulty" in walking

		Performance: 4-Meter Walk			
	Slow†	Quick†	Sensitivity	Specificity	% Agreement	Kappa
---	---	---	---	---	---	---
Yes	85	75	0.60	0.83	78	0.41
No	56	367				

Reported "difficulty" in standing up from a chair

		Performance: 5 Consecutive Rises from a Chair			
	Unable	Able	Sensitivity	Specificity	% Agreement	Kappa
---	---	---	---	---	---	---
Yes	71	41	0.63	0.92	86	0.55
No	42	455	(0.54–0.72)‡	(0.89–0.94)‡	(83–89)‡	(0.47–0.63)‡

*Sensitivity and specificity were calculated considering the physical performance test as the "gold standard."

†"Slow" and "quick" were defined according to whether the subject walked 4 meters in more or less than 7.5 seconds, respectively.

‡Confidence interval for these estimates are presented and their calculation illustrated in Appendix A, Sections A.10 and A.12.

Source: Data from M Ferrer et al, Comparison of Performance-Based and Self-Related Functional Capacity in Spanish Elderly, *American Journal of Epidemiology,* Vol 149, pp 228–235, © 1999, The Johns Hopkins University School of Hygiene & Public Health.

Extensions of the kappa statistic to evaluate the agreement between multiple ratings (or multiple repeat measurements) are available.[36] An example of this application of kappa can be found in a study assessing the reliability of diagnostic classification of emergency visits and its implications for studies of air pollution.[44] The agreement (kappa) between the diagnosis obtained from the hospital database and that made by six external raters (full-time emergency physicians) according to diagnostic category and day's pollution level was efficiently displayed by the authors (as shown in Figure 8–7).

Weighted Kappa

When study results can be expressed by more than two categories, certain types of disagreement may be more serious than others; in this situation, consideration should be given to the use of the weighted kappa. An example of its application is the comparison between self-reported and measured BMI, previously discussed (see Table 8–6). When the kappa statistic for these data was calculated above ($\kappa = 0.75$), it was assumed that only total agreement (the diagonal in Table 8–6) was worth considering: that is, any type of disagreement, regardless of its magnitude, was regarded as such. An alternative approach when calculating the value for kappa is to assign different weights to different levels of disagreement and thus to assume that they represent some sort of "partial" agreement. For example, Table 8–14 shows the same data as in Table 8–6 but also indicates that full weight (1.0) was assigned to the diagonal cells representing perfect agreement, a weight of 0.75 to disagreement between adjacent categories, a weight of 0.5 for disagreement corresponding to a "distance" of two categories, and a weight of 0 for disagreement of three categories. The calculation of the *observed agreement* in Table 8–14 is analogous to the calculation of a weighted mean in that it consists of merely multiplying the number in each cell by the corresponding weight, summing up all products, and dividing the sum by the grand total. Starting in the first row with the cell denoting "Underweight" for both assays, and proceeding from left to right in each row, the observed agreement (P_{ow}, in which the letters o and w denote "observed" and "weighted," respectively) is

$$P_{ow} = (462 \times 1 + 178 \times 0.75 + 0 + 0 + 72 \times 0.75 + 2868 \times 1 + 505 \times 0.75 + 2 \times 0.5 + 0 + 134 \times 0.75 + 2086 \times 1 + 280 \times 0.75 + 0 + 0 + 59 \times 0.75 + 809 \times 1)/7455 = 0.959$$

The calculation of P_{ow} can be simplified by rearranging this equation, grouping the cells with equal weights (and omitting those with zeros):

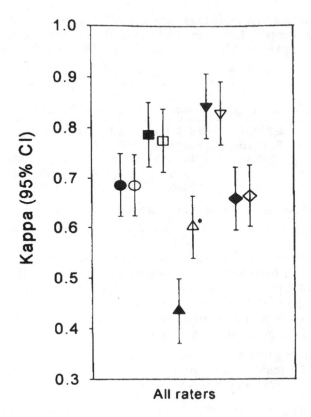

All raters

Figure 8–7 Reliability of diagnostic classification of emergency visits by diagnostic category: ratings by hospital database and six external raters. Saint John Regional Hospital emergency department database, Saint John, New Brunswick, Canada, 1994. Shaded symbols represent high-pollution days and open symbols represent low-pollution days. *, *P* (high- vs low-pollution days) = 0.0002. ●, asthma; ■, chronic obstructive pulmonary disease; ▲, respiratory infection; ▼, cardiac diseases; ◆, other. *Source:* Reprinted with permission from DM Stieb et al, Assessing Diagnostic Classification in an Emergency Department: Implications for Daily Time Series Studies of Air Pollution, *American Journal of Epidemiology,* Vol 148, pp 666–670, © 1998, The Johns Hopkins University School of Hygiene & Public Health.

$$P_{ow} = [(462 + 2868 + 2086 + 809) \times 1 + (178 + 72 + 505 + 134 + 280 + 59) \times 0.75 + (2) \times 0.5]/7455 = 0.959$$

The calculation of the *chance agreement* (P_{ew}, in which the letter e denotes "expected" by chance alone) in this example is done as fol-

Table 8–14 Calculation of Weighted Kappa: Cross-Tabulation of Self-Reported and Measured Four Body Mass Index (BMI) Categories among 7455 Adult Participants of the Lipid Research Clinics Family Study, 1975–1978 (See Table 8–6)

BMI Based on Self-Reports	Measured BMI Category				
	Underweight	Normal	Overweight	Obese	Total
Underweight	462 (1.0)*	178 (0.75)	0 (0.5)	0 (0)	640
Normal	72 (0.75)	2868 (1.0)	505 (0.75)	2 (0.5)	3447
Overweight	0 (0.5)	134 (0.75)	2086 (1.0)	280 (0.75)	2500
Obese	0 (0)	0 (0.5)	59 (0.75)	809 (1.0)	868
Total	534	3180	2650	1091	7455

*Observed number (weight for the calculation of kappa).

lows: (1) multiply the marginal totals corresponding to cells showing a weight of 1.0; then sum these products, and multiply this sum by the weight of 1.0; (2) do the same for the cells with weights of 0.75 and for the cells with weights of 0.5 (ie, including those with observed value of 0); and (3) sum all of the above, and divide the sum by the square of the grand total, as follows:

$$P_{ew} = [(534 \times 640 + 3180 \times 3447 + \ldots) \times 1 + (534 \times 3447 + \ldots) \times 0.75 + (2650 \times 640 + 1091 \times 3447 + 534 \times 2500 + 3180 \times 868) \times 0.5]/7455^2 = 0.776$$

Once the *weighted* observed and chance agreement values are obtained, the formula for the weighted kappa (κ_w) is identical to that for the unweighted kappa:

$$\kappa_w = \frac{P_{ow} - P_{ew}}{1.0 - P_{ew}}$$

Using this formula to calculate a weighted kappa for Table 8–14 yields

$$\kappa_w = \frac{0.959 - 0.776}{1.0 - 0.776} = 0.82$$

Note that in the above example, the weight of 0.5 assigned to a disagreement of two categories was used only as a hypothetical example for the calculation of weighted kappa; in real life, one would be unlikely to assign any weight at all to disagreements between such extreme categories as "obese" vs "normal" or "overweight" vs "underweight." In general, the weights assigned to cells, although somewhat arbitrary, should be chosen on the basis of the investigators' perception of how serious the disagreement is *in the context of how the data will be used.* For example, in a clinical setting where a confirmatory breast cancer diagnosis from biopsy specimens may be followed by mastectomy, nothing short of perfect agreement may be acceptable. (In practice, in this situation disagreement between two observers is usually adjudicated by an additional observer or observers.) As a different example, the inclusion of either "definite" or "probable" myocardial infarction cases in the numerator of incidence rates for analyzing associations with risk factors in a cohort study (see, eg, White et al[5]) may well be acceptable, thus justifying the use of a weighting score similar to that shown in Table 8–15 for the calculation of kappa between two raters. Note that in this example the weighting scheme was set up recognizing that the disagreement between "probable" or "definite" on the one hand and "absent" on the other is deemed to be more serious than that between "definite" and "probable." Obviously, the investigator should assign more weight to the less than to the more extreme disagreements. In the hypothetical example shown in Table 8–15, perfect agreement in myocardial infarction diagnoses between two observers was assigned a weight of 1.0 (as in the calculation of the unweighted kappa); the "definite" versus "probable" disagreement was arbitrarily assigned an "agreement" weight of 0.75, which recognized its lesser seriousness vis-à-vis the weight of 0 assigned to the disagreement between the "absent" and the other categories. If an additional and even "softer" diagnostic category, "possible," were also used, the disagreement between, for example, "definite" and "possible" might be given a smaller weight (eg, 0.5) than that assigned to the "definite-probable" cells. A similar approach could be used for the data shown in Table 8–10, in which the disagreement between the readings "plaque + shadowing" and "plaque" might not be considered as severe as that between either of the two and "normal."

Table 8–15 Agreement Weights for Calculation of Kappa: A Hypothetical Example of Classification of Myocardial Infarction by Certainty of Diagnosis

	Observer No. 1		
Observer No. 2	*Definite*	*Probable*	*Absent*
Definite	1.0	0.75	0
Probable	0.75	1.0	0
Absent	0	0	1.0

In any event, the value of weighted kappa will obviously depend on the weighting scheme that is chosen. This arbitrariness has been criticized and is one of the weaknesses of weighted kappa,[45] particularly when continuous variables are grouped into multiple ordinal categories (eg, the BMI categories in Table 8–6). In the latter case, it will be best to use certain weighting schemes for kappa* that are equivalent to the intraclass correlation coefficient described in Section 8.4.2.

Dependence of Kappa on Prevalence

An important limitation of kappa when comparing the reliability of a diagnostic procedure in different populations is its dependence on the prevalence of true "positivity" in each population.[37] Following is an example that illustrates how differences in prevalence affect the values of kappa.

Consider a given condition Y, which is to be screened independently by two observers (A and B) in two different populations I and II, each with a size of 1000 individuals. Prevalence rates in these populations are, respectively, 5% and 30%, such as can be found in younger and older target populations with regard to hypertension. Thus, the numbers of true positives are 50 for population I and 300 for population II. The sensitivity and specificity of each observer (assumed not to vary with the prevalence of Y) are, for observer A, 80% and 90%, respectively, and for observer B, 90% and 96%, respectively.

These sensitivity levels can be applied to the true positives in populations I and II to obtain the results shown in Table 8–16. For example, for population I, as seen in the row total, the sensitivity of observer A being 0.80, 40 of the 50 true positive subjects are correctly classified by him or her, whereas 10 are mistakenly classified as (false) negatives. For observer B, who has a sensitivity of 0.90, these numbers are, respectively, 45 and 5. Note that the concordance cell—that is, the number of persons who are classified as "positive" by both observers A and B—is merely the joint sensitivity applied to the total group of positive cases: for example, for population I, $(0.80 \times 0.90) \times$

---

*It has been shown (by Fleiss[36]) that for ordinal multilevel variables, when the weights, w_{ij} ($i = 1, \ldots, k; j = 1, \ldots, k$), are defined as

$$w_{ij} = 1 - \frac{(i - j)^2}{(k - 1)^2}$$

where k is the number of categories in the contingency table for the readers indexed by i and j, the value of the weighted kappa is identical to that of the intraclass correlation coefficient (see Section 8.4.2).

Table 8–16 Results of Measurements Conducted by Observers A and B in True Positives in Populations with Different Prevalence Rates of the Condition Measured, Each with a Population Size of 1000

Observer B	Population I (Prevalence = 0.05) Observer A			Population II (Prevalence = 0.30) Observer A		
	Pos	Neg	Total	Pos	Neg	Total
Pos	36**	9	45†	216**	54	270†
Neg	4	1	5	24	6	30
Total	40‡	10	50*	240‡	60	300*

*Number of true positives, obtained by multiplying the prevalence times the total population size: for example, for population I, 0.05 × 1000.

**Obtained by applying the joint sensitivity of observers A and B to the total number of true positives: for example, for population I, (0.80 × 0.90) × 50.

†Obtained by applying the sensitivity level of observer B to the total number of true positives in populations I and II: for example, for population I, 0.90 × 50.

‡Obtained by applying the sensitivity level of observer A to the total number of true positives in populations I and II: for example, for population I, 0.80 × 50.

50 = 0.72 × 50 = 36. With three of these numbers—that is, those classified as "positive" by A, those classified as "positive" by B, and those jointly classified as "positive"—it is possible to calculate the other cells in Table 8–16.

In Table 8–17, similar calculations are done for the true negatives, using the specificity values for observers A and B. Again, the number of true negatives so classified by both observers is obtained by applying the joint probability of both observers detecting a true negative (0.90 for A times 0.96 for B) to the total number of true negatives in each population: for example, in population I, (0.90 × 0.96) × 950 = 821. (Some rounding is used.)

The total results shown in Table 8–18 are obtained by summing the data from Tables 8–16 and 8–17. Kappa calculations for populations I and II, using the data shown in Table 8–18, yield the following values:

Population I

$$\kappa = \frac{0.862 - 0.804}{1.0 - 0.804} = 0.296$$

Population II

$$\kappa = \frac{0.830 - 0.577}{1.0 - 0.577} = 0.598$$

Thus, for the same sensitivity and specificity of the observers, the kappa value is greater (about twice in this example) in the population in which the prevalence of positivity is higher (Population II) than in

Table 8–17 Results of Measurements Conducted by Observers A and B in True Negatives in Populations with Different Prevalence Rates of the Condition Measured, Each with a Population Size of 1000

| | Population I (Prevalence = 5%) | | | Population II (Prevalence = 30%) | | |
| | Observer A | | | Observer A | | |
Observer B	Pos	Neg	Total	Pos	Neg	Total
Pos	4	34	38	3	25	28
Neg	91	821**	912†	67	605**	672†
Total	95	855‡	950*	70	630‡	700*

*Number of true negatives, obtained by subtracting the number of true positives (Table 8–16) from the total population size: for example, for population I, 1000 − 50.

**Obtained by applying the joint specificity of observers A and B to the total number of true negatives: for example, for population I, (0.90 × 0.96) × 950. (Results are rounded.)

†Obtained by applying the specificity level of observer B to the total number of true negatives in populations I and II: for example, for population I, 0.96 × 950.

‡Obtained by applying the specificity level of observer A to the total number of true negatives in populations I and II: for example, for population I, 0.90 × 950.

that in which it is lower (Population I). A formula that expresses the value of kappa as a function of prevalence and the sensitivity/specificity of both observers has been developed,[37] demonstrating that, for fixed sensitivity and specificity levels, kappa tends toward 0 as the prevalence approaches either 0 or 1.

An additional problem is that, paradoxically, high values of kappa can be obtained when the marginals of the contingency table are unbalanced;[46,47] thus, kappa tends to be higher when the positivity prevalence is different between observers A and B than when both observers report similar prevalence. Thus, kappa unduly rewards a differential assessment of positivity between observers.

The discussion above suggests that comparisons among populations or across different manifestations of a condition (eg, symptoms) may be unwarranted; it follows that using a specific kappa value obtained in a given target population to predict the value for another population is warranted only if prevalence rates of the condition(s) of interest are similar in both populations *and* if different raters (or repeat readings) provide reasonably similar prevalence estimates of positivity. For example, in the ARIC carotid ultrasound reliability study,[31] the authors assessed the reliability of plaque identification (with or without shadowing) not only in the carotid

Table 8–18 Results of Measurements by Observers A and B for Total Populations I and II Obtained by Combining Results from Tables 8–16 and 8–17

	Population I (Prevalence = 5%)			Population II (Prevalence = 30%)		
	Observer A			*Observer A*		
Observer B	*Pos*	*Neg*	*Total*	*Pos*	*Neg*	*Total*
Pos	40	43	83	219	79	298
Neg	95	822	917	91	611	702
Total	135	865	1000	310	690	1000

bifurcation (see Table 8–10) but also in the common and the internal carotid sites. The weighted kappa results for the three arterial segments are shown in Table 8–19. Note that both readings resulted in reasonably similar prevalence percentages of plaque for all carotid artery sites. However, note that for each reading there are important differences in plaque prevalence across sites. Thus, in comparing these kappa values across arterial segments, the authors aptly noted that "the low weighted kappa coefficient . . . in the common carotid artery may be partially due to the low prevalence of lesions in this segment."[31(pp796–797)] (On the other hand, although the prevalence is almost as low in the internal carotid as in the common carotid, the highest kappa is found in the former, probably as a function of the fact that the actual images in the internal carotid were of better quality than those in the other sites.)

Notwithstanding these limitations, kappa does provide a useful estimate of the degree of agreement between two observers or tests over and above the agreement that is expected to occur purely by chance, which explains its popularity. Furthermore, under certain conditions, and partly because of its dependence on prevalence, kappa may be useful as an index to predict the degree to which nondifferential misclassification attenuates the odds ratio:[37] that is, it can be used to assess the validity of the value of the measure of association based on data obtained with a given instrument or test.

In summary, although clearly a useful measure of reliability for categorical variables, kappa should be used and interpreted with caution. Most experts agree in recommending its use in conjunction with other measures of agreement, such as the percent agreement indices described above. When using it, however, it is important to take into consideration its variability as a function of the prevalence of the

Table 8–19 Weighted Kappa and Prevalence of Plaque (with or Without Shadowing) in Two Readings of B-Mode Ultrasound Exams in Three Carotid Artery Segments, Atherosclerosis Risk in Communities (ARIC) Study

Carotid Segment	First Reading Prevalence of Plaque %	Second Reading Prevalence of Plaque %	Weighted Kappa
Common carotid	5.0	6.0	0.47
Carotid bifurcation*	21.2	19.5	0.60
Internal carotid	7.7	7.3	0.69

*See data in Table 8–10. Note that this weighted kappa value is slightly greater than the unweighted value of 0.576 (see text).

Source: Data from R Li et al, Reproducibility of Extracranial Carotid Atherosclerosis Lesions Assessed by B-Mode Ultrasound: The Atherosclerosis Risk in Communities Study, *Ultrasound Med Biol*, Vol 22, pp 791–799, © 1996.

condition and of the degree of similarity between observers with regard to the prevalence of positivity.[31,33,41,47]

8.4.2   Indices of Validity/Reliability of Continuous Data

This section describes some of the available methods to evaluate the validity and/or the reliability of a given continuous measurement. The indices most frequently used for these purposes are listed in Table 8–3 and will be briefly described below. As indicated in Table 8–3, some of these indices can be used for the assessment of validity (eg, when measurements in serum samples done in a certain laboratory are compared to measurements in the same samples obtained at a reference laboratory; see Section 8.3.2), whereas others are more often used in reliability studies (eg, for assessment of within-observer, between-observer, or within-individual repeated measurements of a continuous parameter; see Section 8.3.3).

The data shown in Table 8–20 will be used to illustrate the reliability measures discussed in this section. Shown in this table are partial data obtained during a reliability study of polysomnography (PSG) scoring in the Sleep Heart Health Study (SHHS) project, a population-based study of the cardiovascular consequences of sleep-disordered breathing (eg, sleep apnea).[48] In the SHHS, the PSG recordings obtained from 6440 participants in six field centers were sent to a central reading center for scoring (sleep staging and calculation of indices of sleep-disordered breathing). The design and results of the reliability study conducted in the SHHS have been described in detail[49] and have included both the within- and between-scorer reliability of sleep-disordered breathing variables and sleep staging. For the purposes of this example, Table 8–20 shows only data on two measures of sleep-disordered breathing (apnea-hypopnea index, AHI, and arousal index, AI) for 30 PSG studies that were read by two of the scorers (scorers A and B) to assess between-scorer reliability, as well as 10 studies that were read twice by one of the scorers (scorer A) as part of the within-scorer reliability study.

The validity/reliability measures described in the next paragraphs are of one of two types. The first type consists of indices based on assessing the *correlation* between the two sets of values being compared (correlation plot, correlation coefficients). The second type consists of measures based on the *pairwise comparison* of the two measures being compared (mean difference, coefficient of variation, and Bland-Altman plot).

Correlation Graph (Scatter Diagram)

The simplest way to compare two sets of readings is merely to plot the values for each method and carefully examine the patterns observed in the scatter plot. For example, Figures 8–8A and 8–8B show the correlation between the AHI and AI values obtained by scorers A and B. Figures 8–8C and 8–8D correspond to the within-scorer reliability: that is, these charts show the AHI and AI values resulting from the 10 repeat readings done by scorer A. They show that AHI readings (Figures 8–8A and 8–8C) are strongly correlated (as expressed by their being almost perfectly superimposed to the 45° lines, which corresponds to a perfect agreement). For AI, although there appears to be a correlation, a significant scatter is seen around the ideal 45° lines. (The diagonals or identity lines in Figure 8–8 (going through the origin with a 45° slope) are equivalent to regression lines (see Chapter 7, Section 7.4.1) with intercept = 0 and regression coefficient = 1.0 unit.)

Although simple correlation graphs are useful to get a sense of the degree of agreement between two measures, they are not as sensitive as alternative graphic techniques (see Bland-Altman plot below) for the detection of certain patterns in the data.

Linear Correlation Coefficient, Rank Correlation, Linear Regression

Pearson's product-moment correlation coefficient (usually denoted by r) is a measure of the degree to which a set of paired observations in a scatter diagram approaches the situation in which every point falls exactly on a straight line.[39,50] The possible range of values of r is

Table 8–20 Data for a Reliability Study of Scoring of Sleep-Breathing Disorders Variables Obtained from Home Polysomnography Recordings

	Apnea-Hypopnea Index*			Arousal Index†		
	Scorer A		Scorer B	Scorer A		Scorer B
Study No.	First Reading	Second Reading		First Reading	Repeat Reading	
1	1.25	0.99	1.38	7.08	7.65	8.56
2	1.61	1.57	2.05	18.60	23.72	19.91
3	5.64	5.60	5.50	20.39	39.18	25.17
4	0.00	0.32	0.00	16.39	26.77	22.68
5	12.51	11.84	11.03	27.95	22.64	17.21
6	22.13	21.64	21.34	29.57	34.20	27.15
7	2.68	1.77	2.39	13.50	14.31	18.66
8	2.19	2.18	2.04	24.50	21.35	20.58
9	8.52	8.67	8.64	14.63	13.42	15.61
10	0.33	0.16	0.16	11.15	13.12	13.10
11	0.00		0.00	19.52		19.05
12	2.70		2.46	18.91		18.59
13	3.03		2.11	17.98		10.78
14	3.49		3.30	15.78		12.64
15	1.12		0.98	0.00		7.04
16	4.94		4.09	8.15		10.75
17	9.52		8.47	20.36		20.61
18	27.90		25.47	36.62		34.90
19	5.58		5.21	18.31		20.84
20	6.59		6.94	17.56		24.28
21	1.08		1.32	8.14		22.94
22	5.46		5.16	17.30		19.38
23	0.00		0.00	16.39		22.68
24	2.32		1.64	29.29		65.09
25	1.93		1.38	18.80		18.75
26	17.68		18.74	10.92		20.97
27	2.54		1.70	12.53		13.38
28	6.50		6.34	24.94		43.92
29	2.09		2.35	18.66		18.02
30	11.09		9.25	12.50		23.25

└---Within scorer---┘   └---Within scorer---┘
└-----------Between scorer---------------┘   └-------------Between scorer---------------┘

Note: Partial data obtained as part of a formal reliability study in the Sleep Heart Health Study.[48,49] These data, kindly provided by the SHHS investigators, are presented for didactic purposes. Derived validity/reliability indices are not to be interpreted as an accurate and complete representation of the reliability of the scoring procedures in the SHHS, for which readers are referred to the original report.[49]

*Apnea-hypopnea index: average number of apnea and hypopnea episodes per hour of sleep (apnea, cessation of airflow for ≥10 seconds; hypopnea, decrease in airflow or thoracoabdominal excursion of ≥30% for ≥10 seconds, accompanied by a ≥4% decrease in oxygen saturation).

†Arousal index: average number of sleep arousals per hour of sleep.

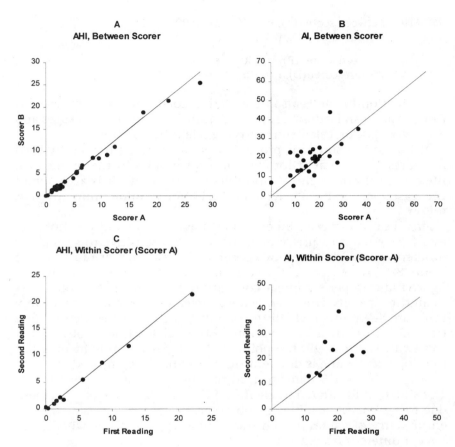

Figure 8–8 Scatter diagrams for between- and within-scorer reliability for data shown on Table 8–20. A: between-scorer AHI values (scorers A and B); B: between-scorer AI values (scorers A and B); C: within-scorer AHI values for repeat readings by scorer A; D: within-scorer AI values for repeat readings by scorer A. The straight diagonal lines in these plots represent the identity lines, that is, where the points would be if agreement was perfect. AHI and AI are expressed as the averge number of episodes per hour of sleep.

from -1 (when there is a perfect negative correlation between the two observers) to 1 (when there is a perfect positive correlation). The closer the r values are to 0, the weaker the correlation (either negative or positive) between the two sets of values. For example, the r values for the scatter diagrams in Figure 8–8 are

AHI: Between scorer (A), n = 30: $r = 0.995$
     Within scorer (C), n =10: $r = 0.999$

AI: Between scorer (B), n =30: $r = 0.655$
    Within scorer (D), n =10: $r = 0.710$

Calculation of the Pearson correlation coefficient is fairly straightforward and can be done using most available statistical packages and even most pocket calculators carrying scientific functions.

Although Pearson's r is probably one of the most frequently used measures of agreement for continuous variables in the biomedical literature (in both validity and reliability studies), it is also one of the least appropriate.[51-54] Its main limitations can be summarized as follows.

First, Pearson's r is an index of linear association, but it is not necessarily a good measure of agreement. It is insensitive to systematic differences (bias) between two observers or readings, as illustrated in Figure 8–9. The values of the correlation coefficients ($r = 1.0$) in this figure indicate perfect linear correlation between the two observers in all three panels. However, perfect agreement of values occurs only in Figure 8–9A, in which all the observations fall in the identity line (ie, for each pair of observations, observer B value = observer A value). In Figure 8–9B, the points fall in a perfect straight line, but the slope of the line is different from 1.0: that is, compared with observer A, observer B tends to read the higher values at lower levels. The situation illustrated in Figure 8–9C also shows lack of agreement due to systematic readings by observer B at higher levels across the entire range of values (which results in a regression line with an intercept different from zero).

The latter situation (Figure 8–9C) is particularly likely in the presence of systematic differences among readers, drifts over time in the readers' ability to apply the study criteria, wearing out of reactives used in certain laboratory techniques, and so forth. In these situations, the exclusive use of Pearson's r may produce a misleading assessment of agreement. A real-life example relates to the LRC data (see Tables 8–6 and 8–7), in which the Pearson correlation coefficient between "self-reported" and "measured" BMI was found to be 0.96. Other studies have shown similarly strong correlations between these approaches of measuring BMI, leading some authors to conclude that "self-reported weights were remarkably accurate across all these variables . . . and may obviate the need for measured weights in epidemiological investigations."[55] This conclusion may be misleading, however, because even though the correlation is high, there is a

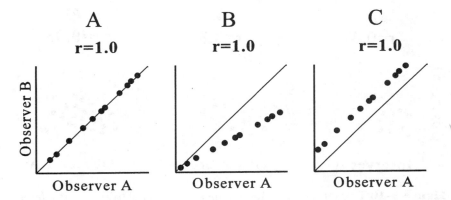

Figure 8–9 Correlation coefficients are equally high when both observers read the same value (A) and when there is a systematic difference between observers but readings vary simultaneously (B and C).

systematic tendency of individuals to underestimate their weights (usually paralleled by an overestimation of their heights). As a result, in Table 8–6 there is a larger number of individuals above (and to the right) of the perfect agreement diagonal than below it. It follows that if the BMI based on self-reports is to be used to define categorical variables of obesity or relative weight, this systematic error will result in less than perfect agreement (and thus misclassification), as indicated by the values of sensitivity and kappa calculated from data from the LRC study in Table 8–6.

Second, the value of r is very sensitive to the range of values. The influence of the range of values on the Pearson's r is illustrated in Figures 8–10A and 8–10B. In this hypothetical example, both readers are assumed to be similarly reliable. Nonetheless, because sample values have a broader distribution in Figure 8–10B than in Figure 8–10A, the correlation coefficients will be higher for the former. This can also be illustrated using real data from Figure 8–8B. As mentioned above, Pearson's r for the total set of 30 repeat readings of AI by scorers A and B was 0.655. If, however, this set is split into two subsets, one including the studies in which scorer B read values of AI < 15 per hour (n = 8) and another in which scorer B read values of AI > 15 per hour (n = 22), the correlation coefficients are estimated at 0.59 and 0.51, respectively: that is, *both r's* are *smaller* than the r based on the entire set of 30 observations, which does not make a lot of intuitive sense.

As a corollary of its dependence on the range of values, Pearson's correlation coefficient is unduly sensitive to extreme values (outliers).

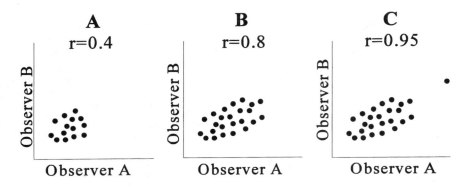

Figure 8–10 Pearson's correlation coefficient is very sensitive to the range of values and to the presence of outliers (extreme values). Hypothetical examples.

Thus, for example, Figure 8–10C is a repetition of Figure 8–10B, but with one additional observation with an extreme value; this outlier has an enormous influence in defining the regression line and the value of the correlation coefficient, which increases from 0.8 in Figure 8–10B to 0.95 in Figure 8–10C.

Despite its undesirable properties, Pearson's correlation coefficient is often used as the main, if not the sole, measure of reliability reported in biomedical or epidemiologic studies. This may have to do with tradition, pattern recognition, and imitation ("Everybody uses it").[52] Some argue that r is an appropriate measure for reliability studies when the objective is to see whether two different sets of readings would classify (order) subjects in the same manner; thus, if Pearson's r is high, it would be justified to use the distribution of study values to classify subjects. If that is the case, however, the *Spearman correlation coefficient* (also called "ordinal" or "rank correlation coefficient" and denoted by r_S) is more appropriate. This coefficient takes the value of $+1$ when the paired ranks are exactly in the same order, a value of -1 when the ranks are exactly in an inverse order, and a value of 0 when there is no correlation between the ordering of the two sets of paired values. For example, the r_S values for the scatter diagrams in Figure 8–8 are 0.984 (AHI, between), 0.58 (AI, between), 0.976 (AHI, within), and 0.757 (AI, within). Although more congruous with the goal of assessing consistency of the ranking and less influenced by outlying values, the Spearman correlation coefficient does not address the other limitation discussed above for Pearson's r, namely its insensitivity to lack of agreement due to systematic differences in values between the readers.

Finally, because of its relatively frequent occurrence in the biomedical literature, it is worth discussing the use of statistical significance testing to evaluate a correlation coefficient (Pearson or Spearman) in the context of validity/reliability studies. The calculation of a P value for a correlation coefficient (ie, evaluating the null hypothesis H_0: $r = 0.0$) is not useful in this context for both theoretical and practical reasons: (1) the null hypothesis—that there is *no relation* between two tests (or two observers) supposedly measuring the *same* variable or construct is illogical, so demonstrating that it can be rejected is not very informative; (2) even when the reliability is fairly poor (eg, $r \leq 0.3$ or 0.4), the corresponding P value may well be "significant" if the sample size is reasonably large. Thus, a highly significant P value may be mistakenly interpreted as evidence of "high reliability" when in fact its only interpretation is that it is relatively safe to reject a (meaningless, anyway) null hypothesis. Testing the hypothesis of quasi-perfect correlation (eg, H_0: $r = 0.95$) has been proposed as an alternative and more useful approach.[53] Another logical alternative is to calculate confidence limits for the value of the correlation coefficient rather than its associated P value.

The preceding discussion suggests that the correlation coefficient should be used judiciously. More specifically, its interpretation is greatly enhanced by a consideration of possible systematic differences between measurements. The use of a scatter diagram of the data is helpful in detecting these systematic differences, the presence of outlying values, and differences between variables with regard to the range of their values. Other indices of reliability that avoid some of the pitfalls inherent to Pearson's r are discussed next.

An alternative to Pearson's r is *linear regression,* which provides a measure of the regression function's intercept and slope (see Chapter 7, Section 7.4.1), thus allowing the assessment of situations such as those illustrated in Figure 8–9, in which the intercept is not zero or in which there is a systematic difference between readers. Linear regression, however, is not problem-free when used to analyze reliability data: for example (and importantly), it neglects the fact that measurement errors occur in this case for both dependent and independent variables.[51] (In ordinal linear regression, the so-called "independent" variable, x, is assumed to be error-free, and only errors (statistical variability) in the "dependent" variable are considered; see Chapter 7, Section 7.4.1.) Linear regression is more useful for "calibration" purposes than to assess reliability: that is, it is more useful to predict outcomes or to obtain "corrected" values once a systematic difference is identified and quantified.

Intraclass Correlation Coefficient

The intraclass correlation coefficient (ICC) or reliability coefficient (R) is an estimate of the fraction of the total measurement variability due to variation among individuals.[36,54] Ideally, an epidemiologic study should use highly standardized procedures and data collection methods known to be valid and reliable. Under these optimal circumstances, most of the variability can be attributed to differences among study participants (between-individual variability) (see Section 8.3.3).

The general formula for the ICC is thus

$$ICC = \frac{V_b}{V_T} = \frac{V_b}{V_b + V_e}$$

in which V_b = variance between individuals, V_t = total variance, which includes both V_b and V_e, and V_e = unwanted variance ("error"). V_e will include different components depending on the design of the study (see Figure 8–3). For example, in a within-laboratory reliability study, it will include the variance due to laboratory/method error. In a within-individual reliability study (ie, repeat readings or determinations by the same reader or technique obtained in the same individual), it will be the estimated variance within individuals. It can also be combinations of these, as, for example, in a study assessing both the laboratory and within-individual variability of hemostasis and inflammation plasma parameters.[55]

The ICC is equivalent to the kappa statistic for continuous variables and has the same range of possible values (from −1.0—or more realistically, from 0—to +1.0, in case of perfect agreement). It has the advantage over the Pearson's or Spearman's correlation coefficient in that it is a true measure of agreement, combining information on both the correlation and the systematic differences between readings.[54] However, as in the case of Pearson's correlation coefficient, ICC is affected by the range of values in the study population. Note in the above formula that when V_b is small, ICC also will be small. This is particularly important in studies within populations in which the exposure values are either very high or very low. For example, a high intake of animal fat in some populations may result in uniformly high serum cholesterol levels. A low reliability coefficient resulting from a small variability of the exposure levels may negatively influence the power of an epidemiologic study and thus make it difficult to assess an association. Obviously, the ICC will also be low when there is substantial intraindividual variability of the factor of interest, as in the case of gonadal hormone levels in premenopausal women.

ICC can be calculated from an analysis of variance (ANOVA) table, although a more simple formula based on the standard deviations of the two sets of observations and the sum and the standard deviation of the paired differences has been provided[54] (see Appendix E). Based on this formula, for example, the ICC for the between-reader reliability study data shown in Table 8–20 can be estimated as 0.99 for AHI and 0.58 for AI. Like kappa, the ICC can also be extended to calculate the reliability between more than two observers or readings. For example, in the actual (full) reliability study of sleep scoring in the SHHS,[49] the reported ICC between the three scorers was 0.99 for AHI and 0.54 for AI.

As an additional example, Table 8–21 shows the ICC for three lipid measurements in a sample of the Atherosclerosis Risk in Communities (ARIC) study cohort baseline examination.[23] The high ICC obtained for total cholesterol and total HDL cholesterol in this study suggests that the proportion of the variance due to within-individual variability or laboratory problems for these analytes is small; on the other hand, the ICC for an HDL fraction (HDL_2) was found to be much lower.

Table 8–21 Intraclass Correlation Coefficients (ICCs) and Coefficients of Variation (CVs) for Selected Analytes in the Atherosclerosis Risk in Communities (ARIC) Study

Analyte	ICC	CV (%)*
Total cholesterol	0.94	5.1
HDL cholesterol	0.94	6.8
HDL_2	0.77	24.8

*Includes both within-individual and laboratory variability.

Source: Data from LE Chambless et al, Short-Term Intraindividual Variability in Lipoprotein Measurements: The Atherosclerosis Risk in Communities (ARIC) Study, *American Journal of Epidemiology*, Vol 136, pp 1069–1081, © 1992, The Johns Hopkins University School of Hygiene & Public Health.

Mean Difference and Paired t Test

The average of the differences between the two values of the pairs of observations is a measure of the degree of *systematic* differences between the two sets of readings. A paired *t*-test statistic* can be performed to calculate the statistical significance of the calculated difference.

This index is typically used when assessing *validity*, as it provides a direct estimate of the degree of *bias* for one of the sets of measurements when it is justified to use the other set as a gold standard. On the other hand, it can be also used in the context of paired *reliability* studies, as when assessing systematic differences between readers of a test. For example, for the between-reader reliability study in Table 8–20, the mean differences between the first readings by scorer A and scorer B's readings were 0.367 (SD = 0.703) for AHI and –3.327 (SD = 8.661) for AI. Although their magnitude is rather small, particularly for AHI, both differences are statistically significant at conventional levels ($P < 0.05$), thus suggesting the existence of systematic between-scorer variability. In Whitney et al's report[49] this index was used to assess within-scorer reliability.

Caution should be exercised when using the mean difference as a measure of validity or reliability without a careful examination of the data (eg, looking at a scatter diagram or a Bland-Altman plot; see below), as its value can be heavily dependent on extreme values.

Coefficient of Variability

Another index of reliability often used in epidemiologic studies is the coefficient of variability (CV), which is the standard deviation expressed as a percentage of the mean value of two sets of paired observations. In an analysis of reliability data, it is calculated for each pair of observations and then averaged over all pairs of original and replicate measures. Its estimation is very straightforward. The variance of each pair of measurements is

$$V_i = \sum_{j=1}^{2} (x_{ij} - \bar{x}_i)^2$$

in which i is a given pair of repeat measurements (indexed by j) on the same sample or individual, x_{i1} and x_{i2} are the values of these two measurements, and $\bar{x}_i$ is their mean.

---

*A paired *t*-test statistic can be calculated simply by dividing the mean value of all paired differences by its standard error (ie, the standard deviation over the square root of the sample size):

$$t \text{ test} = \frac{\bar{x}_{1-2}}{s_{1-2}/\sqrt{n}}$$

The standard deviation (SD) for each pair of observations is the square root of V_i, so for each pair of measurements, the CV (expressed as a percentage) is

$$CV_i = \frac{SD_i}{\overline{x}_i} \times 100$$

For example, for the last pair (pair no. 30) of between-scorer readings of AHI in Table 8–20 (11.09 and 9.25, mean 10.17), these calculations are as follows:

$$V_{30} = (11.09 - 10.17)^2 + (9.25 - 10.17)^2 = 1.693$$

with the resulting coefficient of variability for that pair,

$$CV_{30} = \frac{\sqrt{1.693}}{10.17} \times 100 = 12.8\%$$

This calculation would have to be repeated for all pairs of measurements, and the overall coefficient of variation would be the average of all pairwise CVs. The lower the CV, the less variation there is between the replicate measurements. Obviously, if there were no differences whatsoever between paired values (perfect agreement), the CV value would be zero. For example, the overall between-scorer CV values for all 30 paired observations shown in Table 8–20 are 10.1% for AHI and 22.8% for AI. In addition to the ICCs discussed previously, Table 8–21 shows the CVs for serum total cholesterol, HDL cholesterol, and HDL_2 in the ARIC cohort reliability study.[23] Consistently with the ICCs, CVs are fairly low for total cholesterol and total HDL but high for the HDL fraction, HDL_2, indicating substantial imprecision in the measurement of the latter fraction.

Bland-Altman Plot

This is a very useful graphical technique that is a good complement to the ordinary scatter diagram (see above) for the examination of patterns of disagreement between repeated measurements (or between a given measurement and the "gold standard"). It consists of a scatter plot where the difference between the paired measurements ($A - B$ in the ordinate) is plotted against their mean value [$(A + B)/2$, in the abscissa]. From this plot, it is much easier than in a regular scatter diagram to assess the magnitude of disagreement (including systematic differences), spot outliers, and to see whether there is any trend.[51,52] For example, Figures 8–11A and 8–11B show the Bland-Altman plots for the between-scorer measurements of AHI and AI data from Table 8–20. Note that, compared with the corresponding scatter diagrams (Figures 8–8A and 8–8B), these pictures reveal more clearly some interesting features of the data:

- There is a slight systematic difference between the two measurements, as represented by the departure from zero of the horizontal line corresponding to the mean difference.
- Outliers may be present: in Figure 8–11, there is one measurement with mean AHI greater than 25 and one with mean AI greater than 40 that are clearly outside the range of mean difference ±2 SD.
- The graphs provide a clearer idea of the magnitude of disagreement in comparison with the actual measurement. In Figure 8–11A, for example, all but one (or perhaps two or three) AHI mean differences are within the (mean ±2 SD) range, which spans approximately 3 AHI units; the latter is a relatively low value in the range of AHI values in the abscissa. In contrast, the (mean difference ±2 SD) range for AI (Figure 8–11B), while containing also all but one observation, spans almost 35 AI units, which is practically the entire range of AI values observed in these individuals.
- The AHI plot in Figure 8–11A suggests that disagreement between the scorers increases as the actual value of AHI increases. This pattern is not as evident for AI, however (Figure 8–11B).

Notice that if this graphic approach is used when one of the measurements can be considered a gold standard, one may want to repre-

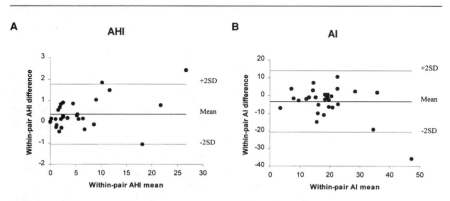

Figure 8–11 Bland-Altman plots for AHI and AI for the between-scorer reliability study data from Table 8–20. The horizontal lines represent the mean within-pair difference (0.367 and −3.327, for AHI and AI, respectively) and the mean ±2 standard deviations (1 SD = 0.703 for AHI and 8.661 for AI). AHI and AI are expressed as the average number of episodes per hour of sleep.

sent the latter in the abscissa instead of the mean of both measurements. In this case, the vertical departure from zero will represent the magnitude of bias of the test value with respect to the gold standard.

8.5 REGRESSION TO THE MEAN

The phenomenon known as *regression to the mean* permeates many of the problems and analytical approaches described in the previous sections and deserves a brief discussion here. This is a well known phenomenon, aptly discussed by Oldham in 1962,[56] which expresses the tendency for high values of continuous variables (eg, blood pressure) measured at any given point in time to decrease, and for low values to increase, when repeated measurements are done. This tendency may result from either intra-individual variability (as illustrated in Figure 8–2) or random measurement errors. As an example, when measurements of blood pressure levels in a group of individuals are repeated, many values converge (*regress*) toward the mean. A corollary of this is that caution is needed when analyzing data on repeated measurements over time and when analyzing data correlation with baseline values.[57] In addition, regression to the mean underscores the desirability of using the average of repeated measurements rather than single measurements for physiological parameters that fluctuate (as is the case of blood pressure, among many other examples). This is particularly important in studies in which a cutoff point is used as a study inclusion criterion, such as the cutoff to define hypertension in clinical trials of hypertension management. Many individuals eligible on the basis of one measurement would not be eligible if the mean of repeated measurements of systolic blood pressure was used instead. Regression to the mean also may occur in other situations, such as in a case-control study in which cases are individuals classified as hypertensive and controls are those classified as normotensive. If the classification of cases and controls was based on a single blood pressure measurement for each individual, misclassification because of regression to the mean might ensue and result in *regression dilution bias* (see Chapter 4, Section 4.3.3).

REFERENCES

1. Kahn HA, Sempos CT. *Statistical Methods in Epidemiology.* New York, NY: Oxford University Press; 1989.
2. Whitney CW, Lind BK, Wahl PW. Quality assurance and quality control in longitudinal studies. *Epidemiol Rev.* 1998;20:71–80.

3. ARIC Investigators. The Atherosclerosis Risk in Communities (ARIC) study: design and objectives. *Am J Epidemiol.* 1989;129:687–702.

4. Prineas RJ, Crow RS, Blackburn H. *The Minnesota Code Manual of Electrocardiographic Findings.* Littleton, Mass: John Wright PSG; 1982.

5. White AD, Folsom AR, Chambless LE, et al. Community surveillance of coronary heart disease in the Atherosclerosis Risk in Communities (ARIC) study: methods and initial two years' experience. *J Clin Epidemiol.* 1996;49:223–233.

6. Sudman S, Bradburn NM. *Asking Questions.* San Francisco, Calif: Jossey-Bass Publishers; 1982.

7. Converse JM, Presser S. *Survey Questions: Handcrafting the Standardized Questionnaire.* Newbury Park, Calif: Sage Publications; 1986.

8. Rose GA. Chest pain questionnaire. *Milbank Mem Fund Q.* 1965;43:32–39.

9. Comstock GW, Tockman MS, Helsing KJ, et al. Standardized respiratory questionnaires: comparison of the old with the new. *Am Rev Respir Dis.* 1979;119:45–53.

10. Burt VL, Culter JA, Higgins M, et al. Trends in the prevalence, awareness, treatment, and control of hypertension in the adult US population: data from the health examination surveys, 1960 to 1991. *Hypertension.* 1995;26:60–69.

11. Block G, Hartman AM, Dresser CM, et al. A data-based approach to diet questionnaire design and testing. *Am J Epidemiol.* 1986;124:453–469.

12. Willett WC, Sampson L, Stampfer MJ, et al. Reproducibility and validity of a semiquantitative food frequency questionnaire. *Am J Epidemiol.* 1985;122:51–65.

13. Dickersin K, Berlin JA. Meta-analysis: state-of-the-science. *Epidemiol Rev.* 1992;14: 154–176.

14. Gordis L. *Epidemiology.* Philadelphia, Pa: WB Saunders; 1996.

15. Lippel K, Ahmed S, Albers JJ, et al. External quality-control of cholesterol analyses performed by 12 lipid research clinics. *Clin Chem.* 1978;24:1477–1484.

16. Burke GL, Sprafka JM, Folsom AR, et al. Trends in serum cholesterol levels from 1980 to 1987: the Minnesota Heart Survey. *New Engl J Med.* 1991;324:941–946.

17. Brinton LA, Hoover RN, Szklo M, et al. Menopausal estrogen use and risk of breast cancer. *Cancer.* 1981;47:2517–2522.

18. Vargas CM, Burt VL, Gillum RF, Pamuk ER. Validity of self-reported hypertension in the National Health and Nutrition Survey III, 1988–91. *Prev Med.* 1997;26: 678–685.

19. Nieto-García FJ, Bush TL, Keyl PM. Body mass definitions of obesity: sensitivity and specificity using self-reported weight and height. *Epidemiology.* 1990;1:146–152.

20. Copeland KT, Checkoway H, McMichael AJ, et al. Bias due to misclassification in the estimation of relative risk. *Am J Epidemiol.* 1977;105:488–495.

21. Block G. A review of validation of dietary assessment methods. *Am J Epidemiol.* 1982;115:492–505.

22. Martin-Moreno JM, Boyle P, Gorgojo L, Maisonneuve P, Fernandez-Rodriguez JC, Salvini S, Willett WC. Development and validation of a food frequency questionnaire in Spain. *Int J Epidemiol.* 1993;22:512–519.

23. Chambless LE, McMahon RP, Brown SA, Patsch W, Heiss G, Shen Y-L. Short-term intraindividual variability in lipoprotein measurements: the Atherosclerosis Risk in Communities (ARIC) study. *Am J Epidemiol.* 1992;136:1069–1081.

24. Colditz GA, Willet WC, Stampfer MJ, Sampson L, Rosner B, Hennekens CH, Speizer FE. The influence of age, relative weight, smoking, and alcohol intake on the reproducibility of a dietary questionnaire. *Int J Epidemiol.* 1987;16:392–398.

25. Sackett DL. *Clinical Epidemiology: A Basic Science for Clinical Medicine.* Boston, Mass: Little, Brown; 1991.

26. Fletcher RH, Fletcher SW, Wagner EH. *Clinical Epidemiology: The Essentials.* 2nd ed. Baltimore, Md: Williams & Wilkins; 1988.

27. Ransohoff DF, Feinstein AR. Problems of spectrum and bias in evaluating the efficacy of diagnostic tests. *N Engl J Med.* 1978;299:926–930.

28. Brenner H, Gefeller O. Variation of sensitivity, specificity, likelihood ratios and predictive values with disease prevalence. *Stat Med.* 1997;16:981–991.

29. Fikree FF, Gray RH, Shah F. Can men be trusted? A comparison of pregnancy histories reported by husbands and wives. *Am J Epidemiol.* 1993;138:237–242.

30. Youden WJ. Index for rating diagnostic tests. *Cancer.* 1950;3:32–35.

31. Li R, Cai J, Tegeler C, et al. Reproducibility of extracranial carotid atherosclerosis lesions assessed by B-mode ultrasound: the Atherosclerosis Risk in Communities study. *Ultrasound Med Biol.* 1996;22:791–799.

32. van der Kooy K, Rookus MA, Peterse HL, van Leeuwen FE. p53 protein overexpression in relation to risk factors for breast cancer. *Am J Epidemiol.* 1996;144:924–933.

33. Cicchetti DV, Feinstein AR. High agreement but low kappa: II. Resolving the paradoxes. *J Clin Epidemiol.* 1990;43:551–558.

34. Chamberlain J, Ginks S, Rogers P, et al. Validity of clinical examinations in mammography as screening tests for breast cancer. *Lancet.* 1975;2:1026–1030.

35. Cohen JA. A coefficient of agreement for nominal scales. *Educ Psychol Meas.* 1960; 20:37–46.

36. Fleiss JL. *Statistical Methods for Rates and Proportions.* 2nd ed. New York, NY: John Wiley and Sons; 1981.

37. Thompson WD, Walter SD. A reappraisal of the kappa coefficient. *J Clin Epidemiol.* 1988;41:949–958.

38. Landis JR, Koch GG. The measurement of observer agreement for categorical data. *Biometrics.* 1977;33:159–174.

39. Altman DG. *Practical Statistics for Medical Research.* London, England: Chapman and Hall; 1991.

40. Byrt T. How good is agreement. *Epidemiology.* 1996;7:561.

41. Siegel DG, Podgor MJ, Remaley NA. Acceptable values of kappa for comparison of two groups. *Am J Epidemiol.* 1992;135:571–578.

42. Klebanoff MA, Levine RJ, Clemens JD, et al. Serum cotinine concentration and reported smoking among pregnant women. *Am J Epidemiol.* 1998;148:259–262.

43. Ferrer M, Lamarca R, Orfila F, Alonso J. Comparison of performance-based and self-rated functional capacity in Spanish elderly. *Am J Epidemiol.* 1999;149:228–235.

44. Stieb DM, Beveridge RC, Rowe BH, et al. Assessing diagnostic classification in an emergency department: implications for daily time series studies of air pollution. *Am J Epidemiol.* 1998;148:666–670.

45. Maclure M, Willett WC. Misinterpretation and misuse of the kappa statistic. *Am J Epidemiol.* 1987;126:161–169.

46. Feinstein AR, Cicchetti DV. High agreement but low kappa: I. The problems of two paradoxes. *J Clin Epidemiol*. 1990;43:543–549.

47. Byrt T, Bishop J, Carlin JB. Bias, prevalence and kappa. *J Clin Epidemiol*. 1993;46: 423–429.

48. Quan SF, Howard BV, Iber C, et al. The Sleep Heart Health Study: design, rationale and methods. *Sleep*. 1997;20:1077–1085.

49. Whitney CW, Gottlieb DJ, Redline S, et al. Reliability of scoring disturbance indices and sleep staging. *Sleep*. 1998;21:749–757.

50. Armitage P, Berry G. *Statistical Methods in Medical Research*. 3rd ed. London: Blackwell; 1994.

51. Altman DG, Bland JM. Measurement in medicine: the analysis of method comparison studies. *Statistician*. 1983;32:307–317.

52. Bland JM, Altman DG. Statistical methods for assessing agreement between two methods of clinical measurement. *Lancet*. 1986;1:307–310.

53. Hebert JR, Miller DR. The inappropriatenesss of conventional use of the correlation coefficient in assessing validity and reliability of dietary assessment methods. *Eur J Epidemiol*. 1991;7:339–343.

54. Deyo RA, Diehr P, Patrick DL. Reproducibility and responsiveness of health statistics measures: statistics and strategies for evaluation. *Controlled Clin Trials*. 1991;12:142S–158S.

55. Sakkinen PA, Macy EM, Callas P, et al. Analytical and biologic variability in measures of hemostasis, fibrinolysis, and inflammation: assessment and implications for epidemiology. *Am J Epidemiol*. 1999;149:261–267.

56. Oldham PE. A note on the analysis of repeated measurements of the same subjects. *J Chron Dis*. 1962;15:969–977.

57. Nieto-García FJ, Edwards LA. On the spurious correlation between changes in blood pressure and initial values. *J Clin Epidemiol*. 1990;43:727–728.

PART V

Issues of Reporting

CHAPTER 9

Communicating Results of Epidemiologic Studies

9.1 INTRODUCTION

Oral and written communication of research results is not only frequently full of specialized jargon but also often characterized by systematic mistakes that might properly be classified as biases. The present chapter reviews some basic concepts and approaches relevant to the reporting of epidemiologic results and discusses common mistakes made when communicating empirical findings. Although some of these mistakes may be a function of errors made during the design and conduct of the study and are thus difficult, if not impossible, to rectify, many can be prevented during the preparation of the report of study results. This chapter is not meant to be prescriptive but rather to discuss some issues that should be considered when preparing a report of epidemiologic findings.

9.2 WHAT TO REPORT

Notwithstanding the necessary flexibility in style and content of reports of epidemiologic studies, Exhibit 9–1 summarizes some of the key issues that are worth considering when preparing such reports. Obviously, not all the items listed in Exhibit 9–1 are relevant to all reports of empirical findings. In the following paragraphs, selected is-

Exhibit 9–1 Issues To Be Considered When Preparing Epidemiologic Reports

---

1. *Introduction*
   a. Succintly review rationale for study: • biologic plausibility*
                                               • what is new about study
   b. State hypothesis/hypotheses (specify interaction(s), if part of the hypothesis).
2. *Methods*
   a. Describe study population characteristics (eg, age, gender), setting (eg, hospital patients, population-based sample), and time frame of the study.
   b. Describe inclusion and exclusion criteria.
   c. Describe data collection procedures; give accuracy/reliability figures for these procedures, if known.
   d. Specify criterion/criteria for identification of confounding variables.
   e. Describe statistical methods; explain criterion/criteria for categorization of study variables.
   f. Give rationale for believing that the assumptions underlying the selected model are reasonable (eg, for the use of the Cox model, that the hazard ratio is constant over the follow-up time).
3. *Results*
   a. Present data with minimum modeling (frequency distributions, medians, means, unadjusted differences).
   b. Present stratified data.
   c. Present data using more complex models, but use the most parsimonious model warranted by the data (eg, Mantel-Haenszel-adjusted odds ratio if only one or two categorical variables need to be adjusted for).
   d. When postulating interactions a priori (or exploring their presence a posteriori), consider assessing both multiplicative and additive interactions.
4. *Discussion*
   a. Review main results of study, and emphasize similarities and dissimilarities with the literature.
   b. Review strengths and limitations of study. Consider bias and confounding as alternative explanations for the results. Comment on possible misclassification of data in the context of the known or estimated validity and reliability of the data collection instruments used in the study.
   c. Suggest specific ways to rectify some of the shortcomings of previous research and the present study, so as to help future investigators to address the same question(s).

---

continues

Exhibit 9–1 continued

d. If appropriate and warranted by the data, discuss the implications for medical pratice or public health policy of the study results.

*"Biologic" if the disease process investigated is biological or physiological in nature. For epidemiologic studies dealing with psychosocial aspects, for example, the relevant aspects will be based on the psychosocial theoretical model underlying the phenomenon under study.
Source: Data from HA Kahn and CT Sempos, *Statistical Methods in Epidemiology,* © 1989, Oxford University Press.

sues summarized in Exhibit 9–1 that are often neglected when describing the study rationale, design, and results are briefly discussed.

9.2.1 Study Objectives and/or Hypotheses Developed at the Inception of the Study

The study objectives and hypotheses that guided the conduct of the study need to be explicitly stated, usually at the end of the Introduction section. One common way to structure the Introduction section of the paper is to link previous evidence on the subject (from epidemiologic and other studies, such as animal experiments) with the specific questions that justify the present study.

If the study does not have specific hypotheses—that is, it is an exploratory study of multiple exposure-outcome relationships (ie, a "fishing expedition" in the epidemiology jargon)—this too should be clearly stated in the Introduction. In many large epidemiologic studies and surveys, dozens or hundreds of variables can be cross-tabulated in search of possible associations. For example, up to 1000 two-by-two tables showing pooled data can be generated from a survey with information on 100 two-level exposure variables and 10 possible binary outcomes (eg, the prevalence of 10 different diseases). Theoretically, even if none of these exposure variables is truly associated with the outcomes, chance alone will determine that in approximately 50 of the 1000 cross-tabulations a statistical association will be found to be significant at $P \leq 0.05$ level. Selective publication of only these "significant" findings will lead to publication bias (see Chapter 4, Section 4.5).

For example, Friedman et al[1] published a paper reporting for the first time a strong graded relationship between leukocyte count and risk of myocardial infarction. In their discussion of these findings, then unexpected, Friedman et al aptly opened their Discussion section with the following statement: "Our finding that the leukocyte count is a predictor of myocardial infarction should be viewed in the context of the exploratory study that we have been carrying out. In searching through approximately 750 assorted variables for new predictors of infarction. . . ."[1(p1278)]

In fact, these results were subsequently replicated in a number of other studies, although the causal nature of the association remains controversial.[2] On the other hand, how many other findings in the medical/epidemiologic literature are just the product of a chance finding in a "fishing expedition," create a one-time uproar in the mass media (Figure 9–1), and are then never replicated?

The above argument also applies to the reporting of interactions. Because effect modification may occur by chance (see Chapter 6, Section 6.10), the reader needs to consider whether a reported interaction was a chance event resulting from multiple stratified cross-tabulations between the study variables, rather than an expected finding based on a previously established and plausible hypothesis.

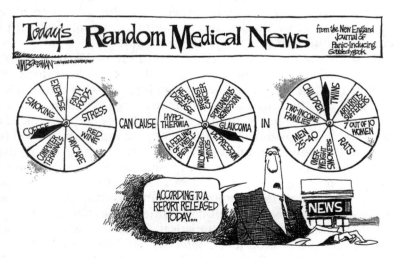

Figure 9–1 Uncritical publication of findings based on "fishing expeditions" sends confusing and sometimes contradictory messages to the population and results in cynical views of medical and epidemiologic research. *Source:* Jim Borgman, The Cincinnati Enquirer, King Features Syndicate. Reprinted with permission of King Features Syndicate.

9.2.2 Description of Validity and Reliability of Data Collection Instruments

When describing the data collection procedures, it is important to report the corresponding measures of validity and reliability whenever possible (see Chapter 8). Avoid statements such as "The validity/reliability of [the questionnaire] has been reported elsewhere [Reference]," as such wording is not informative for the reader without time or access to the source article. Moreover, the statement above may be interpreted as meaning that the instrument is "valid" and "reliable," when in fact it frequently refers to questionnaire items with poor to moderate validity/reliability (eg, Kappa or intraclass correlation coefficients of 0.20–0.40, as seen in validation studies of dietary data, for example). In the case of questionnaires, a special problem is that their validity and reliability may be a function of the characteristics of the study population (eg, educational level): that is, validity/reliability figures obtained from a given population may not be applicable to another population (see Chapter 8, Sections 8.3.2 and 8.3.3). Similarly, as discussed in Chapter 8, the validity/reliability of certain instruments or tests may be different between populations as a function of the underlying distribution of the trait. It is therefore important not only that results of validity/reliability studies be reported but also that a summary of the characteristics of the individuals who participated in these studies be provided. Obviously, reports of study findings should also include internal results of the quality control substudies, if available (see Chapter 8).

9.2.3 Rationale for the Choice of Confounders

Reports of epidemiologic observational studies frequently fail to describe the criteria for selection of confounding variables. For example, was the choice of potentially confounding variables initially based on the literature and subsequently verified in the study data? Were new potential confounders explored in the study that had not been considered in previous studies? And if so, which analytic approaches were used to examine confounding? (See Chapter 5, Section 5.3.)

9.2.4 Criteria for Selection of the Cutoff Points When Establishing Categories for Continuous or Ordinal Variables

Common approaches for categorizing continuous or ordinal variables are the use of either established standards (eg, "abnormal" ST-T segment elevations observed in an electrocardiogram tracing to define myocardial ischemia) or study data distributions (eg, use of percentiles as cutoff points). On occasion, investigators choose cutoff points that have been widely used for clinical purposes or in previous epidemiologic research (eg, defining hypertension as values of ≥ 140 mm Hg systolic or ≥ 90 mm Hg diastolic blood pressure levels, or defining hypercholesterolemia as serum cholesterol levels ≥ 240 mg/dL). When no such cutoff points exist, and particularly when investigating novel risk factor–disease associations, the investigator may be interested in using exploratory techniques for optimizing and exploring the consequences of different cutoff choices for categorical[3] or ordinal[4] regression analyses. In any case, the report should explicitly describe the criteria or method used for this purpose; failure to clearly define criteria for selection of categories of the variables of interest may suggest that data were regrouped over and over again until the results were to the investigator's liking (eg, until they achieved statistical significance).

9.2.5 Unmodeled and Parsimoniously Modeled Versus Fully Modeled Data

To provide adequate background information to put the study findings in proper perspective, unmodeled and parsimoniously modeled results should be presented, including the characteristics of the study population and both univariate and stratified distributions of key study variables. Authors should avoid the temptation of reporting only the results of full statistical modeling. Because unadjusted results undergo minimum modeling and are thus more "representative" of the study population, it could even be argued that, if adjusted and unadjusted results are similar, only the latter should be presented. Otherwise, it is advantageous to show unadjusted along with adjusted results (see also Chapter 5, Section 5.3); this strategy not only allows additional insight into the strength of the confounding effect but also may help in elucidating underlying mechanisms. An illustration of the advantage of showing both unadjusted and adjusted measures of association is given by a study of the relationship of social class to carotid atherosclerotic disease.[5] The weakening of the relationship resulting from adjustment for major cardiovascular risk factors (eg, hypertension, smoking, and hypercholesterolemia) gives a measure of the importance of these factors as mediating factors. Because the relationship may indeed be explained (at least partly) by these risk factors, it is inappropriate to show only the adjusted results.

Another example is that, assuming no measurement errors, the difference in the magnitude of birth weight–adjusted and unadjusted associations of maternal smoking with perinatal mortality reflects the importance of low birth weight as a mechanism explaining the association (Chapter 5, Figures 5–4 and 5–5). Ideally, the role of each individual potential confounder should be assessed so as to pinpoint the exact source of confounding and/or to assess the mechanism linking the risk factor to the outcome. Formulas for evaluating the influence of a given variable reflecting a mechanism linking the risk factor of interest to the outcome or the degree of positive confounding were given in Chapter 5, Section 5.2.3.

9.2.6 Assessment of Interaction

All too often, the widespread use of logistic regression, Cox regression, and related models results in an almost exclusive focus on multiplicative interaction. However, as discussed in Chapter 6, the evaluation of additive interaction is of importance to public health practitioners[6,7] and should be carried out regardless of the statistical model used to analyze epidemiologic data. It is important to bear in mind that the use of logistic regression or other "multiplicative" models does not preclude the assessment of additive interaction.[8]

9.3 HOW TO REPORT

9.3.1 Avoiding Scientific Arrogance

When reporting results of individual studies, particularly those of observational studies, epidemiologists frequently do not sufficiently recognize that no study can stand alone and that replication is needed to minimize the effects of chance or design problems. One individual study supplies at best only one piece of a huge, almost limitless puzzle. Thus, in general, it is advisable to avoid "definitive" statements, such as "This study unequivocally demonstrates that . . . ," when interpreting the results of a single observational study. In general, caution is called for when interpreting results of observational research.

9.3.2 Avoiding Verbosity

As in all scientific communication, it is important to be as concise as possible when reporting results from epidemiologic studies. In an editorial written a few years ago, Friedman[9] underscored the possibility of conveying the same ideas in an abbreviated form without loss of meaning or clarity. Consider the 73-word paragraph that follows; it comes from a paper submitted to an epidemiology journal:[9]

> Other investigations exploring the association between multiparity and scleroderma have obtained information on multiparity using surrogate measures. The amount of money spent on diapers, without consideration of inflation, has been used as a proxy by several groups of investigators, and all have reported that no significant differences were observed once the data were stratified by age at last full time pregnancy. Similar results were found in the analysis reported here.

A significant reduction of its length (to about 40 words) recommended by Friedman[9] not only preserved the paragraph's meaning but may well have improved its clarity:

> Other investigators have used surrogate measures of multiparity, such as the amount of money spent on diapers, without consideration of inflation. As with our study, all revealed no significant differences once the data were stratified by age at last full time pregnancy.

9.3.3 Improving Readability

Another way to make communication of epidemiologic findings more efficient, particularly when it is expected that some of the readers will lack familiarity with the terms used in the article, is to use as simple a language as possible. Several readability formulas are available to determine the educational grade level of the intended readership.[10,11] Consider, for example, applying the SMOG grading formula for tailoring an English-written report to the educational level of the readers[12]—an approach that reminds us of the need to keep the language simple when communicating with the public at large. The formula is easy to apply: (1) Select 30 sentences from the paper's text—10 at the beginning of the text, 10 at the middle, and 10 near the end; (2) count words with three or more syllables; (3) take the square root of this count; and (4) add 3 to this square root to obtain the US-equivalent grade level needed for understanding the report. For example, if there are 100 such words, the educational level needed will be,

$$\text{SMOG index} = \sqrt{100} + 3 = 13$$

that is, at least completion of high school. By applying this formula, Freimuth[10] concluded that patients receiving educational pamphlets about mammography from the Fox Chase Cancer Center would need to have at least 2 years of high school to be able to understand them. Although there is an obvious difference in the educational level of readers of scientific papers and that of the usual target readers of health education pamphlets, the SMOG formula and related formulas may be useful to epidemiologists who need to interface with the lay public—for example, to communicate with the press or to have their views understood in a court of law.

In view of their culture specificity, and assuming that epidemiologic literature is read all over the world, jargon and abbreviations should be avoided or used sparingly only when they achieve a universal acceptance/permanence status, as in the case of the terms DNA or IgG. Widely used abbreviations such as CHD (for coronary heart disease), SES (for socioeconomic status), or HIV (for human immunodeficiency virus) may be acceptable, provided that they are properly spelled out at their first appearance in the article. However, even the widespread use of these commonly recognized abbreviations may lead to some confusion: for example, in Spanish-speaking countries, the abbreviation *AIDS* for "acquired immunodeficiency syndrome" becomes *SIDA* (*síndrome de inmunodeficiencia adquirida*), which in turn may be regarded by English-speaking readers as a misspelling of the abbreviation *SIDS*, denoting "sudden infant death syndrome." In any case, authors should always be reminded that the abuse of abbreviations, while shortening the length of the manuscript, tends to decrease its readability, particularly for readers not entirely familiar with the specific research topic. Consider the following paragraph, taken from the (structured) abstract of a paper published in a major medical journal,[13] that the use of abbreviations makes virtually incomprehensible to the average reader:

> ***Methods and Results***—Relative LV myocardial MMP activity was determined in the normal (n = 8) and idiopathic DCM (n = 7) human LV myocardium by substrate zymography. Relative LV myocardial abundance of interstitial collagenase (MMP-1), stromelysin (MMP-3), 72 kD gelatinase (MMP-2), 92 kD gelatinase (MMP-9), TIMP-1, and TIMP-2 were measured with quantitive immunoblotting. LV myocardial MMP zymographic activity increased with DCM compared with normal (984 ± 149 versus 413 ± 64 pixels, $P < .05$). With DCM, LV myocardial abundance of MMP-1 decreased

to $16 \pm 6\%$ (P < .05), MMP-3 increased to $563 \pm 212\%$ (P < .05), MMP-9 increased to $422 \pm 64\%$ (P < .05), and MMP-2 was unchanged when compared with normal. LV myocardial abundance of TIMP-1 and TIMP-2 increased by >500% with DCM. A high-molecular-weight immunoreactive band for both TIMP-1 and TIMP-2, suggesting a TIMP/MMP complex, was increased >600% with DCM.

9.3.4 Deriving Appropriate Inferences

Common inferential mistakes in epidemiologic reports include the implication that a statistical association can be automatically interpreted as causal, the use of statistical significance as the main criterion to judge whether an association is present, and the comparison of the "strength" of associations for different risk factors using the size of the regression coefficients or derived risk estimates.

The Presence of an Association (Even If Statistically Significant) Does Not Necessarily Reflect Causality

That statistical associations are not necessarily causal is extensively discussed in basic epidemiology and statistics textbooks (eg, Gordis,[14] Armitage and Berry[15]) and Chapters 4 and 5 in this textbook. However, epidemiologists often use the word *effect* (or otherwise imply causality from statistical associations: eg, "A decrease in X led to a decrease in Y"), even if it is not warranted given that most etiologic studies are observational in nature.[16]

Even more troubling because of its frequent occurrence is the implicit assumption that an adjusted estimate is free of confounding. Caution about inferring that confounding has been eliminated is crucial because even if multivariate models are used as an attempt to adjust for all known confounding variables, the possibility of residual confounding must almost always be explicitly considered (as discussed in detail in Chapter 7, Section 7.5).

Statistical Significance Is Not a Measure of the Strength of an Association

It is a common mistake to describe an association that is not statistically significant as nonexistent. For example, it may be correctly reported in a paper's abstract that a *statistically significant* association has not been found between depressed mood and subsequent breast cancer, as the estimated relative risk was 1.5, with the lower 95% confidence limit barely overlapping the null hypothesis. Yet it would be erroneous if this finding was subsequently interpreted by other authors as evidence of lack of association. Similarly, on the basis of the hypothetical results shown in Table 9–1, particularly because of the suggestion of a dose response for every outcome examined, it would be a mistake to conclude that smoking was related to mortality due to lung cancer and coronary heart disease *but not to mortality from stroke*. It is important to remember that statistical significance and the width of the confidence limits are strongly dependent on the sample size; a smaller number of stroke deaths, compared to coronary disease deaths, could explain why the latter but not the former association was found to be statistically significant in a situation such as that shown in the hypothetical example in Table 9–1.

The inference that there is no association when the association is not statistically significant (or when the confidence interval overlaps the null hypothesis value) fails to consider the important fact that the likelihood of the values within the confidence interval is maximum for the point estimate.[17] It is our impression that many authors who publish in the medical (and even in the epidemiologic) literature view the 95% confidence interval as some kind of *flat* (and *closed*) range of possible values of the parameter of interest. In other words, all these "possible values" included in the range are assumed to be equally likely (Figure 9–2A). Thus, in the above hypothetical example (estimated relative risk [RR] for current smoking and stroke = 2.1; 95% confidence interval: 0.9, 4.9), because the 95% confidence interval includes the null hypothesis (ie, the value RR = 1.0 is "possible"), this result may be mistakenly interpreted as reflecting lack of association. This is a mistaken interpretation because the likelihood of any given value of the true parameter being estimated is not uniform across the range of values contained in the confidence interval. It is *maximum at the point estimate* (eg, RR = 2.1) and declines as the values move away from it (Figure 9–2B). The value RR = 0.9 (the lower bound of the

---

Table 9–1 Age-Adjusted Mortality Rate Ratios for Current and Former Cigarette Smokers Versus Nonsmokers, According to Cause of Death, Hypothetical Example

Cause of Death	*Mortality Rate Ratio (95% Confidence Interval)*		
	Current Smokers	*Former Smokers*	*Nonsmokers*
Lung cancer	8.0 (3.0, 21.3)	2.5 (0.9, 6.9)	1.0
Coronary heart disease	2.3 (1.6, 3.3)	1.5 (1.1, 2.0)	1.0
Stroke	2.1 (0.9, 4.9)	1.4 (0.8, 2.5)	1.0

418   EPIDEMIOLOGY

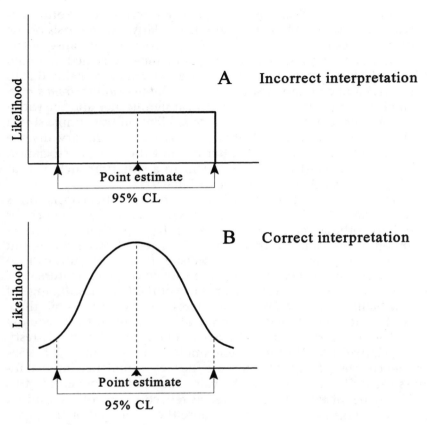

Figure 9–2 Incorrect and correct interpretation of the confidence limits (CL): the likelihood of any given value within the range is not uniform (as shown in **A**); it is maximum at the point estimate of the parameter being measured and declines as values move away from it (**B**). (Likelihood is a measure of the *support* provided by a body of data for a particular value of the parameter of a probability model. For more details on this fundamental statistical concept, the reader should refer to more specialized textbooks (eg, Clayton and Hills[18]).

confidence interval) is very unlikely (as is the uppermost value—RR = 4.9). Moreover, values *outside* the 95% confidence limits are also possible (albeit less likely). If the sample size in the study had been larger, the same estimate of the RR = 2.1 might have been associated with a 95% confidence interval not including the null hypothesis value (eg, 1.1, 2.7). The confidence interval merely expresses the statistical uncertainty of the point estimate and should not be mechanically and erroneously interpreted as a range of equally likely possible values.

The Magnitude of the Association Estimates Across Variables May Not Be Directly Comparable

The issue of comparing different variables with regard to the strength of their association with a given outcome has been introduced in Chapter 3, Section 3.5, to which the reader is referred. An extension of that discussion follows.

For an example of a situation in which it is inappropriate to compare the values of a measure of association between variables, consider the results of the logistic regression analysis shown in Chapter 7, Table 7–17: the inference that the association for gender is stronger than that for age, based on the fact that the odds ratio is higher for the former (3.70) than for the latter (1.011) variable, is clearly unwarranted in view of the striking difference in the nature and width of the units used (in the example shown in that table, male/female versus 1 year of age). While this example highlights the difficulties when comparing discrete with continuous variables, the comparison between continuous variables, too, is a function of the width of unit used for each variable; thus, in Table 7–17, it would be unwarranted to compare the increase in coronary heart disease odds related to a change in total serum cholesterol of 1 mg/dL (odds ratio = 1.007) with that related to a change of 1 kg/m^2 in body mass index (odds ratio = 1.024), since these "units" (the "width" for which the odds ratio in this case is calculated) are rather arbitrary. For example, if instead of 1 mg/dL one were to adopt 1 cg/mL (ie, 10 mg/dL) as the unit for serum cholesterol, the corresponding odds ratio (based on Table 7–17 results) would be $e^{(10 \times 0.0074)} = 1.08$: that is, larger than the odds ratio for 1 kg/m^2 in body mass index.

On occasion, authors attempt to overcome this problem by calculating the so-called "standardized" regression coefficients for continuous variables. These are obtained by using one standard deviation as the unit for each variable (or simply multiplying each regression coefficient by its standard deviation); it is argued that this strategy permits comparing different variables within a study or the same variable across studies.[19] This approach, however, has serious problems,[20] including the following: (1) when different variables in the same study are compared, smaller standard deviation units will result from variables with less variability than from those with more variability; and (2) when the same variable is compared across different studies, the fact that a standard deviation is heavily dependent on the distribution of the variable and design characteristics of each study results in the regression coefficients' not being "standardized" at all and thus not comparable across studies.

An additional and more fundamental problem is that these comparisons do not take the biologic nature of each factor into consideration.[21] As discussed in Chapter 3, Section 3.5, the unique biological nature of each variable makes it difficult to compare its association strength with that of other variables. Consider, for example, a study in which a 1-mg/dL change in total serum cholesterol is compared with a blood pressure change of 1 mm Hg with regard to coronary disease risk; because the mechanisms by which these variables produce both the underlying disease process (atherosclerosis) and its clinical manifestation (eg, myocardial infarction) may be quite different, this comparison would be difficult, if not impossible, to justify.

In Chapter 3, Section 3.5, an approach was suggested for comparing different variables that consisted of estimating the exposure intensity necessary for each risk factor of interest to produce an association of the same magnitude as that of well-established risk factors. In addition, Greenland et al[22] have suggested a method that compares the increase in the level of each factor needed to change the risk of the outcome by a certain fixed amount, such as +50%.

9.3.5   Tables and Figures

There is no standard way of reporting findings in text and tabular form, and the need to address different audiences (eg, peers vs the lay public) and use different vehicles (eg, scientific journals vs newsletters) calls for flexibility. However, there seem to be some simple rules that, if not always followed, should be systematically considered.

Tables

The following are general guidelines concerning the presentation of tables:

- *Labels and headings.* Tables should be clearly labeled, with self-explanatory titles. Optimally, readers should be able to understand the table even if it is examined in isolation. Regrettably, however, to understand and interpret tables published in the literature, often the entire paper or at least the Methods section must also be read (eg, the relevant subgroups are not well defined, or the outcome is not specified or defined in the table). Generous use of footnotes to render the table self-explanatory is recommended.

- *Units.* Categories for discrete variables and units for continuous variables should be specified. For example, an odds ratio next to the variable "age" is meaningless unless it is also stated whether the unit is 1 year of age or some other age grouping. Likewise, an odds ratio next to the variable "race" is not very informative unless the categories being compared are explicitly stated.
- *Comparability with other reports.* Often it is useful to present results in a way that would make them comparable with results of most previous reports. For example, it may be more useful to present age using conventional (eg, 25–34, 35–44, etc) than unconventional groupings (eg, 23–32, 33–42, etc).
- *Comparing statistics between groups.* Another useful strategy, and one that facilitates grasping the meaning of the results, is to present side by side the statistics that provide the main comparison(s) of interest. For example, when one is presenting cohort study results, the ease of comparing rate/person-years side by side makes the (blank) Table A below more "reader friendly" than Table B.

Table A Preferred presentation

No. of Person-Years		Rate/Person-Years	
Exposed	Unexposed	Exposed	Unexposed

Table B Less desirable presentation

Exposed		Unexposed	
No. of Person-Years	Rate/ Person-Years	No. of Person-Years	Rate/ Person-Years

The same principle applies to frequency distributions. Data on diabetes according to smoking status[23] can be presented as shown on the right-hand side of Table 9–2 or, in a less desirable format, on the left.

- *Avoidance of redundancy.* Although there is some controversy regarding the advantages of reporting statistical testing results vis-à-vis precision estimates (ie, confidence intervals),[24] avoidance of redundancy is not controversial; thus, it is usually undesirable to show in the same table values for chi square, standard error, and *P* values. Another type of redundancy is the text's repetition of all or most of the table results, often including *P* values or confidence limits. Whereas some repetition of this sort may be useful,

Table 9–2 Number and Percent Distributions of Individuals with and Without Diabetes Mellitus, According to Smoking at Baseline

| | Less Desirable Presentation | | | | Preferred Presentation | | | |
| | Diabetes | | No Diabetes | | No. | | % | |
Smoking	No.	%	No.	%	Diabetes	No Diabetes	Diabetes	No Diabetes
Current	90	19.6	2307	18.2	90	2307	19.6	18.2
Former	70	12.7	1136	9.1	70	1136	12.7	9.1
Never	155	27.0	2553	20.4	155	2553	27.0	20.4
Unknown	287	40.7	6566	52.3	287	6566	40.7	52.3

Source: Data from ES Ford and F DeStefano, Risk Factors for Mortality from All Causes and from Coronary Heart Disease among Persons with Diabetes. Findings from the National Health and Nutrition Examination Survey I, *American Journal of Epidemiology,* Vol 133, pp 1220–1230, © 1991, The Johns Hopkins University School of Hygiene & Public Health.

the text ought to emphasize mainly the patterns of associations, rather than repeating what is clearly seen in the tables.

- *Shifting denominators.* In most studies, the number of individuals for whom information is missing differs from variable to variable. When this situation occurs, totals should be given for each variable so as to allow the reader to judge whether the magnitude of the loss is such as to cast doubt on the precision and accuracy of the information. A useful strategy is to add a "not stated" or "unknown" category for each variable; alternatively, the apparent inconsistencies in the denominators can be explained in footnotes.
- *Presenting data parsimoniously.* A choice often exists between presenting an "intermediate" statistic or a more easily interpretable one. For example, given the choice of presenting either a beta coefficient from a logistic regression model or the corresponding odds ratio, the latter is usually preferable, particularly when the purpose of the communication is to present an adjusted measure of association rather than a formula needed for prediction. Another example is the customary reporting of a beta coefficient for an "interaction term," which is difficult to interpret outside the predictive context of the regression formula, and which may imply that there are "main effects" even in the presence of interaction (Table 9–3A). It is usually more useful to show stratified results (Table 9–3B).

Table 9–3 Colon Cancer Incidence Rates per 1000 per 5 Years among 1963 Census Participants 45 to 64 Years of Age at Baseline, by Sex and Residence, Washington County, Maryland, 1963–1975

A

Characteristic	No.	Colon Cancer Incidence Rates/1000	
		Crude	*Adjusted*
Total	17,968	6.5	6.5
Sex			
Men	8674	5.5	5.2
Women	9294	7.3	5.6
Residence			
Rural	8702	7.6	9.7
Urban	9266	5.4	4.5
Interaction term			
(sex × residence)			−4.6

B

Sex	No.	Colon Cancer Incidence Rates/1000			
		Crude		*Adjusted*	
		Rural	*Urban*	*Rural*	*Urban*
Men	8674	5.5	5.6	5.9	5.6
Women	9294	9.7	5.2	10.1	5.2

Source: Unpublished data from GW Comstock.

Some of the principles just discussed are illustrated in the hypothetical example shown in Table 9–4A and Table 9–4B (preferred). In Table 9–4A, beta coefficients rather than relative risks are given, no units for the variables are shown, and three statistics are given (standard error, chi square, and *P* values). In Table 9–4B, on the other hand, the units that correspond to the relative risks are given, and, instead of the three (somewhat redundant) statistics, only 95% confidence intervals are shown.

Figures

The rules that guide presentation of data in tabular form generally also apply to figures. Some of the issues that should be considered

Table 9–4 Multiple Risk Equation for Coronary Artery Disease: Cox Regression Model Relating Baseline Risk Factors to the Incidence of Coronary Heart Disease

A

Variable	Beta Coefficient	Standard Error	χ^2	P Value
Age	0.149	0.027	29.97	0.0000
Cholesterol	0.013	0.003	15.36	0.0001
Smoking	0.380	0.125	9.28	0.0020
Parental history of coronary heart disease	0.152	0.392	0.15	0.7000

B

Variable	Risk Comparison	Risk Ratio	95% Confidence Interval
Age	10-year difference	4.5	2.6–7.6
Cholesterol	40 mg/dL difference	1.7	1.3–2.2
Smoking	20 cigarettes/day vs nonsmokers	2.1	1.3–3.5
Parental history of coronary heart disease	Present vs absent	1.2	0.5–2.5

specifically when preparing figures for presentation are discussed next.

- *Use of figure format.* Avoid abusing figures and graphs: that is, displaying data in a graphical format when they could be easily reported in the text. An example of this type of superfluous graphical display is illustrated in Figure 9–3. The information in this figure obviously could be succinctly described in the text. Figure 9–3 exemplifies what Tufte[25] has called a "low data-ink ratio": too much ink for very little data.
- *Titles and labels.* As with tables, titles should be as self-explanatory as possible. Ordinates and abscissas should be labeled in their units. When the plot includes several lines, it is useful to organize and place the legends in a manner as closely related as possible to the order and place of the corresponding categories in the actual figure. For example, in Figure 9–4A, the legend for each of the curves is under the figure, and the reader has to go back

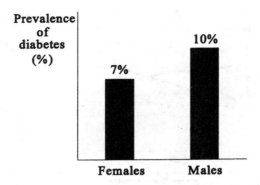

Figure 9–3 Example of superfluous use of a figure. The only two data points (prevalence in males and prevalence in females) could be easily described in the text.

and forth from the graph to the legend to correlate each curve with the corresponding group. On the other hand, in Figure 9–4B, the legend is next to the curves, but the order in which the curves appear and the order for the race/sex legends are opposite. By placing the sex/race identification next to the actual curves, Figure 9–4C seems to be the most readily understandable.

- *Ordinate scale.* The scale in the ordinate should be consistent with the measure being plotted. For example, when plotting relative measures of association (eg, relative risks or odds ratios) with bar charts, a baseline value of 1.0 and a logarithmic scale should be used. An example is shown in Figure 9–5, in which three alternative ways to plot the relative risks corresponding to two different levels associated with a certain variable (RR = 0.5 and RR = 2.0) are compared. In Figure 9–5A, in which the baseline value is 0 (an "unreal" value in a relative scale), the visual impression conveyed by the bars is that the relative risk on the right-hand side is four times higher than that on the left-hand side, which is senseless in view of the fact that these two relative risks go in opposite directions. The plot in Figure 9–5B, although an improvement over that shown in Figure 9–5A in that its baseline corresponds to the correct null relative risk value (RR = 1.0), is still a distorted representation of the magnitude of the relative risks, as it uses an arithmetic scale on the ordinate. The height of the bar corresponding to the relative risk of 2.0 is twice that corresponding to a relative risk of 0.5, when in fact, both relative risks are of the same magnitude, albeit in opposite directions. The correct repre-

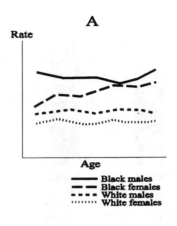

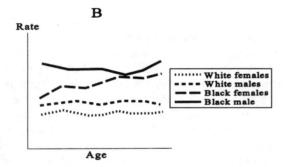

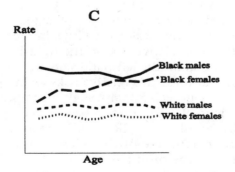

Figure 9–4 Examples of ways to label curves in a figure

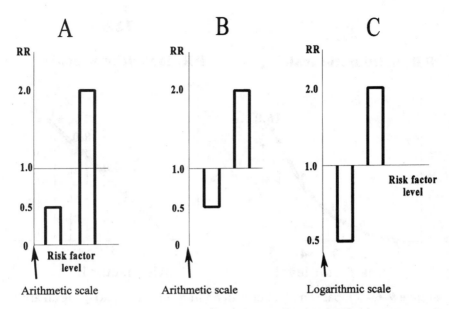

Figure 9–5 Graphic representation of relative risks with arithmetic scales (**A**, origin at 0; **B**, origin at 1.0) or logarithmic scale (**C**)

sentation is seen in Figure 9–5C, in which a logarithmic scale is used in the ordinate. Even if all relative risks are in the same direction, the use of an arithmetic scale in the ordinate is inappropriate when the main focus is the assessment of linear trends in relative differences (ratios). An example is given in Figure 9–6. In Figure 9–6A, in which an arithmetic scale is used, the visual impression is that the relative risk increases more rapidly at the higher levels of variable X. When a logarithmic scale is used instead (Figure 9–6B), the correct impression is obtained: the relative risk increase is linear. The curvature in Figure 9–6A is the product of the exponential nature of all relative measures of effect. Although the trained eye may correctly infer that the pattern in Figure 9–6A is linear in an exponential scale, the use of a logarithmic scale on the ordinate, as seen in Figure 9–6B, is less prone to misinterpretation. (A possible exception to the rule that relative risks or odds ratios are best reported using a log scale in a figure is perhaps when assessing additive interaction in a graphic form, as illustrated in Figure 6–2 of Chapter 6. In this situation,

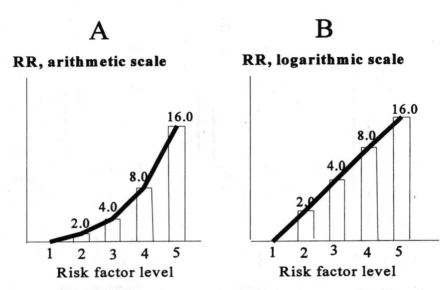

Figure 9–6 Comparison of a linear trend in relative risk (RR) using an arithmetic scale (**A**) and a logarithmic scale (**B**)

relative risks or odds ratios are used as proxies for attributable risks, and thus the focus is on absolute, rather than relative, excesses.)

Sometimes, the use of a logarithmic ordinate scale may be pragmatically necessary so as to include all data in the graph, as illustrated in Figure 1–7, Chapter 1. The use of a logarithmic rather than an arithmetic scale in the ordinate allows plotting the wide range of rates included in the analysis of age, cohort, and period effects (from 2–3 per 100,000 in those 40–44 years old from the 1920–1930 birth cohorts, to 200–500 per 100,000 in those ≥80 years old from the 1905–1910 birth cohorts). It must be emphasized that when a log scale is used, a given difference should be interpreted as a relative difference (ratio) between the rates; in the example shown in Figure 1–7, the fact that the slope of each line tends to be steeper for the older than for the younger age groups in men (with the exception of the 40–44 age group) means that the relative increase (rate ratio, see Chapter 3) from older to recent birth cohorts tends to be larger in older than in younger men (the opposite seems to be true among women).

9.4 CONCLUSION

Epidemiologists must communicate results of empirical research not only to their peers but also to other consumers of epidemiologic data, including practicing physicians, public health personnel, lawyers, and the general public. Scientific journals with a readership traditionally formed by clinical practitioners, such as the *New England Journal of Medicine* and the *Journal of the American Medical Association,* are devoting more and more pages to epidemiologic studies. The use of epidemiologic data by the legal profession is also on the increase. Christoffel and Teret,[26] for example, found that the number of times a word starting with *"epidemiol. . ."* appeared in federal or state courts increased from close to zero in 1970 to more than 80 in 1990. It is virtually certain that this increase has been continuing ever since. Thus, epidemiologists should concern themselves not only with the conduct of scientifically valid studies but also with clearly expressing their results to audiences with varying degrees of scientific sophistication. Epidemiologic papers using simple, unambiguous language are likely to be more easily understood by individuals both inside and outside the discipline and are thus more likely to perform their major function: to be used.

REFERENCES

1. Friedman GD, Klatsky AL, Siegelaub AB. The leukocyte count as a predictor of myocardial infarction. *N Engl J Med* 1974;290:1275–1278.
2. Nieto FJ, Szklo M, Folsom AR, et al. Leukocyte count correlates in middle-aged adults: the Atherosclerosis Risk in Communities (ARIC) Study. *Am J Epidemiol.* 1992;136:525–537.
3. Wartenberg D, Northridge M. Defining exposure in case-control studies: a new approach. *Am J Epidemiol.* 1991;133:1058–1071.
4. Pastor R, Guallar E. Use of two-segmented logistic regression to estimate change-points in epidemiologic studies. *Am J Epidemiol.* 1998;148:631–642.
5. Diez-Roux AV, Nieto FJ, Tyroler HA, et al. Social inequalities and atherosclerosis: the Atherosclerosis Risk in Communities Study. *Am J Epidemiol.* 1995;141:960–972.
6. Saracci R. Interaction and synergism. *Am J Epidemiol.* 1980;112:465–466.
7. Rothman KJ, Greenland S, Walker AM. Concepts of interaction. *Am J Epidemiol.* 1980;112:467–470.
8. Thompson WD. Statistical analysis in case-control studies. *Epidemiol Rev.* 1994; 33–50.
9. Friedman GD. Be kind to your reader. *Am J Epidemiol.* 1990;132:591–593.
10. Freimuth VS. Assessing the readability of health education messages. *Public Health Rep.* 1979;94:568–570.

11. Johnson ME, Mailloux SL, Fisher DG. The readability of HIV/AIDS educational materials targeted to drug users. *Am J Public Health*. 1997;87:112–113.

12. McLaughlin GH. SMOG grading: a new readability formula. *J Reading*. 1969;12: 639–646.

13. Thomas CV, Coker ML, Zellner JL, et al. Increased matrix metalloproteinase activity and selective upregulation in LV myocardium from patients with end-stage dilated cardiomyopathy. *Circulation*. 1998;97:1708–1715.

14. Gordis L. *Epidemiology*. Philadelphia, Pa: W.B. Saunders; 1996.

15. Armitage P, Berry G. *Statistical Methods in Medical Research*. 3rd ed. London, England: Blackwell; 1994.

16. Pettiti DB. Associations are not effects. *Am J Epidemiol*. 1991;133:101–102.

17. Rothman KJ, Lanes S, Robins J. Causal inference. *Epidemiology*. 1993;4:555–556.

18. Clayton D, Hills M. *Statistical Models in Epidemiology*. New York, NY: Oxford University Press; 1993.

19. Newman TB, Browner WS. In defense of standardized regression coefficients. *Epidemiology*. 1991;2:383–386.

20. Greenland S, Maclure M, Schlesselman JJ, et al. Standardized regression coefficients: a further critique and review of some alternatives. *Epidemiology*. 1991;2: 387–392.

21. Criqui MH. On the use of standardized regression coefficients. *Epidemiology*. 1991; 2:393.

22. Greenland S, Schlesselman JJ, Criqui MH. The fallacy of employing standardized regression coefficients and correlations as measures of effect. *Am J Epidemiol*. 1986;123:203–208.

23. Ford ES, DeStefano F. Risk factors for mortality from all causes and from coronary heart disease among persons with diabetes: findings from the National Health and Nutrition Examination Survey I. *Am J Epidemiol*. 1991;133:1220–1230.

24. Savitz DA, Tolo KA, Poole C. Statistical significance testing in the *American Journal of Epidemiology*, 1970–1990. *Am J Epidemiol*. 1994;139:1047–1052.

25. Tufte ER. *The Visual Display of Quantitative Information*. Cheshire, Conn: Graphics Press; 1983.

26. Christoffel T, Teret SP. Epidemiology and the law: courts and confidence intervals. *Am J Public Health*. 1991;81:1662.

APPENDIX A

Standard Errors, Confidence Intervals, and Hypothesis Testing for Selected Measures of Risk and Measures of Association

CONTENTS

Introduction 432
A.1   Cumulative Survival Estimate 433
A.2   Incidence Rate (per Person-Time). 435
A.3   Relative Risk and Rate Ratio 436
A.4   Odds Ratio (Unmatched and Matched) 440
A.5   Attributable Risk 443
A.6   Difference Between Two Adjusted Rates or Probabilities
       (Direct Method) 445
A.7   Standardized Mortality Ratio 447
A.8   Mantel-Haenszel Odds Ratio (and Rate Ratio) 448
A.9   Regression Coefficient 450
A.10   Sensitivity, Specificity, and Percent Agreement 452
A.11   Youden's *J* Statistic 454
A.12   Kappa 454

INTRODUCTION

In this appendix, methods for calculating confidence intervals for selected measures of risk and measures of association presented in this textbook are described. For some of the measures, common methods for hypothesis testing are also presented.

This appendix is not intended to represent a comprehensive review of all the statistical inference methods used in epidemiology. Methods for only some of the epidemiologic parameters are presented, and only one commonly used method for the calculation of standard error is described for each—sometimes among other alternatives. Moreover, it is not our intention to discuss the methodological and conceptual limitations of these methods, which have been thoroughly discussed elsewhere.[1,2] Our intention is pragmatic: to provide a brief description of the methods of statistical inference that we believe are most commonly used in relation to the epidemiologic parameters presented in this textbook.

It is assumed that the reader of this appendix is familiar with basic biostatistical concepts, including standard normal distribution (z score), t test, standard deviation, standard error, confidence intervals, hypothesis testing, and the P value. (For a review of these basic concepts, the reader should refer to biostatistics books such as Armitage and Berry[3] or Altman.[4])

The general purpose for the calculation of confidence intervals and hypothesis testing is to estimate the statistical uncertainty around the measure of risk or association obtained in the study (the so-called *point estimate*) in relation to the (unknown) true value of the *parameter* in the reference population. Although shortcuts are provided in specific cases, the general structure of the presentation for most of these measures is as follows:

1. The method for calculating the *variance* and/or its square root, the *standard error,* of the estimate is presented in most instances. However, in cases where the calculation of the standard error is more mathematically cumbersome (eg, for regression coefficients), it is assumed that the standard error can be obtained from a computer-assisted statistical analysis, and thus this step is skipped.
2. Based on the point estimate of the parameter in question and its standard error (SE), the formula for the 95% confidence interval is provided. The general structure of this formula is as follows:

Point estimate $\pm$ [1.96 $\times$ SE (estimate)]

Notice that 1.96 is the *z* score (standard normal score) corresponding to the 95% confidence level (ie, an alpha error of 5%). Confidence intervals for different levels of alpha error can be obtained by simply replacing this value with the corresponding *z* score value (eg, 1.64 for 90% confidence intervals, 2.58 for 99% confidence intervals, etc).

3. The test of the null hypothesis is presented for some of the indices (depending on our assessment of its relevance in each particular case and the frequency of its use in the literature). The logic and structure of these tests of hypothesis are also fairly homogeneous across different measures. The standard test of hypothesis is designed to test the *null hypothesis*—that is, the absence of a difference (absolute or relative) or a correlation. Thus, for *absolute* measures of association (eg, a difference between two means or two rates), the null hypothesis is formulated as follows:

$$H_0 : \text{True parameter} = 0$$

For *relative* measures of association (eg, a relative risk, a rate ratio, an odds ratio), the null hypothesis is formulated as

$$H_0 : \text{True parameter} = 1$$

Specific formulations for statistical testing approaches are presented in a few cases. In others, the general approach for a test of hypothesis is to calculate a *z* score by dividing the point estimate by its standard error:

$$\frac{\text{Point estimate}}{\text{SE (estimate)}} \approx z \text{ score}$$

Or equivalently, the square of the *z* score has a distribution approximate to a chi-square with 1 degree of freedom.

4. An example of each of the above calculations (usually based on one of the examples in the textbook) is presented in most cases.

Finally, a note on "notation": throughout this appendix, the symbol "log x" refers to the natural logarithm of x—that is, the logarithm on base *e*. The corresponding antilog is the exponential function, which is denoted by either exp[x] or e^x.

A.1 CUMULATIVE SURVIVAL ESTIMATE

As described in Chapter 2, Section 2.2.1, the cumulative survival estimate is the product of the conditional survival probabilities for all preceding intervals (in the case of the classical actuarial life table) or for all preceding events (in the case of the Kaplan-Meier method; see Chapter 2, Table 2–3).

Variance and Standard Error (Greenwood Formula)

In 1926, Greenwood[5] described the following formula, which approximates the variance of a cumulative survival estimate at time i:

$$\text{Var } (S_i) \approx (S_i)^2 \times \sum_{j=1}^{i} \left(\frac{d_j}{n_j (n_j - d_j)} \right)$$

where j indexes all the previous event times (or intervals) up to and including time i, d is the number of deaths at each time (typically 1 in the Kaplan-Meier method, any number in the classical life table), and n is the denominator—that is, the number of individuals at risk at each time (or the "corrected" denominator in the life table—see Equation 2.1 in Chapter 2, Section 2.2.1).

The standard error (SE) can be obtained as the square root of the variance:

$$\text{SE } (S_i) \approx S_i \times \sqrt{\sum_{j=1}^{i} \left(\frac{d_j}{n_j (n_j - d_j)} \right)}$$

95% Confidence Interval

This can be obtained from the point estimate (S_i) and the SE (S_i) as follows:

$$S_i \pm [1.96 \times \text{SE}(S_i)]$$

Example

To calculate the standard error for the cumulative survival estimate at time 9 months in Chapter 2, Table 2–3, we need the estimate of S_9 from the table (0.675) and the number of events and individuals at risk at all previous times up to 9 months (ie, 1, 3, and 9 months):

$$\text{SE}(S_9) \approx 0.675 \times \sqrt{\left(\frac{1}{10(10 - 1)} + \frac{1}{8(8 - 1)} + \frac{1}{7(7 - 1)} \right)} = 0.155$$

Thus, the 95% confidence interval can be obtained as follows:

$$0.675 \pm (1.96 \times 0.155) = 0.675 \pm 0.304$$

or 0.371 to 0.979.

A.2   INCIDENCE RATE (PER PERSON-TIME)

A person-time incidence rate is obtained by dividing the number of events by the sum of person-time units contributed to by all individuals in the study population over the time interval of interest. Because rates are usually calculated for rare events (ie, the numerator is usually a small number compared to the denominator), the number of events can be assumed to follow a Poisson distribution.[3] Procedures to calculate variance and standard error of the rate are based on this assumption.

95% Confidence Interval

A simple way to calculate the confidence limits for a rate is based on the table provided by Haenszel et al[6] (see also Breslow and Day[7(p70)]):

Tabulated Values of 95% Confidence Limit Factors
for a Poisson-Distributed Variable

Observed No. of Events on Which Estimate Is Based	Lower Limit Factor	Upper Limit Factor	Observed No. of Events on Which Estimate Is Based	Lower Limit Factor	Upper Limit Factor	Observed No. of Events on Which Estimate Is Based	Lower Limit Factor	Upper Limit Factor
1	.0253	5.57	21	.619	1.53	120	.833	1.200
2	.121	3.61	22	.627	1.51	140	.844	1.184
3	.206	2.92	23	.634	1.50	160	.854	1.171
4	.272	2.56	24	.641	1.49	180	.862	1.160
5	.324	2.33	25	.647	1.48	200	.868	1.151
6	.367	2.18	26	.653	1.47	250	.882	1.134
7	.401	2.06	27	.659	1.46	300	.892	1.121
8	.431	1.97	28	.665	1.45	350	.899	1.112
9	.458	1.90	29	.670	1.44	400	.906	1.104
10	.480	1.84	30	.675	1.43	450	.911	1.098
11	.499	1.79	35	.697	1.39	500	.915	1.093
12	.517	1.75	40	.714	1.36	600	.922	1.084
13	.532	1.71	45	.729	1.34	700	.928	1.078
14	.546	1.68	50	.742	1.32	800	.932	1.072
15	.560	1.65	60	.770	1.30	900	.936	1.068
16	.572	1.62	70	.785	1.27	1000	.939	1.064
17	.583	1.60	80	.798	1.25			
18	.593	1.58	90	.809	1.24			
19	.602	1.56	100	.818	1.22			
20	.611	1.54						

Source: Data from W Haenszel, DB Loveland, and MG Sirken, Lung Cancer Mortality as Related to Residence and Smoking Histories, I. White Males, *Journal of the National Cancer Institute,* Vol 28, pp 947–1001, 1962.

The process involves two steps:

1. Estimate a confidence interval for the number of events (the numerator of the rate): multiply the number of observed events times the lower and upper limit factors shown in the table. (Note that, for large numbers, an approximate interpolation can be made—eg, if the number of events is 95, the limit factors would approximately be .813 and 1.23.)
2. Use these lower and upper limits of the number of events to calculate the confidence limits of the rate, using the number of person-time units as the denominator.

Example

In the hypothetical example cited in Chapter 2, at the beginning of Section 2.2.2, 12 events are observed for a total follow-up time of 500 days. The incidence rate in this example is $12/500 = 0.024$ per person-day, or 2.4 per 100 person-days. The 95% confidence limits for that count, assuming a Poisson distribution, are

Lower $= 12 \times 0.517 = 6.2$

Upper $= 12 \times 1.75 = 21.0$

Thus, the 95% confidence limits for the rate are

Lower $= 6.2/500 = 0.0124$ per person-day

Upper $= 21/500 = 0.042$ per person-day

That is, the 95% confidence interval for the observed rate (2.4 per 100 person-days) is 1.24 to 4.2 per 100 person-days.

A.3   RELATIVE RISK AND RATE RATIO

Relative Risk (Ratio of Probabilities)

The relative risk is the ratio of two incidence cumulative probabilities: the ratio of the proportion of exposed individuals with the event of interest out of the total exposed divided by the proportion of unexposed individuals with the event out of the total number of unexposed subjects (see Chapter 3, Table 3–2, Equation 3.1). Consider the notation in the following:

	Diseased	Nondiseased	Total
Exposed	a	b	$a + b$
Unexposed	c	d	$c + d$
Total	$a + c$	$b + d$	T

The relative risk (RR) (from Equation 3.1) is

$$RR = \frac{q_+}{q_-} = \frac{\dfrac{a}{a + b}}{\dfrac{c}{c + d}}$$

Standard Error

Because the relative risk is a multiplicative measure and thus asymmetrically distributed, its standard error (SE) needs to be calculated in a logarithmic scale. Thus, the standard error of the logarithm of the relative risk is[8]

$$SE(\log RR) = \sqrt{\frac{b}{a(a + b)} + \frac{d}{c(c + d)}}$$

95% Confidence Interval

The 95% confidence interval should be also calculated in the logarithmic scale:

$$95\%CI(\log RR) = \log RR \pm 1.96 \times SE(\log RR)$$

$$= \log RR \pm \left(1.96 \times \sqrt{\frac{b}{a(a + b)} + \frac{d}{c(c + d)}}\right)$$

The confidence interval for the relative risk can be obtained taking the antilog (exponentiation) of these numbers:

$$95\%CI(RR) = \exp\left\{\log RR \pm \left[1.96 \times \sqrt{\frac{b}{a(a + b)} + \frac{d}{c(c + d)}}\right]\right\}$$

Note: A shortcut for this calculation is as follows:

Lower Limit 95%CI(RR) $= RR \times e^{-[1.96 \times SE(\log RR)]}$

Upper Limit 95%CI(RR) $= RR \times e^{[1.96 \times SE(\log RR)]}$

Hypothesis Testing

The null hypothesis is

$$H_0: RR = 1$$

Use usual chi-square or Fisher's exact test for two-by-two contingency tables.

n < s

Example

From the data in Chapter 3, Table 3–3, the relative risk of myocardial infarction is estimated as

$$RR = \frac{0.018}{0.003} = 6.0$$

1.8%

.390

more events, less error

The standard error of the log of this estimate is

$$SE(\log RR) = \sqrt{\frac{9820}{180(10,000)} + \frac{9970}{30(10,000)}} = 0.197$$

less events, more error

Thus, the 95% confidence interval can be obtained as follows:

$$95\%CI(RR) = \exp[\log(6.0) \pm (1.96 \times 0.197)] = \exp[1.792 \pm 0.386]$$

$$\text{Lower Limit} = \exp[1.406] = 4.08$$

$$\text{Upper Limit} = \exp[2.178] = 8.83$$

Note: The alternative shortcut is

$$\text{Lower Limit } 95\%CI(RR) = 6.0 \times e^{-[1.96 \times 0.197]} = 4.08$$

$$\text{Upper Limit } 95\%CI(RR) = 6.0 \times e^{[1.96 \times 0.197]} = 8.83$$

Rate Ratio (Ratio of Incidence Densities)

Approximate procedures to calculate the confidence interval of a rate ratio have been proposed by Ederer and Mantel.[9] Definitions for the notations that will be used are

O_1 = observed events in group 1

O_2 = observed events in group 2

L_1 = person-time observed in group 1

L_2 = person-time observed in group 2

$R_1 = O_1/L_1$ = event rate in group 1

$R_2 = O_2/L_2$ = event rate in group 2

$RR = R_1/R_2$

95% Confidence Interval

Perform the following two steps:

1. Set limits on the ratio of observed events in one group (eg, group 1) to the total number of observed events:

$$\hat{P} = \frac{O_1}{O_1 + O_2}$$

Using the general formula for the standard error of a binomial proportion, the lower (P_L) and upper (P_U) limits of the 95% confidence interval for this ratio are

$$P_L = \hat{P} - \left[1.96 \times \sqrt{\frac{\hat{p}(1-\hat{p})}{O_1 + O_2}} \right]; \quad P_U = \hat{P} + \left[1.96 \times \sqrt{\frac{\hat{p}(1-\hat{p})}{O_1 + O_2}} \right]$$

2. Convert to limits on rate ratio:

$$RR_L = \left[\frac{P_L}{1 - P_L} \right] \times \frac{L_2}{L_1}; \quad RR_U = \left[\frac{P_U}{1 - P_U} \right] \times \frac{L_2}{L_1}$$

Hypothesis Testing

For testing H_0: RR = 1, an approximate chi-square test with 1 degree of freedom can be used:

$$\chi_1^2 = \frac{(O_1 - E_1)^2}{E_1} + \frac{(O_2 - E_2)^2}{E_2}$$

where

$$E_1 = (O_1 + O_2) \times \frac{L_1}{L_1 + L_2}$$

$$E_2 = (O_1 + O_2) \times \frac{L_2}{L_1 + L_2}$$

Example

$O_1 = 60, L_1 = 35,000, R_1 = 0.00171$

$O_2 = 45, L_2 = 30,000, R_2 = 0.0015$

$RR = 0.00171/0.0015 = 1.14$

$$\hat{P} = \frac{60}{105}$$

The 95% confidence limits are

$$P_L = \frac{60}{105} - \left(1.96 \times \sqrt{\frac{60}{105} \times \frac{45}{105} \times \frac{1}{105}} \right) = 0.4768$$

$$P_U = \frac{60}{105} + \left(1.96 \times \sqrt{\frac{60}{105} \times \frac{45}{105} \times \frac{1}{105}} \right) = 0.6661$$

$$RR_L = \frac{0.4768}{0.5232} \times \frac{30,000}{35,000} = 0.78$$

$$RR_U = \frac{0.6661}{0.3339} \times \frac{30,000}{35,000} = 1.71$$

Hypothesis testing is performed as follows:

$$E_1 = (60 + 45) \times \frac{35,000}{65,000} = 56.54$$

$$E_2 = (60 + 45) \times \frac{30,000}{65,000} = 48.46$$

$$\chi_1^2 = \frac{(60 - 56.54)^2}{56.54} + \frac{(45 - 48.46)^2}{48.46} = 0.46; P > 0.5$$

A.4   ODDS RATIO (UNMATCHED AND MATCHED)

Unmatched Case-Control Study

Based on the notation from Chapter 3, Table 3–6 (or from the table in Section A.3, assuming a case-control sampling scheme), in which the controls (cells b and d) are a sample of noncases, the odds ratio can be calculated as the cross-product ratio:

$$OR = \frac{a \times d}{b \times c}$$

Standard Error

As with the relative risk (see Section A.3), because of its multiplicative nature, the standard error for the odds ratio is calculated in a logarithmic scale, as described by Woolf[10]:

$$SE(\log OR) = \sqrt{\frac{1}{a} + \frac{1}{b} + \frac{1}{c} + \frac{1}{d}}$$

95% Confidence Interval

The 95% confidence interval is also calculated in the logarithmic scale:

95%CI(log OR) = log OR ± [1.96 × SE(log OR)]

$$= \log OR \pm \left(1.96 \times \sqrt{\frac{1}{a} + \frac{1}{b} + \frac{1}{c} + \frac{1}{d}} \right)$$

The confidence limits for the odds ratio can be obtained taking the antilog of (exponentiating) these numbers:

$$95\%CI(OR) = \exp \left[\log OR \pm \left(1.96 \times \sqrt{\frac{1}{a} + \frac{1}{b} + \frac{1}{c} + \frac{1}{d}} \right) \right]$$

Note: a shortcut for these calculations is as follows:

Lower 95% Confidence Limit = OR × $e^{-[1.96 \times SE(\log OR)]}$

Upper 95% Confidence Limit = OR × $e^{[1.96 \times SE(\log OR)]}$

Hypothesis Testing

For testing H_0: OR = 1, the usual chi-square or Fisher's exact test for two-by-two contingency tables can be used.

Example

From the data in Chapter 3, Table 3–6:

$$OR = \frac{180 \times 997}{982 \times 30} = 6.09$$

The standard error of the logarithm of this estimate is

$$SE(\log OR) = \sqrt{\frac{1}{180} + \frac{1}{982} + \frac{1}{30} + \frac{1}{997}} = 0.202$$

The 95% confidence interval can be obtained as follows:

95%CI(OR) = exp [log 6.09 ± (1.96 × 0.202)] = exp [1.807 ± 0.396]

Lower Limit = exp [1.411] = 4.10

Upper Limit = exp [2.203] = 9.05

Note: The alternative shortcut is

Lower Limit 95%CI(RR) = 6.09 × $e^{-[1.96 \times 0.202]}$ = 4.10

Upper Limit 95%CI(RR) = 6.09 × $e^{[1.96 \times 0.202]}$ = 9.05

Matched Case-Control Study

In a case-control study in which cases and controls are individually matched (paired), the odds ratio is estimated as the number of pairs in which the case is exposed and the control is not exposed, divided by the number of pairs in which the case is unexposed and the control is exposed. Thus, based on the notation in Chapter 7, Table 7–12:

$$OR = \frac{b}{c}$$

Standard Error

The standard error for the logarithm of the paired odds ratio is

$$SE(\log OR) = \sqrt{\frac{1}{b} + \frac{1}{c}}$$

95% Confidence Interval

The 95% confidence interval is also calculated in the logarithmic scale:

$$95\%CI(\log OR) = \log OR \pm [1.96 \times SE(\log OR)]$$

$$= \log OR \pm \left(1.96 \times \sqrt{\frac{1}{b} + \frac{1}{c}} \right)$$

The confidence limits for the OR can be obtained, taking the antilog of (exponentiating) these numbers:

$$95\%CI(OR) = \exp \left[\log OR \pm \left(1.96 \times \sqrt{\frac{1}{b} + \frac{1}{c}} \right) \right]$$

The same shortcut as for the unmatched OR can be used.

Hypothesis Testing

For testing H_0: OR = 1, use McNemar's chi-square test (corrected for continuity), with 1 degree of freedom:

$$\chi_1^2 = \frac{(|b - c| - 1)^2}{b + c}$$

Example

From the data in Chapter 7, Table 7–12:

$$OR = \frac{65}{42} = 1.55$$

The standard error of the logarithm of estimate is

$$SE(\log OR) = \sqrt{\frac{1}{65} + \frac{1}{42}} = 0.198$$

The 95% confidence interval is obtained as follows:

95%CI(OR) = exp [log 1.55 ± (1.96 × 0.198)] = exp [0.438 ± 0.388]

Lower Limit = exp [0.050] = 1.05

Upper Limit = exp [0.826] = 2.28

Note: The alternative shortcut is

Lower Limit 95%CI(OR) = 1.55 × $e^{-[1.96 \times 0.198]}$ = 1.05

Upper Limit 95%CI(OR) = 1.55 × $e^{[1.96 \times 0.198]}$ = 2.28

Hypothesis testing is performed as follows:

$$\chi_1^2 = \frac{(|65 - 42| - 1)^2}{65 + 42} = 4.52, P < 0.05$$

A.5 ATTRIBUTABLE RISK

Attributable Risk in the Exposed

For the simple excess attributable fraction—that is, the difference in incidence between exposed and unexposed individuals (Chapter 3, Equation 3.4)—the variance can be estimated as the sum of the variances of each of the incidence estimates. For example, if the incidence estimates are based on cumulative survival, the variance of the attributable risk will be the sum of the individual variances obtained using Greenwood's formula (see Section A.1). The standard error is then the square root of the variance, from which 95% confidence limits can be estimated and hypothesis testing can be done using the general approach outlined in the Introduction to this appendix.

Percent Attributable Risk in the Exposed (% AR_{exp})

Because the %AR_{exp} (Chapter 3, Equation 3.5) reduces to the following equation (Equation 3.6):

$$\%AR_{exp} = \frac{q_+ - q_-}{q_+} \times 100 = \frac{RR - 1}{RR} \times 100$$

this measure is a function of only one parameter (the relative risk, RR). Thus, an estimate of the confidence interval for %AR$_{exp}$ can be based on the confidence interval of RR (see Section A.3).

Percent Population Attributable Risk (%Pop AR)

Levin's formula for the calculation of the %Pop AR, based on data from a cohort study (Chapter 3, Equation 3.10), is

$$\%\text{Pop AR} = \frac{p_e(\text{RR} - 1)}{p_e(\text{RR} - 1) + 1} \times 100$$

where RR is the estimated relative risk and p_e is the proportion of individuals exposed in the population [ie, based on the notation in the table in Section A.3, $p_e = (a + b)/T$]. In a case-control study, assuming that the disease is rare and that the controls are reasonably representative of the total reference population, the relative risk in Levin's formula can be replaced by the odds ratio (see Chapter 3, Section 3.2.2), and p_e can be estimated from the prevalence of exposure in controls.

Standard Error

The following formulas, proposed by Walter,[11] are based on the notation in the table in Section A.3. For %Pop AR calculated from cohort data:

$$\text{SE(\%Pop AR)} = \sqrt{\frac{cT[ad(T - c) + bc^2]}{(a + c)^3 \, (c + d)^3}} \times 100$$

For %Pop AR calculated from case-control data:

$$\text{SE(\%Pop AR)} = \sqrt{\left(\frac{c(b + d)}{d(a + c)}\right)^2 \left(\frac{a}{c(a + c)} + \frac{b}{d(b + d)}\right)} \times 100$$

95% Confidence Interval

The 95% confidence interval can be calculated using the point estimate and the above standard errors:

$$95\%\text{CI(\%Pop AR)} = \%\text{Pop AR} \pm 1.96 \times \text{SE(\%Pop AR)}$$

Hypothesis Testing

For testing H_0: %Pop AR = 0, the z score is obtained:

$$\frac{\%\text{Pop AR}}{\text{SE(\%Pop AR)}} \approx z \text{ score}$$

Example

According to the hypothetical cohort study data in Chapter 3, Table 3–3, the relative risk of myocardial infarction is 6.0, comparing severe hypertensives to nonhypertensives; the prevalence of exposure (severe systolic hypertension) is 50%. Thus, the population attributable risk is

$$\%\text{Pop AR} = \frac{0.5(6.0 - 1)}{0.5(6.0 - 1) + 1} \times 100 = 71.4\%$$

The standard error of this estimate is

$$\text{SE}(\%\text{Pop AR}) = \sqrt{\frac{30 \times 20{,}000 \times [180 \times 9970 \times 19{,}970 + 9820 \times 30^2]}{210^3 \times 10{,}000^3}} \times 100$$

$$= 4.82\%$$

The 95% confidence interval is obtained as follows:

$$95\%\text{CI}(\%\text{Pop AR}) = 71.4 \pm (1.96 \times 4.82) = 71.4 \pm 9.4$$

Lower Limit = 62.0%

Upper Limit = 80.8%

Hypothesis testing is performed as follows:

$$\frac{71.4}{4.82} = 14.8, P < 0.001$$

A.6 DIFFERENCE BETWEEN TWO ADJUSTED RATES OR PROBABILITIES (DIRECT METHOD)

Define $d = I^*_A - I^*_B$—that is, the difference between two adjusted probabilities (see Chapter 7, Section 7.3.1, Table 7–3).

Standard Error

An approximate standard error for d (d being an estimated adjusted difference [eg, excess incidence] based on $i = 1 \ldots k$ strata) is obtained using the formula[12]:

$$\text{SE}(d) = \frac{\sqrt{\sum_{i=1}^{k} w_i^2 p_i(1 - p_i)\left(\frac{1}{n_{iA}} + \frac{1}{n_{iB}}\right)}}{\sum_{i=1}^{k} w_i}$$

where p_i are the overall stratum-specific rates (both study groups combined):

$$p_i = \frac{x_{iA} + x_{iB}}{n_{iA} + n_{iB}}$$

and w_i are the standard population weights used to adjust the study group rates. Note that if the minimum variance method is used (ie, if these weights are calculated as follows; see Chapter 7, Section 7.3.1),

$$w_i = \frac{n_{iA} \times n_{iB}}{n_{iA} + n_{iB}}$$

the above formula is substantially simpler:

$$SE(d_{\text{min variance}}) = \frac{\sqrt{\sum_{i=1}^{k} w_i p_i (1 - p_i)}}{\sum_{i=1}^{k} w_i}$$

95% Confidence Interval

The 95% confidence interval can be obtained using the general approach outlined in the introduction to this appendix:

$$d \pm [1.96 \times SE(d)]$$

Hypothesis Testing

Hypothesis testing also uses the general approach (see above):

$$\frac{d}{SE(d)} \approx z \text{ score}$$

Example

The data for this example come from the study by Pandey et al[13] on the comparison of mortality according to dietary vitamin intake in the Western Electric Company Study cohort. These data were used as an example for the techniques to evaluate confounding in Chapter 5 (Tables 5–1 through 5–5). For the purpose of the current example, the category "moderate" is ignored, and the purpose is to calculate the smoke-adjusted difference in mortality rates between the *high* and *low* vitamin intake categories, as well as the corresponding confidence interval for such adjusted difference. Based on the numbers presented in the tables mentioned above, the following working table for the calculation of the adjusted difference (using direct adjustment with the minimum variance method) and its standard error was con-structed:

	Low Vitamin Intake*		High Vitamin Intake*		Total			Minimum Variance Standard		
Smoking	N	Rate	N	Rate	N	Rate (p_i)	N $(w_i)^\dagger$	Expected No. of Deaths $(Low)^\dagger$	Expected No. of Deaths $(High)^\dagger$	$w_i p_i (1 - p_i)^\dagger$
No	4260	.0134	5143	.0103	9403	.0117	2330.020	31.1763	24.0115	26.9386
Yes	6447	.0214	6233	.0178	12680	.0196	3169.097	67.8355	56.4367	61.0102
Sum							5499.117	99.0118	80.4482	87.9488

*See Table 5–4, Chapter 5.

†The expected numbers shown in the table are exact and may differ slightly from those obtained using the rates shown for low and high because the latter have been rounded.

Thus, the adjusted rates are:

- For the low vitamin intake group: 99.0118/5499.117 = 0.0180.
- For the high vitamin intake group: 80.4482/5499.117 = 0.0146.

The adjusted difference between the high and the low vitamin in-take groups is therefore: $d = 0.0146 - 0.018 = -0.0034$, or -3.4 per 1000.

The standard error of this estimate can be calculated as:

$$SE(d_{\text{min variance}}) = \frac{\sqrt{87.9488}}{5499.117} = 0.0017$$

The 95% confidence interval is as follows:

$-0.0034 \pm 1.96 \times 0.0017$

Lower Limit $= -0.0034 - 0.0033 = -0.0067$

Upper Limit $= -0.0034 + 0.0033 = -0.0001$

A.7 STANDARDIZED MORTALITY RATIO

The standardized mortality ratio (SMR) and related measures such as the standardized incidence ratio (SIR) are defined as the number of observed events (eg, deaths, incident cases) in a given population (O) divided by the expected number of events (E) if the study population had the same rates as those in a reference population (see Chapter 7, Section 7.3.2):

$$SMR = \frac{O}{E}$$

95% Confidence Interval

Assuming that the number of expected events is not subject to random variability, an easy way to obtain the 95% confidence interval for an SMR is to calculate the lower and upper limits for the observed number of events, O (see Section A.2), and then to substitute in the SMR formula. (For alternative methods, see Breslow and Day.[7])

Example

Based on the hypothetical data in Chapter 7, Table 7–8, 70 deaths were observed in study group B. The number of expected events obtained by applying the rates of an external reference population is 110. Thus, the estimated SMR for study group B is $70/110 = 0.64$. According to the table in Section A.2, the lower and upper limit factors for a rate based on 70 observed events (O) are, respectively, 0.785 and 1.27. Thus, the 95% confidence interval limits for O are $O_L = 70 \times 0.785 = 54.95$, and $O_U = 70 \times 1.27 = 88.9$. The resulting 95% confidence limits for the SMR are thus

$$SMR = \frac{54.95}{110} = 0.50$$

$$SMR = \frac{88.9}{110} = 0.81$$

A.8 MANTEL-HAENSZEL ODDS RATIO (AND RATE RATIO)

Standard Error

For two-by-two contingency tables stratified in k strata ($i = 1, \ldots k$), an approximate formula for the standard error (SE) of the Mantel-Haenszel estimate of the adjusted log odds ratio (OR), based on the notation in Chapter 7, Table 7–9, has been given by Robins et al[14]:

$$SE(\log OR_{MH}) = \sqrt{\frac{\sum\limits_{i=1}^{k}(P_i R_i)}{2\left(\sum\limits_{i=1}^{k} R_i\right)^2} + \frac{\sum\limits_{i=1}^{k}(P_i w_i + Q_i R_i)}{2\left(\sum\limits_{i=1}^{k} R_i\right)\left(\sum\limits_{i=1}^{k} w_i\right)} + \frac{\sum\limits_{i=1}^{k}(Q_i w_i)}{2\left(\sum\limits_{i=1}^{k} w_i\right)^2}}$$

where

$$P_i = \frac{a_i + d_i}{N_i}$$

$$Q_i = \frac{b_i + c_i}{N_i}$$

$$R_i = \frac{a_i \times d_i}{N_i}$$

$$w_i = \frac{b_i \times c_i}{N_i}$$

(Note: Greenland and Robins[15] have derived an analogous equation for the calculation of the SE of the Mantel-Haenszel estimate of the adjusted rate ratio for stratified cohort data—see Chapter 7, Section 7.3.3.)

95% Confidence Interval

The same approach described for the unadjusted OR in Section A.4 should be used: that is, the calculation of the confidence limits in a log scale and the exponentiation of the results to obtain the confidence interval for the OR_{MH}.

Hypothesis Testing

Again, following the notation in Chapter 7, Table 7–9, an approximate chi-square test with 1 degree of freedom (regardless of the number of strata involved) can be calculated as follows[16]:

$$\chi_1^2 = \frac{\left(\left|\sum_{i=1}^{k} a_i - \sum_{i=1}^{k} E_i\right| - 0.5\right)^2}{\sum_{i=1}^{k}\left(\frac{n_{1i}n_{2i}m_{1i}m_{2i}}{N_i^2(N_i - 1)}\right)}$$

where E_i is the expected value in the "a" cell in each stratum, calculated from the values in the margins as in any chi-square test (eg, $n_{i1} \times m_{i1}/N_i$).

Example

From the stratified results in Chapter 7, Table 7–1, the estimate of the OR_{MH} was 1.01. The following working table was set to apply the SE formula:

Sex	Case	Cont	N	OR	P	Q	R	w	PR	Pw+QR	Qw
Stratum 1											
M	53	15	81	1.06	0.691	0.309	1.963	1.852	1.357	1.886	0.572
F	10	3									
Stratum 2											
M	35	53	219	1.00	0.521	0.479	12.626	12.584	6.572	12.604	6.034
F	52	79									
		SUM =					14.589	14.436	7.929	14.490	6.605

Thus:

$$\text{SE(log OR}_{\text{MH}}) = \sqrt{\frac{7.929}{2 \times 14.589^2} + \frac{14.490}{2 \times 14.589 \times 14.436} + \frac{6.605}{2 \times 14.436^2}}$$

$$= 0.262$$

The 95% confidence limits can be obtained as follows:

95%CI(OR) = exp [log 1.01 ± (1.96 × 0.262)]

Lower Limit = exp [−0.504] = 0.60

Upper Limit = exp [0.525] = 1.69

(Note: The same shortcut for the direct calculation of the confidence limits of the OR as that shown for the crude OR—Section A.4—can be used.)

Hypothesis testing is performed as follows:

$$\chi_1^2 = \frac{\left(\left| (53 + 35) - \left(\frac{63 \times 68}{81} + \frac{87 \times 88}{219} \right) \right| - 0.5 \right)^2}{\dfrac{63 \times 18 \times 68 \times 13}{81^2(81 - 1)} + \dfrac{87 \times 132 \times 88 \times 131}{219^2(219 - 1)}} = 0.008$$

Thus, in this example, the OR_{MH} is not statistically significant.

A.9   REGRESSION COEFFICIENT

In Chapter 7, Section 7.4, several regression models for multivariate analysis of epidemiologic data (linear, logistic, Cox, Poisson) are described. These regression analyses are typically conducted with the help of computers and statistical packages, which provide the estimates of the regression coefficients (b) and of their standard error ($\text{SE}(b)$). On the basis of these estimates, and following the general approach described in the introduction to this appendix, it is possible to obtain confidence limits and carry out hypothesis testing.

95% Confidence Interval

The 95% confidence interval for a regression coefficient can be obtained with the following formula:

$b \pm [1.96 \times SE(b)]$

Hypothesis Testing

The null hypothesis is formulated as follows:

$H_0 : \beta = 0$

where β denotes the true value of the parameter in the reference population.

The test statistic in this context is known as the Wald statistic:

$$\frac{b}{SE(b)} \approx z \text{ score}$$

Examples

Linear Regression

From the value of the regression coefficient and standard error for systolic blood pressure (10 mm Hg increase) in Chapter 7, Table 7–16, the 95% confidence intervals can be calculated as

$0.040 \pm (1.96 \times 0.011)$

That is, the estimated 95% confidence interval for the increase in leucocyte count per 10 mm Hg increase in systolic blood pressure is 0.018 to 0.062 thousand per mm^3.

The Wald statistic, which approximates the z score, is calculated as

$$z \approx \frac{0.040}{0.011} = 3.64$$

This value is associated with $P < 0.001$, which allows rejecting the null hypothesis with an alpha error probability lower than 1/1000.

Logistic Regression

In the example in Chapter 7, Table 7–18, the estimated logistic regression coefficient associated with hypertension is 0.5103, which translates into an estimated odds ratio of coronary disease of $e^{0.5103} = 1.67$, comparing hypertensives with nonhypertensives (adjusted for all the other variables displayed in Table 7–18). The standard error

SE

corresponding to the estimated regression coefficient is 0.1844 (not shown in Table 7–18). Thus, the 95% confidence interval for the regression coefficient is calculated as follows:

$$0.5103 \pm (1.96 \times 0.1844)$$

or 0.1489 (lower limit) and 0.8717 (upper limit). The corresponding confidence interval (CI) of the odds ratio (OR) estimate can be obtained by exponentiating these confidence limits, which can be done in just one step, as follows:

Lower Limit = exp [0.5103 − (1.96 × 0.1844)] = 1.16

Upper Limit = exp [0.5103 + (1.96 × 0.1844)] = 2.39

The corresponding Wald statistic for the regression coefficient estimate is

$$z \approx \frac{0.5103}{0.1844} = 2.767$$

The associated *P* value for this *z* score is 0.006. Note that this statistic tests the null hypothesis (H_0: $b = 0$, or the equivalent H_0: OR = 1).

The same approach can be used to obtain confidence limits and conduct hypothesis testing for regression coefficients and derived measures of association from Cox and Poisson regression models.

Wald Statistic for Interaction

If the model contains an interaction term (eg, the product of two *x* variables; see Chapter 7, Section 7.4.2, Equation 7.4), the statistical significance of the corresponding regression coefficient estimate (Wald statistic) is a formal test for the interaction between the two variables. In the example in Equation 7.4, which is a variation of model 2 in Table 7–15, allowing for an interaction between age and systolic blood pressure, the estimated β_3 is 0.0000503, with a standard error of 0.0000570, which corresponds to a Wald statistic of 0.882 (not statistically significant). Thus, these data do not support the hypothesis that there is an interaction between age and systolic blood pressure in relation to carotid intimal-medial thickness.

A.10 SENSITIVITY, SPECIFICITY, AND PERCENT AGREEMENT

Statistical inference procedures for these three measures are the same as those for any other simple proportion.

Standard Error, 95% Confidence Interval

The standard formulation to calculate the standard error of a proportion (p) calculated in a sample of N individuals can be used:

$$SE(p) = \sqrt{\frac{p(1-p)}{N}}$$

Once the standard error is calculated, the general approach for obtaining confidence limits outlined in the introduction to this appendix can be used.

Examples

The following examples are all based on the data from a validation study of self-reported "difficulty in standing up from a chair"[17] (Chapter 8, Table 8–13).

Sensitivity

The estimated sensitivity is $71/(71 + 42) = 0.628$. To calculate the standard error, use as N the total number of true positives ($N = 113$, the denominator for sensitivity):

$$SE(\text{sensitivity}) = \sqrt{\frac{0.628(1-0.628)}{113}} = 0.0455$$

Thus, the 95% confidence limits are

Lower = $0.628 - (1.96 \times 0.0455) = 0.539$

Upper = $0.628 + (1.96 \times 0.0455) = 0.717$

Specificity

The estimated specificity is $455/(455 + 41) = 0.917$. To calculate the standard error, use as N the total number of true negatives ($N = 496$, the denominator for specificity):

$$SE(\text{specificity}) = \sqrt{\frac{0.917(1-0.917)}{496}} = 0.0124$$

Thus, the 95% confidence limits are

Lower = $0.917 - (1.96 \times 0.0124) = 0.893$

Upper = $0.917 + (1.96 \times 0.0124) = 0.941$

Percent Agreement

The estimated percent agreement is $[(71 + 455)]/(609) = 0.864$. To calculate the standard error, use as N the total number in the table ($N = 609$):

$$SE(\%\text{Agreement}) = \sqrt{\frac{0.864(1 - 0.864)}{609}} = 0.0139$$

Thus, the 95% confidence limits (using percentage values) are

Lower = 86.4 − (1.96 × 1.39) = 83.7%

Upper = 86.4 + (1.96 × 1.39) = 89.1%

A.11   YOUDEN'S *J* STATISTIC

Standard Error, Confidence Interval

Youden's *J* statistic is based on the sum of two proportions (sensitivity and specificity) (see Chapter 8, Section 8.4.1). Assuming that these are independent, the standard error (SE) can be calculated as

$$SE(J) = \sqrt{\frac{\text{Sens}(1 - \text{Sens})}{N_{\text{true} +}} + \frac{\text{Spec}(1 - \text{Spec})}{N_{\text{true} -}}}$$

Once the standard error is calculated, the general approach for obtaining confidence limits outlined in the introduction to this appendix can be used.

Examples

The following example is based on the data from Chapter 8, Table 8–5. The estimated Youden's *J* statistic is $(18/19) + (11/30) - 1 = 0.314$. Using the above formula, the standard error is as follows:

$$SE(J) = \sqrt{\frac{\frac{18}{19} \times \frac{1}{19}}{19} + \frac{\frac{11}{30} \times \frac{19}{30}}{30}} = 0.102$$

Thus, the 95% confidence limits are

Lower = 0.314 − (1.96 × 0.102) = 0.114

Upper = 0.314 + (1.96 × 0.102) = 0.514

A.12   KAPPA

The kappa statistic is a useful measure of reliability of categorical variables (see Chapter 8, Section 8.4.1). Formulas for the calculation of the standard error and 95% confidence interval for the *unweighted* kappa are provided as follows.

Standard Error and 95% Confidence Interval

Formulas for the calculation of the standard error of kappa have been published.[18] Consider a situation in which two replicate readings (eg, readings by two raters, A and B) of a given set of test values have been done. The outcome of the test has k possible values. The following table defines the notation for the observed proportions (p) in each cell and marginal of the resulting contingency table of both sets of readings.

RATER B

		1	2	...	k	Total
RATER A	1	p_{11}	p_{12}	...	p_{1k}	$p_{1\cdot}$
	2	p_{21}	p_{22}	...	p_{2k}	$p_{2\cdot}$
	...	...	...	...	...	...
	k	p_{k1}	p_{k2}	...	p_{kk}	$p_{k\cdot}$
	Total	$p_{\cdot1}$	$p_{\cdot2}$	...	$p_{\cdot k}$	1

Based on the above notation, the SE of the estimated kappa can be obtained as follows:

$$SE(\hat{K}) = \frac{1}{(1 - p_e) \times \sqrt{n}} \times \sqrt{p_e + p_e^2 - \left[\sum_{i=1}^{k} p_{i\cdot} \times p_{\cdot i} \times (p_{i\cdot} + p_{\cdot i})\right]}$$

where p_e is the total expected chance agreement, which is calculated from the product of the symmetrical marginal proportions (see Chapter 8, Section 8.4.1):

$$p_e = \sum_{i=1}^{k} p_{i\cdot}p_{\cdot i}$$

Note: Formulas for the standard error of *weighted* kappa have also been derived; see, eg, Fleiss.[18]

Example

The following example is based on the data from a study of self-reported "difficulty in standing up from a chair"[17] (Chapter 8, Table 8–13) (see also Section A.10):

	Observed Difficulty		
Reported Difficulty	Yes	No	Total
Yes	71	41	112
No	42	455	497
Total	113	496	609

Source: Data from M Ferrer et al, Comparison of Performance-Based and Self-Rated Functional Capacity in Spanish Elderly, *American Journal of Epidemiology,* Vol 149, pp 228–235, © 1999, The Johns Hopkins University School of Hygiene & Public Health.

Dividing numbers in the table by the total ($N = 609$), the following table shows the proportions as in the notation table shown previously.

Reported Difficulty	Observed Difficulty		Total
	Yes	No	
Yes	0.1166		0.1839
No		0.7471	0.8161
Total	0.1856	0.8144	1

Note: The proportions in the discordant cells are not shown because they are not used in the calculations that follow.

Source: Data from M Ferrer et al, Comparison of Performance-Based and Self-Rated Functional Capacity in Spanish Elderly, *American Journal of Epidemiology*, Vol 149, pp 228–235, © 1999, The Johns Hopkins University School of Hygiene & Public Health.

The observed agreement is

$$p_0 = \sum_{i=1}^{k} p_{ii} = 0.1166 + 0.7471 = 0.8637$$

The expected (chance) agreement is

$$p_e = \sum_{i=1}^{k} p_{i.}p_{.i} = (0.1865 \times 0.1839) + (0.8144 \times 0.8161) = 0.6989$$

Thus, the estimated kappa for these data is

$$\hat{K} = \frac{p_0 - p_e}{1 - p_e} = \frac{0.8637 - 0.6989}{1 - 0.6989} = 0.547$$

Using the above formula, the standard error is as follows:

$$\frac{1}{(1 - 0.6989)\sqrt{609}}\sqrt{0.6989 + 0.6989^2 - \left(\begin{array}{c}0.1839 \times 0.1856 \times (0.1839 + 0.1856) + \\ 0.8161 \times 0.8144 \times (0.8161 + 0.8144)\end{array}\right)} = 0.041$$

Thus, the 95% confidence interval limits are

Lower $= 0.547 - (1.96 \times 0.041) = 0.467$

Upper $= 0.547 + (1.96 \times 0.041) = 0.627$

REFERENCES

1. Goodman SN. P values, hypothesis tests, and likelihood: implications for epidemiology of a neglected historical debate. *Am J Epidemiol.* 1993;137:485–496.

2. Royal R. *Statistical Evidence: A Likelihood Primer.* London: Chapman and Hall; 1997.

3. Armitage P, Berry G. *Statistical Methods in Medical Research.* 3rd ed. London, England: Blackwell; 1994.

4. Altman DG. *Practical Statistics for Medical Students.* London, England: Chapman and Hall; 1991.

5. Greenwood M. A report on the natural duration of cancer. *Rep Public Health Med Subjects.* 1926;33:1–26.

6. Haenszel W, Loveland DB, Sirken MG. Lung cancer mortality as related to residence and smoking histories. I. White Males. *J Natl Cancer Inst.* 1962;28:947–1001.

7. Breslow NE, Day NE. *Statistical Methods in Cancer Research. Vol 2. The Design and Analysis of Cohort Studies.* Lyon, France: IARC Scientific Publications; 1987.

8. Katz D, Baptista J, Azen SP, et al. Obtaining confidence intervals for the risk ratio in cohort studies. *Biometrics.* 1978;34:469–474.

9. Ederer F, Mantel N. Confidence limits on the ratio of two Poisson variables. *Am J Epidemiol.* 1974;100:165–167.

10. Woolf B. On estimating the relation between blood group and disease. *Ann Hum Genet.* 1955;19:251–253.

11. Walter SD. Calculation of attributable risks from epidemiological data. *Int J Epidemiol.* 1978;7:175–182.

12. Kahn HA, Sempos CT. *Statistical Methods in Epidemiology.* New York, NY: Oxford University Press; 1989.

13. Pandey DK, Shekelle R, Selwyn BJ, et al. Dietary vitamin C and β-carotene and risk of death in middle-aged men: the Western Electric study. *Am J Epidemiol.* 1995;142:1269–1278.

14. Robins J, Greenland S, Breslow NE. A general estimator for the variance of the Mantel-Haenszel odds ratio. *Am J Epidemiol.* 1986;124:719–723.

15. Greenland S, Robins JM. Estimation of a common effect parameter from sparse follow-up death. *Biometrics.* 1985;41:55–68.

16. Mantel N, Haenszel W. Statistical aspects of the analysis of data from retrospective studies of disease. *J Natl Cancer Inst.* 1959;22:719–748.

17. Ferrer M, Lamarca R, Orfila F, Alfonso J. Comparison of performance-based and self-rated functional capacity in Spanish elderly. *Am J Epidemiol.* 1999;149: 228–235.

18. Fleiss JL. *Statistical Methods for Rates and Proportions.* 2nd ed. New York, NY: John Wiley and Sons; 1981.

APPENDIX B

Test for Trend
(Dose Response)

When exposure is categorized into multiple *ordinal* categories, it may be of interest to assess whether the observed relation between increasing (or decreasing) levels of exposure and the risk (or odds) of disease follows a *linear* dose-response pattern. One example was provided in Chapter 3 at the end of Section 3.4.1, Table 3–11, in which the odds ratios of craniosynostosis seemed to increase in relation to increasing maternal age in a dose-response fashion.[1] A statistical test to assess whether the observed trend is statistically significant (ie, whether the null hypothesis that there is no linear trend can be rejected) was developed by Mantel.[2] The formulation below is based on the following notation:

Stratum (i)	Score (x_i)	No. of Cases (a_i)	No. of Controls (b_i)	Total (n_i)
1	x_1	a_1	b_1	n_1
2	x_2	a_2	b_2	n_2
.	.	.	.	.
.	.	.	.	.
k	x_k	a_k	b_k	n_k
Total		A	B	N

The following statistic has a chi-square distribution with 1 degree of freedom:

$$\chi^2_1 = \frac{\left[\sum_{i=1}^{k}\left(a_i x_i - \frac{n_i x_i A}{N}\right)\right]^2}{\left(\frac{A \times B \times \left[\left(N \times \sum_{i=1}^{k} n_i x_i^2\right) - \left(\sum_{i=1}^{k} n_i x_i\right)^2\right]}{N^2(N-1)}\right)}$$

459

where the scores (x_i) are values that represent the level of exposure in each subsequent ordinal category (see below).

EXAMPLE

To illustrate the application of Mantel's trend test, the data from the example in Chapter 3, Table 3–11, are used. For the purpose of making the calculations easier, these data are rearranged in the following work table:

Age (yr)	i	x_i	a_i	b_i	n_i	$a_i x_i - \dfrac{n_i x_i A}{N}$	$n_i x_i$	$n_i x_i^2$
<20	1	1	12	89	101	−6.748	101	101
20–24	2	2	47	242	289	−13.290	578	1156
25–29	3	3	56	255	311	−5.186	933	2799
>29	4	4	58	173	231	60.485	924	3696
Total			173	759	932	35.262	2536	7752

Source: Data from BW Alderman et al, An Epidemiologic Study of Craniosynostosis: Risk Indicators for the Occurrence of Craniosynostosis in Colorado, *American Journal of Epidemiology,* Vol 128, pp 431–438, © 1988, The Johns Hopkins University School of Hygiene & Public Health.

Thus, applying the above formula:

$$\chi_i^2 = \frac{[35.262]^2}{\left(\dfrac{173 \times 759 \times [(932 \times 7752) - 2536^2]}{932^2(932 - 1)}\right)} = 9.65$$

corresponding to a P value of 0.0019.

NOTES

The null hypothesis corresponding to this trend test is that there is no linear association, or, in other words, that the *slope* of the association with increasing levels of exposure is zero (flat). Thus, a significant P value from this test means that the data do not support the hypothesis of a zero slope. Such a result should not replace the examination of the actual odds ratio estimates in order to judge whether a linear trend is indeed present. As for any other statistical test, the P value depends strongly on the sample size; thus, if the sample size is large, a J-type or a threshold-type association may result in a significant trend test, even though the association is not linear. For example, suppose that the estimated odds ratios for five increasing ordinal categories of a given exposure (eg, quintiles of a continuous variable) are 1.0 (reference), 0.9, 1.1, 1.0, and 3.0. If the sample size is sufficiently large, the trend test may yield a highly significant result, which simply indicates that the null hypothesis ("slope" = 0) can be rejected with a certain level of confidence, notwithstanding the fact that, in this example, the pattern of the association is practically flat, except for the high odds ratio in the top quintile that is an increase in odds limited to the individuals in the top fifth of the distribution. This phenomenon is analogous to the issues discussed in Chapter 7 on the use of linear models to analyze nonlinear patterns (Section 7.4.7).

The above trend test is analogous to the Wald test for a linear regression coefficient (see Section 7.4.8), except that it is based on a small number of data points (four in the above example), which are *weighted* according to the number of subjects in the corresponding category. Thus, the same limitations and care that should be taken when using linear regression models apply when interpreting the results of a trend test.

Alternative formulations of the trend test described above have been proposed, based on assessing the linear trends in proportions (see for example, Cochran[3]). Given the arithmetical equivalence between proportions and odds, all these alternative tests lead to similar results; for additional references and discussion, see Fleiss[4] or Schlesselman.[5]

In the above example, the scores were arbitrarily set as 1, 2, 3, and 4. Note that the exact same chi-square value will be obtained using the scores -1, 0, 1, and 2, while the calculations (if done by hand) will be considerably easier. In the case of ordinal categorizations based on a continuous variable (such as age in the example above), instead of these completely arbitrary scores, it may be more appropriate to choose as scores the midpoints for the variables that define each category. For example, assuming that the ranges for the top and bottom open-ended categories above were 10 to 19 years and 30 to 39 years, respectively, the scores would be 15, 22.5, 27.5, and 35, with the following result:

Age (yr)	i	x_i	a_i	b_i	n_i	$a_i x_i - \dfrac{n_i x_i A}{N}$	$n_i x_i$	$n_i x_i^2$
<20	1	15	12	89	101	-101.22	1515	22,725
20–24	2	22.5	47	242	289	-149.51	6502.5	146,306.3
25–29	3	27.5	56	255	311	-47.535	8552.5	235,193.8
>29	4	35	58	173	231	529.244	8085	282,975
Total			173	759	932	230.982	24,655	687,200

Source: Data from BW Alderman et al, An Epidemiologic Study of Craniosynostosis: Risk Indicators for the Occurrence of Craniosynostosis in Colorado, *American Journal of Epidemiology*, Vol 128, pp 431–438, © 1988, The Johns Hopkins University School of Hygiene & Public Health.

In this example, the resulting chi-square is 10.08, $P = 0.0015$. (Alternatively, the score for each category could be the mean or median value for the variable in question for all the individuals included in each respective category.)

MULTIVARIATE TREND TEST

As stated previously, the statistical test for trend is the analogue to the Wald test assessing the statistical significance of a linear regression coefficient (see Chapter 7, Section 7.4.8 and Appendix A.9). In fact, a regression approach can be used to test the statistical significance of a linear dose-response trend (using odds ratios or another measure of association, depending on the statistical model at hand; see Chapter 7, Table 7–14) corresponding to an ordinal variable *while adjusting for additional covariates* included in the model. For example, it may be of interest to assess whether the risk of craniosynostosis increases linearly with age (categorized as above) while adjusting for additional covariates (eg, socioeconomic status, family history). In that situation, to carry out the multivariate analogue of the above trend test in the example, a logistic regression model can be used entering the variable AGEGROUP as a single ordinal term (with values 1, 2, 3, and 4, or any other meaningful alternative, as discussed above), along with any other variables in the model that need to be controlled for. The Wald statistic for the regression coefficient corresponding to this variable can be interpreted as a statistical test for linear dose response for adjusted data. As for the trend test for unadjusted data, it is important to examine whether there is an actual dose response trend by inspection of stratum-specific estimates (eg, by examining the estimates based on a model using dummy variables) before interpreting this statistical trend test on the basis of regression (see Chapter 7, Section 7.4.7).

REFERENCES

1. Alderman BW, Lammer EJ, Joshua SC, et al. An epidemiologic study of craniosynostosis: risk indicators for the occurrence of craniosynostosis in Colorado. *Am J Epidemiol.* 1998;128:431–438.
2. Mantel N. Chi-square tests with one degree of freedom: extensions of the Mantel-Haenszel procedure. *J Am Stat Assoc.* 1963;58:690–700.
3. Cochran WG. Some methods for strengthening the common chi-square tests. *Biometrics.* 1954;10:417–451.
4. Fleiss JL. *Statistical Methods for Rates and Proportions.* 2nd ed. New York, NY: John Wiley and Sons; 1981.
5. Schlesselman JJ. *Case Control Studies.* New York, NY: Oxford University Press; 1982.

APPENDIX C

Test of Homogeneity of Stratified Estimates (Test for Interaction)

As discussed in Chapter 6, interaction or effect modification is present when the association between a given exposure and an outcome is modified by the presence or level of a third variable (the *effect modifier*). The different aspects that need to be considered when judging whether an observed heterogeneity of the association is truly interaction or is due to random variability of the stratum-specific estimates were discussed in Chapter 6 (Sections 6.9 and 6.10.1). In this appendix, a general procedure to assess the hypothesis of homogeneity (ie, lack of interaction) is described. As with any hypothesis testing, the P value resulting from this homogeneity testing is strongly dependent on sample size. This problem is especially important when stratified data are evaluated. Epidemiologic studies are typically designed to optimize the statistical power to detect associations based on pooled data from the total study sample. However, the power to detect interaction is often limited by insufficient stratum-specific sample sizes.[1]

Consider a situation in which a given measure of association R between exposure and outcome is estimated across k strata of a suspected effect modifier. The general form of a statistical test of the homogeneity hypothesis (ie, H_0: the strength of association is homogeneous across all strata) is analogous to a familiar type of statistical test to compare stratified survival data (log rank test) and adopts the following general form[1]:

$$\chi^2_{k-1} = \sum_{i=1}^{k} \frac{(R_i - \hat{R})^2}{V_i}$$

where R_i is the stratum-specific measure of association (for $i = 1$ to k strata), V_i is the corresponding variance, and $\hat{R}$ is the estimated "common" underlying value of the measure of association under the null hypothesis. The latter is usually estimated using one of the approaches to obtain weighted averages of stratum-specific estimates of association described in Section 7.3 of Chapter 7 (eg, direct adjustment, indirect adjustment, Mantel-Haenszel). This test statistic has a chi-square distribution with as many degrees of freedom as the number of strata minus 1.

One important consideration is that for multiplicative (relative) measures of association (eg, relative risk, odds ratio, rate ratio), the logarithm of the ratio (not the ratio itself) is used in the above equation for R_i and $\hat{R}$; consequently, the corresponding variance, V_i, is the variance of the log (ratio).

EXAMPLE: TEST OF HOMOGENEITY OF STRATIFIED ODDS RATIOS

This test uses the following formula:

$$\chi^2_{k-1} = \sum_{i=1}^{k} \frac{(\log OR_i - \log \widehat{OR})^2}{var(\log OR_i)}$$

The following example of the application of this test uses data from Table 7–2, which displayed the association between oral contraceptive use and myocardial infarction stratified by age.[2] The Mantel-Haenszel estimate of the overall odds ratio for these data is OR_{MH} = 3.97 (Section 7.3.3). The following table is organized to facilitate the calculations of the homogeneity test statistic:

Stratum No. (Age, Yr)	OC	No. of Cases (a) (c)	No. of Controls (b) (d)	OR $\frac{(a \times d)}{(b \times c)}$	log OR	Var(log OR) $\left(\frac{1}{a} + \frac{1}{b} + \frac{1}{c} + \frac{1}{d}\right)$*
1 (25–29)	Yes	4	62	7.226	1.978	0.771
	No	2	224			
2 (30–34)	Yes	9	33	8.864	2.182	0.227
	No	12	390			
3 (35–39)	Yes	4	26	1.538	0.431	0.322
	No	33	330			
4 (40–44)	Yes	6	9	3.713	1.312	0.296
	No	65	362			
5 (45–49)	Yes	6	5	3.884	1.357	0.381
	No	93	301			

Note: OC, oral contraceptive use.

*See Appendix A, Section A.4.

Source: Data from S Shapiro et al, Oral-Contraceptive Use in Relation to Myocardial Infarction, *Lancet*, Vol 1, pp 743–747, © 1979.

Thus, applying the above formula:

$$\chi_4^2 = \frac{(1.978 - \log{(3.97)})^2}{0.771} + \frac{(2.182 - \log{(3.97)})^2}{0.227} + \ldots + \frac{(1.357 - (\log{(3.97)})^2}{0.381}$$

$$= 0.4655 + 2.8382 + 2.7925 + 0.0151 + 0.0013$$

$$= 6.113$$

This chi-square value with 4 degrees of freedom is associated with a *P* > 0.10 and thus is nonsignificant at conventional levels.

REFERENCES

1. Rothman KJ, Greenland S. *Modern Epidemiology.* 2nd ed. Philadelphia, PA: Lippincott-Raven; 1998.
2. Shapiro S, Slone D, Rosenberg L, et al. Oral-contraceptive use in relation to myocardial infarction. *Lancet.* 1979;1:743–747.

Quality Assurance and Quality Control Procedures Manual for Blood Pressure Measurement and Blood/Urine Collection in the ARIC Study

The following is a verbatim transcription of two sections of the Atherosclerosis Risk in Communities (ARIC) Study Quality Assurance/Quality Control Manual of operations. These are included as examples for some of the procedures discussed in Chapter 8. For more detail on the ARIC Study design and protocol (including the entire Quality Control Manual and other manuals cited in the following text), see the ARIC Study Web page (http://www.bios.unc.edu/cscc/ARIC).

Source: Reprinted from Atherosclerosis Risk in Communities (ARIC) Study coordinated by the University of North Carolina at Chapel Hill for the National Heart, Lung and Blood Institute, National Institutes of Health.

SITTING BLOOD PRESSURE

1. Brief Description of Sitting Blood Pressure Procedures and Related Quality Assurance and Quality Control Measures

The following equipment is used for measuring sitting blood pressure: a standard Littman stethoscope with bell; standardized Hawksley random-zero instrument; standard Baum manometer for determining peak inflation level; four standardized cuffs (from Baum). After the technician explains the procedure to the participant, measures the arm circumference and wraps the arm with the correct cuff, the participant sits quietly for 5 minutes, and then the technician makes two readings, with at least 30 seconds between reading one measure and beginning the next. The average of the two readings is reported to the participant.

From the detailed protocol for sitting blood pressure in ARIC Manual 11, the various data transfer points and other possible sources of error have been considered, and needed quality assurance and control measures have been derived. Important elements in quality assurance are training and certification programs, observation of data collection by supervisors, biannually simultaneous blood pressure measurements using Y-tubes by two technicians, and standard equipment maintenance procedures performed and entered into logs.

2. Maintenance of Equipment

1) <u>Availability of all sizes cuffs:</u> The field center blood pressure supervisor makes certain that the field center always has the full range of blood pressure cuffs available at each blood pressure station. Field center staff report immediately to the blood pressure supervisor if they cannot find all cuff sizes at the station.

2) <u>Sphygmomanometers:</u> Regular inspections of random-zero and standard sphygmomanometers are described in ARIC Manual 11, Section 1.13.1 and Appendices I, II, and V. A log sheet is kept by the field center blood pressure supervisor, who records the performance of these checks and comments on any problems found (see copy of log sheet in Manual 11, Appendix IV). By the end of each January and July, the summary form for the checklists should be filled and mailed to the Coordinating Center.

3) <u>Measuring tape:</u> Each week the blood pressure supervisor checks the condition of the measuring tape used to measure arm circumfer-

ence at the blood pressure station(s), and replaces any that have become worn. The results of this check are recorded on the anthropometry weekly log. (See the anthropometry section for details.)

3. Field Center Monitoring of Technician Performance

1) Double stethoscoping: To help assess the accuracy and precision of blood pressure measurements, once each January and July each blood pressure technician takes part in measuring blood pressure simultaneously with another technician, using a Y-tube. This procedure should be carried out using volunteers or other field center staff members, not ARIC study participants. The two technicians also perform independent measurements of arm circumference, which they record on the forms. If the two technician measurements lead to a disagreement on which blood pressure cuff to use, then both remeasure the arm together and use the cuff size determined by that measurement. Each records this disagreement on the Sitting Blood Pressure form. Each technician separately records all blood pressure measurements on paper on a standard Sitting Blood Pressure form. The two paper forms are given to the field center blood pressure supervisor, who compares the results.

The field center blood pressure supervisor reviews the results of these duplicate examinations, calculating the disagreement between technicians on the blood pressure measurements and recording it on the form. The two technicians should agree on each of the two measurements of diastolic and systolic blood pressure within 4 mmHg, and their average should agree within 3 mmHg, as is required by the standards for certification. If they do not, further duplicate readings are taken to determine if either or both technicians require recertification. These further measurements should again be recorded as described in the previous paragraph.

The IDs of each set of technicians paired for simultaneous measurement of blood pressure are recorded in the Report on Use of Observation and Equipment Checklist, which is mailed to the Coordinating Center at the end of each January and July.

2) Biannual observation: Once every January and July, the field center's blood pressure supervisor observes each blood pressure technician performing the entire measurement procedure with a study participant. The field center supervisor notes any problems with technique and discusses them with the technician after the examination has been completed. Also, another technician observes the field center blood pressure supervisor perform the entire measurement process. Af-

ter the examination, the two of them discuss any questions that come up in the course of this observation. In performing these observations, the supervisor and technicians use the checklist given in Appendix III of ARIC Manual 11. For each technician, the date that the technician was observed and the observer's ID number are recorded in the Report on Use of Observation and Equipment Checklist.

4. Recording of Participant ID Data

In filling out the Sitting Blood Pressure screen, the technician verifies that the name and ID number on the DES screen which accompanies the participant match the participant's to avoid ID errors. If the PC is down and a paper form is used, the technician verifies the name on the folder accompanying the participant before using the ID labels in the folder on the forms.

5. Measurement of Arm Circumference and Choice of Blood Pressure Cuff

As described above, once every six months duplicate measurements of blood pressure are performed on a volunteer or field center staff member (not an ARIC participant). During the course of this procedure, both technicians measure arm circumference and record their results. The field center blood pressure supervisor compares these results, and if they differ by more than 1 cm, the measurement technique is reviewed with both technicians.

Both the arm measurement and the cuff size chosen are recorded on the SBP form. The data entry system checks for the consistency of cuff size and arm circumference.

6. Participant Posture and Rest Before Blood Pressure Measurement

The field center blood pressure supervisor monitors that the station(s) used for blood pressure measurement continue to meet the conditions specified in the protocol, e.g., that blood pressure measurements are done in a quiet room away from other field center activities. Coordinating Center staff on monitoring visits also take note whether this condition is being maintained.

The field center blood pressure supervisor is responsible for seeing that the protocol is followed by timing blood pressure measurements early in the visit, before blood drawing or other stressful activities.

Each month the field center supervisor reviews a sample of participant itinerary forms for the previous month to confirm that this is done.

To assist in judging that a full five-minute rest is allowed before taking the first blood pressure measurement, the blood pressure technician uses a hand held timer or other means of accurately timing the rest period. Biannually, the field center blood pressure supervisor observes each technician performing the full blood pressure procedure and notes whether the correct rest period is being allowed.

7. Coordinating Center Quality Control Analyses

The Coordinating Center analyzes data from each technician for digit preference in reading systolic or diastolic blood pressure. This check is performed annually, unless problems detected call for more or less intensive monitoring. The Coordinating Center reports these results to the field center, and the field center blood pressure supervisor reviews these results with each technician.

The Coordinating Center checks that correct data entry procedures are used for recording missing data. The Coordinating Center communicates with the field centers when problems are identified.

BLOOD AND URINE COLLECTION AND PROCESSING

1. Brief Description of Blood Collection and Processing and Related Quality Assurance and Quality Control Measures

At the time of the telephone contact participants are requested to fast for 12 hours before field center visit, unless they are diabetics taking insulin or have other medical reasons that make fasting inadvisable. A detailed protocol, set out in ARIC Manual 7 (<u>Blood Collection and Processing</u>) has been developed, which describes the preparation of blood tubes, the anticoagulants to be used for samples for each laboratory, and the specific steps to be taken in blood drawing and processing. After the blood is drawn, the sample tubes go through further processing at the field center. Blood samples used for lipid and hemostasis analyses are frozen at $-70°C$ for weekly shipment to the ARIC central laboratories. Samples for hematology analyses are sent to local laboratories. All shipments to Central Laboratories are by overnight delivery services. All of these steps are performed by technicians trained in the ARIC protocol and certified to have adequately mastered its details.

The first step in quality assurance for blood drawing consists in this training and certification process. Other steps include maintaining logs of equipment checks; observation of technicians (by other technicians and by monitors on visits) as they go through the sequence of steps in blood drawing and processing; review of the condition of samples received at central laboratories for problems in shipment; and periodic analysis of the study data for participant compliance with fasting and for signs of problems in drawing or processing, such as hemolysis or delays in completing processing.

2. Maintenance of Equipment

Each field center performs daily temperature checks on refrigerators, freezers, the refrigerated centrifuge, and the heating block (see ARIC Manual 7). The actual speed of the centrifuge is checked and recorded monthly with a tachometer. The results of these checks are recorded on a log sheet kept at the blood processing station and are summarized onto the Report on the Use of Observation and Equipment Checklist at the end of each January and July. A copy of the report is sent to the Coordinating Center at that time.

3. Participant Compliance with Protocol

In contrast to previous visits, venipuncture is performed on all cohort members, regardless of their fasting status (Manual 2, Section 3.9.2), and includes 3 plasma samples for the Lipid and Hemostasis labs; 2 serum samples for the Hemostasis and Dental labs; and an optional sample for a local Hematology lab. In addition, a second venipuncture is performed on OGTT eligible participants. The post glucola blood draw must occur within 2 hrs. (plus or minus 10 min.) of administration of the glucola drink. Failure to meet criteria can affect the values of various measurements (e.g., lipids, glucose) and compromise their value to the study. ARIC participants should also abstain from smoking and vigorous physical effort before the visit to the field center, since smoking may affect electrocardiograms or blood pressure and vigorous activity may activate fibrinolysis and alter blood levels of tPA and FPB8. Interviewers are trained to explain the importance of compliance with these restrictions. When field centers contact participants before their appointment to remind them about the scheduled visit, they repeat these instructions.

The Coordinating Center analyzes study data for information on length of time fasting and time since smoking and hard exercise, broken down by field center, to obtain the number and percent of participants at each field center each month who do not comply with these restrictions.

4. Maintaining Proficiency

To maintain their proficiency, technicians are urged to perform blood drawing and processing at least once each week (or 8 times each 2 months). The Coordinating Center analyzes the study data to report on the number of times that technicians collect and process blood in the field centers.

5. Periodic Observation

Periodically (each month in the beginning) each field center technician performing blood drawing and processing is observed performing the entire procedure by either another trained technician or a supervisor, using a detailed checklist to verify that the technician is continuing to follow all parts of the ARIC protocol. Carrying out this observation also provides a review of the protocol for the person doing the observation. (See ARIC Manual 7 for further details and for a copy of the ARIC Venipuncture and Processing Procedure Certification Checklist.) This checklist is also used for observations by monitors from the Coordinating Center performing monitoring. The IDs of observer and observed are recorded in the ARIC Venipuncture and Processing Procedure Certification Checklist. They are also recorded on the Report on the Use of Observation and Equipment Checklist, which is mailed to the Coordinating Center by the end of each January and July.

6. The Laboratory Form

To avoid ID errors in which information regarding a given participant's samples is written down on the wrong form, the technician should begin filling out each Laboratory Form (LABB) as the blood is drawn, verifying the ID from the folder which accompanies the participant.

7. Quality Control Replicate Data

The system of drawing extra tubes of blood for QC replicate analysis is fully explained in ARIC Manual 7. In this system specified extra tubes of blood are drawn from a number of participants and matched to one "phantom participant" per week. The post-glucola blood sample is designated as Tube #6 on the Phantom Participant and Non-Participant ID form. See also Chapter 2 of Manual 12 for an explanation of the QC phantom system.

Persons who are non-fasting and indicate that they would like to be rescheduled for another blood draw should never be used as a QC blood phantom.

The field center blood drawing station maintains a schedule of which tubes should be drawn for phantoms each day (see ARIC Manual 7) to help fit the QC phantom sets into the work flow and make it easy to keep track of what is required. The Coordinating Center reviews each month, broken down by field center, the number of QC phantom forms for which blood drawing is indicated. If field centers fail to provide sufficient sets of QC phantom blood, the Coordinating Center contacts the field centers to discuss the problem. To reduce the risk of labeling a QC phantom blood tube with the wrong ID or of recording the wrong match between phantom and participant IDs on the QC Phantom Participant Forms, QC blood is drawn from no more than one member of each pair of participants whose blood is processed together. To help make certain that the correct match is recorded between real participant ID and QC phantom ID, as soon as blood-drawing has been completed an ID label for the real participant ID is added to the appropriate space on the QC Phantom Participant and Non-Participant ID Form in the QC phantom folder.

8. Analysis of Venipuncture and Processing Data for Quality Control

The Coordinating Center analyzes the study data annually to determine the frequencies of filling time, number of stick attempts and reported presence of hemolysis, and selected markers of lack of adherence to protocol during phlebotomy and/or processing of specimens at the field center laboratory. These analyses include field center tabulations by the ID of the technician performing the blood drawing or processing. (Standards for time needed for various processing steps are given in ARIC Manual 7.) Adherence to the 2-hr. post-glucola blood draw window is assessed quarterly and reported to field centers.

9. Packing Samples for Shipment to Laboratories

All vials of blood samples as well as the plastic bags in which the samples for a given participant are packed for shipment to the several laboratories are labeled with the participant's ID. A shipping list is enclosed with each shipment to the Central Laboratories giving the IDs for all sets of samples that are enclosed. The person unpacking these samples at the Central Laboratories verifies that the IDs on the vials match the ID on the plastic bag and checks both against the shipping list. If any discrepancies are detected, the Central Laboratory contacts the field center to resolve the problem.

Blood vials shipped to the Central Laboratories must be packed securely to avoid both breakage and warming. Full instructions for packing samples are specified in ARIC Manual 7, Sections 5.1–5.3. The laboratories monitor the arrival condition of the samples sent from each field center. If problems are encountered, the laboratories notify the field centers involved. If a pattern of sample damage becomes apparent that suggests a need to modify the materials used to ship samples (e.g., excessive leakage of a certain type of vial) or how samples are packed, the Laboratory Subcommittee takes appropriate action.

ARIC blood samples are mailed promptly to the Central Laboratories at the start of the week after they are drawn. The laboratories monitor the dates of blood drawing on samples which they receive and notify the field center and the Coordinating Center if they receive samples that were shipped at a later date than that called for under this schedule. (Note: quality control phantom blood tubes are held over one week before shipping, but the date of drawing on these samples that is reported to the laboratory is altered to conceal their identity as QC.) The field centers should phone the central laboratories to notify them if they are shipping on a day other than Monday.

To avoid delays in transit to the laboratories which might cause samples to be warmed or thawed in shipping, all samples are shipped by an overnight delivery service. To avoid delays over weekends or holidays in delivering samples or in moving them to the Central Laboratory freezer once they are delivered to the receiving area, all samples are shipped out at the beginning of the working week, on Monday or Tuesday. The laboratories notify the Coordinating Center and the field center if a shipment is received that was shipped out on a later day in the week, and the field center reports to the Coordinating Center on the reasons for this deviation from protocol. The laboratories notify the Field Centers if sets of samples are received late. If a pattern of delays is encountered with the delivery service a field center is using, the field center will change to an alternate delivery service.

10. Description of Urine Collection and Processing and Related Measures for Quality Assurance and Quality Control

After a participant is greeted at the clinic, he/she is asked to provide a urine specimen at the participant's convenience (e.g., when the participant expresses the need to void). When the participant is ready to void, a specimen cup (labeled with the participant's ID and TIME VOIDED) is provided, and the participant is instructed to fill the cup if possible. If the sample is insufficient for processing, the participant is requested to void again in a clean container prior to leaving the field center. Prior to processing, the technician records on the participant's Laboratory Form whether a urine sample was obtained, the collection time of the initial (if more than one) urine sample, and adequacy of volume.

11. QC Sample Preparation

The following instructions describe specific additions to urine collection and processing protocols in order to meet QC requirements. These instructions assume that the normal procedures for collecting, processing, and shipping creatinine and albumin samples (see Manual 7, Section 6.0–6.3) are being followed.

12. Urine QC Schedule

The Visit 4 schedule for urine QC sampling parallels the blood QC sampling protocol: a minimum of one sample is required each week. QC specimens should be taken from the first participant either Tuesday or Thursday who provides sufficient urine. If no participant on Tuesday (or Thursday) provides a sufficient amount, the first participant to do so on Wednesday (or Friday) should be selected.

Urine QC sample collection should be added to the weekly checklist maintained by the field center venipuncture technicians. As with blood QC samples, each urine sample should be checked off as it is prepared. On Wednesday or Friday mornings, the checklist is consulted to see if an additional urine sample is still needed.

13. QC Sample Requirements

Each participant's urine specimen is divided into three separate sample tubes and frozen at the field centers until shipping. Aliquots for creatinine and albumin on each participant (3.5 ml each) are shipped to the Minneapolis ARIC Field Center. The 50 ml conical tube (one per participant) for the hemostatic metabolites is shipped to the ARIC Hemostasis Laboratory; this tube must contain a minimum of 40 ml. When the schedule calls for collection of a QC sample (phantom) for creatinine and albumin, the participant's specimen cup must contain at least 54 ml (14 ml for a total of four 3.5 ml vials and one 40 ml hemostasis sample). For a hemostasis laboratory phantom, 87 ml (7 ml for two 3.5 ml vials and two 40 ml hemostasis samples) are needed.

14. Laboratory and Phantom Forms

To ensure that the correct match is recorded between the real participant ID and the QC phantom ID, as soon as it can be ascertained that sufficient urine for a QC sample has been provided, an ID label for the real participant ID is added to the appropriate space on the QC Phantom Participant and Nonparticipant ID Form.

To avoid ID errors in which information regarding a given participant's urine sample is entered on the wrong form, the technician should begin filling out a URINE SAMPLE section of the Laboratory Form for the phantom ID at the same time the participant's URINE SAMPLE section of this form is completed.

15. Sample Preparation

When creatinine and albumin phantom urine specimens are to be prepared, a total of four 3.5 ml aliquoting vials are required. Two vials are labeled with the participant ID and the remaining two with the phantom ID.

The two CREATININE and two ALBUMIN specimen vials are distinguished by cap inserts: YELLOW for CREATININE, and BLUE for ALBUMIN. The creatinine participant and phantom cryovials are filled first by the lab technician. Then the procedure for pH balancing of the albumin sample is executed (Manual 7, Section 6.1.2), and the pH balanced specimen is pipetted into the participant and phantom cryovials.

The phantom hemostasis urine specimen is prepared at the same time and manner as the participant hemostasis urine sample.

16. Procedure for Small Samples

For QC purposes, the pairs of participant and phantom creatinine, albumin, and hemostasis urine samples must come from the same batch. If a single batch is inadequate for both the participant and phantom samples, then the specimens should be combined prior to drawing the samples.

17. Storage Instructions

Storage instructions (Manual 7, Section 6.2) stipulate that samples be packed in the order of the date drawn, putting a single participant's two specimens (CREATINE and ALBUMIN) side by side in the row. Since the phantom and participant specimens are drawn on the same date, they will likely be on the same row, possibly next to each other.

Record the box and position numbers on the participant's Laboratory Form, and be sure to do the same for the phantom.

Finally, record the IDs of all participants and phantoms in each box on a Box Log Form.

18. Quality Assurance and Quality Control

In addition to annual recertification authorized by the Hemostasis Laboratory, protocol adherence in the performance of each procedure is reviewed at least biannually by the lead technician, and annually by Coordinating Center field center monitors. Deviation from protocol and possible remedial actions are discussed with study coordinators and staff at that time. Major deviations are brought to the attention of the Cohort Operation Committee.

The CC will produce reports based on replicate data from the labs. Results of these reports will be examined by the QC Committee, and recommended corrective actions will be implemented. The Coordinating Center will provide to the QC Committee and field centers a report based on the procedural data recorded on the Laboratory Form. This report will evaluate data for consistency, and for missing or out of range values.

Calculation of the Intraclass Correlation Coefficient

The intraclass correlation coefficient (ICC) is the proportion of the total variability in the measured factor that is due to the variability between individuals (see Chapter 8, Section 8.4.2). In this appendix, two approaches for the calculation of the ICC are described: one is based on analysis of variance (ANOVA) results[1] and the other on a shortcut formula described by Deyo et al.[2] Both techniques are illustrated using as an example the between-scorer reliability data from the Sleep Heart Health Study quality control study (see Chapter 8, Table 8–20).

ANALYSIS OF VARIANCE

To carry out an ANOVA on a set of replicate observations (eg, the between-scorer apnea-hypopnea index (AHI) reliability data from Table 8–20), the data need to be arranged so that *all* AHI values (from both sets of replicate observations) are contained in a single variable. Additional indicator variables denote the identifier for both the study number and the scorer. Thus, in this example, the data can be arranged for a total of 60 observations, as follows:

Study No.	Scorer	AHI
1	A	1.25
1	B	1.38
2	A	1.61
2	B	2.05
3	A	5.64
3	B	5.50
.	.	.
.	.	.
.	.	.
29	A	2.09
29	B	2.35
30	A	11.09
30	B	9.25

A similar approach is used to arrange the arousal index (AI) data, also shown in Table 8–20.

An ANOVA of these data can be conducted using any standard statistical package. From the output of the analysis conducted using SAS, Version 6.12 (SAS Institute, Cary, NC), the following tables are obtained:

For AHI:

Source of Variation	Sum of Squares (SS)	Degrees of Freedom (DF)*	Mean Square SS/DF	Label
Observer	2.023	1	2.023	MSO
Study	2477.991	29	85.448	MSS
Error	7.169	29	0.247	MSE

*Degrees of freedom: for *observer*, $k - 1$, where k is the number of times each observation is made; for *study*, $n - 1$, where n is the number of observations; for *error*, $(k - 1) \times (n - 1)$.

For AI:

Source of Variation	Sum of Squares (SS)	Degrees of Freedom (DF)*	Mean Square SS/DF	Label
Observer	166.010	1	166.010	MSO
Study	4436.759	29	152.992	MSS
Error	1087.749	29	37.509	MSE

*Degrees of freedom: for *observer*, $k - 1$, where k is the number of times each observation is made; for *study*, $n - 1$, where n is the number of observations; for *error*, $(k - 1) \times (n - 1)$.

In these tables, "observer" relates to the variability due to the scorer in this example (or to the specific set of repeat readings in a within-observer reliability study), and "study" refers to the variability related to the participant, study, or specimen that is being repeatedly studied, read, or determined.

The formula for the calculation of the ICC is[1]

$$ICC = \frac{MSS - MSE}{MSS + MSE\,(k-1) + k(MSO - MSE)/n}$$

where k is the number of repeated readings (eg, 2 in the above example) and n is the number of individual studies or specimens being studied (eg, 30 in the above example).

Applying this formula to the above data, the following results are obtained:

For AHI:

$$ICC_{AHI} = \frac{85.448 - 0.247}{85.448 + 0.247(2-1) + 2(2.023 - 0.247)/30} = 0.993$$

For AI:

$$ICC_{AI} = \frac{152.992 - 37.509}{152.992 + 37.509(2-1) + 2(166.01 - 37.509)/30} = 0.580$$

DEYO'S METHOD

An equivalent formula described by Deyo et al[2] can be easily applied using a pocket calculator or a standard computer spreadsheet. The layout for this calculation requires obtaining the difference between the values (eg, scores) for each pair of repeated observations, as shown in the following table for both the AHI and AI data from Table 8–20.

Study No.	AHI Scorer A	AHI Scorer B	AHI Difference	AI Scorer A	AI Scorer B	AI Difference
1	1.25	1.38	−0.13	7.08	8.56	−1.48
2	1.61	2.05	−0.44	18.60	19.91	−1.31
3	5.64	5.50	0.14	20.39	25.17	−4.78
.	.	.	.	.	.	.
.	.	.	.	.	.	.
.	.	.	.	.	.	.
29	2.09	2.35	−0.26	18.66	18.02	0.64
30	11.09	9.25	1.84	12.50	23.25	−10.74
Mean	5.748	5.381	**0.367**	17.306	20.632	**−3.327**
s	6.702	6.386	0.703	7.682	11.467	8.661
s²	**44.918**	**40.777**	**0.494**	**59.017**	**131.483**	**75.017**

s: standard deviation.

Deyo's formula uses the numbers shown in bold in the table, namely the mean difference ($\bar{x}_{diff}$), the variances (standard deviations squared) for the measurements by each scorer (s_A^2 and s_B^2), and the variance of the differences (s_{diff}^2):

$$\text{ICC} = \frac{s_A^2 + s_B^2 - s_{diff}^2}{s_A^2 + s_B^2 + \bar{x}_{diff}^2 - s_{diff}^2/n}$$

where n is the total number of studies (paired observations).

For the above data:

$$\text{ICC}_{AHI} = \frac{44.918 + 40.777 - 0.494}{44.918 + 40.777 + 0.367^2 - 0.494/30} = 0.993$$

$$\text{ICC}_{AI} = \frac{59.017 + 131.483 - 75.017}{59.017 + 131.483 + 3.327^2 - 75.017/30} = 0.580$$

These results are identical to the values obtained from the ANOVA, shown above.

REFERENCES

1. Armitage P, Berry G. *Statistical Methods in Medical Research*. 3rd ed. London: Blackwell; 1994.

2. Deyo RA, Diehr P, Patrick DL. Reproducibility and responsiveness of health statistics measures: statistics and strategies for evaluation. *Controlled Clin Trials*. 1991;12:142S–158S.

Index

A

Absolute differences
 additive interaction, 215–216, 220–221
 situations for use, 91, 92
Absolute odds, 106–107
Actuarial life-table. *See* life table
Additive interaction, 212, 215, 220–221
 detection of, 215, 220–221, 229–231
 and matching, 45
 presence of, 215
Adjustment
 meaning of, 258
 multiple-regression methods, 281–328
 overadjustment, 331–333
 residual confounding, 328–331
 stratification-based adjustment,
  258–278
Administrative losses, 66
Age effects, 4–16
 definition of, 10
 importance of, 4
 and prevalence rates, 4–8
Aggregate measures, ecologic studies, 17
Aggregation bias. *See* Ecologic fallacy
Ambidirectional designs. *See* Case-cohort
 studies
Analysis of birth cohorts, 3–4
Analysis of variance (ANOVA), 479–481
Analytical epidemiology, nature of, 3
Antagonistic interaction, meaning of,
 211–212

Arithmetic scale, ordinate of figures,
 427–428
Association measures
 absolute differences, 91, 92
 attributable risk, 98–105
 in case-control studies, 106–118,
  117–118
 in cohort studies, 91–105
 in cross-sectional studies, 105–106
 odds ratio, 93–98, 106–117
 relative differences, 91, 92
 relative risk, 93
 risk ratio, 92–93
 strength of associations, assessment of,
  118–120
Attributable risk, 98–105
 additive interaction, 212, 215
 case-control studies, 117–118
 definition of, 98
 as etiologic fraction, 98
 in exposed individuals, 98–101
 Levin's population attributable risk,
  101–105
 percentage expressed in, 100–101
 standard error estimation, 443–445

B

Berksonian bias. *See* Selection bias
Bias
 compared to confounding, 177–178,
  205–208

compensating bias, 133
definition of, 125–126
duration ratio bias, 156
heterogeneity due to, 246–247
information bias, 127–128, 135–153
interviewer bias, 138–139
lead-time bias, 164–169
length bias, 162–164
medical surveillance bias, 127, 153–155
observer bias, 139–140
point prevalence complement ratio
    bias, 156–157
prevention of, 126
publication bias, 169–173
recall bias, 136–138
regression dilution bias, 401
respondent bias, 140–141
selection bias, 126–127, 128–135
temporal bias, 159–161
Binary linear regression, 297
Binary variable. *See* Dichotomous
variables; Dummy variables
Birth cohorts
in case-control studies, 15
cohort effects, 8–16
data plot with, 6–8
meaning of, 5
See also Cohort effects; Cohort-age-
    period analyses
Bland-Altman plot, validity/reliability
measure, 399–401
Built-in bias, odds ratio, 96

C

Case-based case-control studies, 29–33
choosing population, 31–32
cross-sectionality of, 29–30
features of, 29–31
selection bias, 32
Case-cohort studies, 33–38
advantages of, 112–113
case and noncase strategies, 113–114
controls, selection of, 34–36, 114–115
features of, 33–34
multivariate analysis, 316–317
odds ratio, 111–117
situations for use, 36–38
Case-control studies, 28–38
attributable risk, 117–118
case-based case-control studies, 29–33
case-cohort studies, 33–38

compared to cohort studies, 28–29
features of, 28–29
homogeneity of effects, 225–227
interaction, assessment of, 223–233
interviewer bias, 138–139
Levin's attributable risk formula, 104
matching, 41
medical surveillance bias, 127, 153–155
multiple logistic regression, 305–306
nested-case control design, 115–116
observed/joint effects comparison,
    228–233
observer bias, 140–141
odds ratio, 29, 30, 106–117
recall bias, 136–138
selection bias, 128–134
Case-crossover design, elements of, 40
Categorical dichotomous outcome
variables, definition of, 55
Censored observations
in cumulative incidence, 58–62, 65
reasons for censoring, 65–67
Chamberlain's percent positive
agreement, 375
Chance agreement, 381–382
Classical life table. *See* Life table
Coefficient of variability, validity/
reliability measure, 398–399
Cohort-age-period analysis, 4–16
Cohort effects, 8–16
age/calendar time interaction, 11
cohort-age-period analyses, 11–14
definition of, 10
Cohort studies, 24–28
association measures in, 91–105
compared to case-control studies,
    28–29
concurrent studies, 29
cross-tabulation of exposure, 92–94
interaction, assessment of, 222–223
matching, 41
medical surveillance bias, 153–155
mixed design, 29
multiple logistic regression, 299–304
non-concurrent studies, 29
observer bias, 139–140
respondent bias, 140–141
selection bias, 128–134
selection of population, 91–92
Collinearity, examples of, 188–189
Compensating bias, meaning of, 133

Concurrent studies, cohort studies, 29
Conditional confounding, meaning of, 205
Conditional logistic regression, uses of, 314, 315–316
Conditional probabilities in life table approach, 61
  in Kaplan-Meier approach, 62–63
Confidence interval, estimates of, 328, 432–433
Confounders, in epidemiologic reports, 411
Confounding
  assessment of effects of, 190–198
  in cohort studies, 177, 179
  compared to bias, 177–178, 205–208
  conditional confounding, 205
  definition of, 177
  general rule of causation, 180–184
  heterogeneity based on, 244–246
  and matching, 40
  and misclassification bias, 151
  negative confounding, 200–203
  in observational studies, 178–179
  partial effects of, 198–199
  positive confounding, 200–203
  and prevention, 207–208
  qualitative confounding, 202
  residual confounding, 42, 47, 187, 199–200, 222, 328–331
  statistical significance and assessment of, 203–205
Confounding variables
  and causal pathway of exposure/ outcome, 184–187
  effects of, 40, 177–180
  excessive correlation with exposure, 187–190
  and exposure-outcome associations, 182–184, 190–196
  and interaction, 241–243
  and matching, 40
  misclassification of, 331
  and random associations, 184
  and residual confounding, 329–330, 331
Construct validity, meaning of, 19, 330
Continuous variables
  and linear regression, 282, 302, 308
  and matching, 47
  and stratification, 279

uses of, 55
Control group
  case-based control selection, 132–133
  case-cohort studies, 34–36, 111–113
Correlation coefficient
  intraclass correlation coefficient, 396–397
  Pearson's linear (product moment) correlation coefficient, 283–284, 389–396
  Spearman correlation coefficient, 394–395
Correlation graph. *See* Scatter diagrams
Cox proportional hazards model, 306–310
  basic assumptions in, 307–308
  hazard ratio, 308–309
  uses of, 306, 310
Cross-product ratio
  and odds ratio, 93–94, 106–107
Cross sectional studies, 38–40
  and age associations, 4
  association measures in, 105–106
  features of, 38–39
  incidence-prevalence bias, 155–159
  morbidity surveys, 39
  point prevalence rate ratio, 105–106
  temporal bias, 159–161
Cross-tabulation of exposure and disease. *See* Two-by-two table
Cumulative incidence, 58–67
  censoring and survival, assumption of independence, 65–67
  cumulative probability of event, 60–61, 63
  cumulative probability of survival, 61–64
  joint probability of survival, 61
  for Kaplan-Meier approach, 62–64
  for life table, 59–62
  secular trends, lack of, 67
  uniformity of events/losses in, 64–65
Cumulative lifetime prevalence, meaning of, 85
Cumulative survival, 58, 61–64
  standard error estimation, 433–434

D

Data collection procedures
  quality assurance, 348–349
  validity and reliability, 411

Density sampling, nested-case control design, 115–116
Descriptive epidemiology, nature of, 3
Detection bias. *See* Medical surveillance bias
Deyo's method, 481–482
Dichotomous variable, 55
Differential losses to follow-up, 134–135
Differential misclassification, 145–151
  causes of, 145–146
  examples of, 146–151
Direct adjustment, 265–271
  examples of, 266–268
  procedure in, 265
  standard population in, 269–270
  uses of, 265, 269
Discussion section, epidemiologic reports, 408–409
Dose-response pattern, test for, 459–462
Dummy variables, for nonlinear releationships, 319–325
Duration ratio bias, 156
Dynamic cohorts, 70, 72, 75

E

Ecologic fallacy, definition of, 19
Ecologic studies, 4, 17–23
  aggregate measures, 17
  cross-level inference, 20–21
  ecologic fallacy, 19
  environmental measures, 17
  examples of, 19–20
  global measures, 17
  linear regression, 289–290
  multilevel analyses, 18–19
  as preliminary studies, 21–22
  procedure in, 17–23
Effect modification
  use of term, 211, 212, 213
  See also Interaction
Effect modifier, 211, 212, 213–214
  rationale for use, 213–214
Effects, measurement of, 212
Emergent risk factors, interaction and search for, 249–251
Environmental measures, ecologic studies, 17
Epidemiologic reports
  assessment of interaction, 413
  categorizing continuous/ordinal variables, 411–412

concise presentation in, 413–414
confounders, rationale for choice of, 411
discussion section, 408–409
figures, 423–428
hypotheses development, 408, 409–410
inferences presented in, 416–420
introduction, 408
readability of, 414–416
results section, 408
study objectives, 408, 409
tables, 420–423
unmodeled/parsimoniously modeled/fully modeled data, 412–413
validity/data collection procedures, 411
Epidemiology
  analytical epidemiology, 3
  definition of, 3
  descriptive epidemiology, 3
  observational epidemiology, 4
Etiologic fraction, attributable risk as, 98
Event
  definition of, 56
  examples of, 57
  and incidence, 56
  interval-based probability of, 60–61
  and prevalence, 56
Exact event times approach. *See* Kaplan-Meier approach
Excess fraction, attributable risk as, 98
Exposure, and confounding, 183–190
Exposure disease associations
  case-control studies, 28–38
  See also Association measures
Exposure identification bias
  interviewer bias, 138–139
  recall bias, 127–128, 136–138
Exposure levels, heterogeneity based on, 247

F

False positives/false negatives, 365
Figures, 423–428
  format for, 424
  ordinate scale, 425–428
  titles/labels, 424–425
Force of morbidity, mortality. *See* Hazard rate
Framingham multiple-logistic risk equation, 304
Frequency matching, use of, 42, 314–315

G

Generalized linear models, 281
Global measures, ecologic studies, 17
Gold standard procedures, validity
  studies, 352, 353, 354, 355, 357
Greenwood formula, 434, 443

H

Hazard rate, 83–84
  analogy with Kaplan-Meier approach, 84
  definition of, 83–84
  hazard function, estimation of, 84
  in survival analysis, 84, 85
Hazard ratio, Cox proportional hazards
  model, 308–309
Heterogeneity of effects
  interaction based on, 212
  meaning of, 212
Hierarchical models, 23
  See also Multilevel analysis
Homogeneity of effects
  assessment of, 213–217
  case-control studies, 225–227
  interaction based on, 212
  meaning of, 212
Homogeneity of stratified estimates, test
  of, 463–465
Host factors, and interaction
  interpretation, 247–249
Hypotheses development, epidemiologic
  reports, 408, 409–410

I

Incidence
  cumulative incidence, 58–67
  definition of, 56
  and odds, 94–95
  and prevalence, 85–87
Incidence density
  individuals as basis, 70–71
  meaning of, 69
  sampling, use of, 34–35
Incidence-prevalence bias, 155–159
  causes of, 155–156
  duration ratio bias, 156
  for evaluation of screening, 162–164
  examples of, 157–158
  length bias, 162–164
  point prevalence complement ratio
    bias, 156–157

prevention of, 158–159
Incidence rates, 56, 58–84
  comparison of measures, 81–83
  event in, 56–57
  hazard rate, 83–84
  for individuals at risk, 58–67
  and period effects, 14
  for person-time units, 67–81
  standard error estimation, 435–436
  yearly average rates, 82
  See also Cumulative incidence
Independence of censoring and survival,
  65–67
Indirect adjustment, 271–273
  standard population in, 272–273
  use of, 271–272
Individual matching, use of, 41–42
Individuals at risk, incidence based on,
  58–67
Individuals, studies of
  case-control studies, 28–38
  case-crossover design, 40
  cohort studies, 24–28
  cross-sectional studies, 38–40
  incidence density based on, 70–71
  matching, 40–48
Inferences, in epidemiological reports,
  416–420
Information bias, 135–153
  meaning of, 127–128
  misclassification bias, 141–153
  observer bias, 139–140
  recall bias, 127–128, 136–138
  respondent bias, 140–141
  temporal bias, 159–161
Interaction
  antagonistic interaction, 211–212
  conditions for occurrence of, 212
  and confounding, 241–243
  definitional interchangeability, 233–235
  definitions of, 211, 212
  effect, measurement of, 212
  to find new risk factors, 249–251
  homogeneity of effects, 212
  interaction fallacy, 227
  qualitative interaction, 239–240
  quantitative interaction, 238
  reciprocity of, 240–241
  and representativeness of associations,
    251
  statistical tests for, 243

synergistic interaction, 211
test of homogeneity, 463–465
Interaction assessment
    additive interaction, 212, 215,
        220–221, 229–231
    in case-control studies, 223–233
    choosing model for, 235–237
    in cohort study, 222–223
    homogeneity of effects, 213–217
    multiplicative interaction, 212, 216,
        221–222, 231–233
    observed/joint effects comparison,
        217–222
Interaction interpretation, 243–249
    heterogeneity from bias, 246–247
    heterogeneity from confounding,
        244–246
    heterogeneity from differential
        intensity of exposure, 247
    heterogeneity from random variability,
        244
    and host factors, 247–249
Intercept
    linear regression, 285–287
    logistic regression, 303
    utility of, 287, 303
Intraclass correlation coefficient
    calculation of, 479–482
    validity/reliability measure, 396–397
Inter-observer variability, 358
Interval-based probability of event, 60–61
Interviewer bias, 138–139
    cause of, 138
    prevention of, 138–139
Intra-observer variability, 358
Introduction, epidemiologic reports, 408

K

Kaplan-Meier approach, 58
    analogy with hazard rate, 84
    conditional probabilities in, 62–63
    cumulative incidence based on, 62–64
    procedure in, 62–64
    survival function, 63
Kappa statistic
    applications of, 376–379
    kappa values interpretation, 377
    for multiple ratings, 380
    prevalence, dependence on, 384–388
    standard error estimation, 454–456
    validity/reliability measure, 375–388

weighted kappa, 380–384

L

Language bias, 173
Lead-time bias, 164–169
    cause of, 164–165
Lead-time, estimation of, 166–169
Least squares method, 285–286
Length bias, 162–164
    cause of, 162–164
    prevention of, 164
Levin's population attributable risk
    calculation, 101–105
    and case-control studies, 104
Lexis diagram, 78
Life table, 58–62
    cumulative incidence based on, 59–62
    duration of intervals, 61–62
    terms related to, 58
    uniformity of events/losses, 64–65
Likelihood ratio test (LRT), 328
Linear function, elements of, 281
Linear regression, 281–297
    basic concepts, 282–285
    intercept, 285–287
    least squares method, 285–286, 327–328
    maximum likelihood method (MLE),
        327–328
    multiple linear regression, 290–297
    for nonlinear relationships, 317–325
    Pearson linear correlation coefficient,
        283–285
    regression coefficient, 287–289
    statistical testing, 326–328
    validity/reliability measure, 395–396
Logarithmic scale, ordinate of figures, 13,
    427–428
Logit, 299
Log-linear model, 311
Log odds, 299, 306
Logistic regression. See multiple logistic
    regression
Losses to follow-up
    assumptions related to, 65–67
    and selection bias, 67, 134–135
    types of, 65–67

M

Mantel-Haenszel adjustment method,
    235, 273–278
    adjusted rate ratio, 276–277

odds ratio calculation, 274–276
odds ratio, standard error estimation, 448–450
for paired case-control data, 277–278
Matched case-control studies, multivariate analysis, 314–315
Matched odds ratio, 110, 277–278, 314–315
Matching, 40–48
  advantages of, 43–45
  case-control studies, 41
  cohort studies, 41
  disadvantages of, 45–47
  frequency matching, 42
  individual matching, 41–42
  minimum Euclidean distance measure method, 43
  necessity for, 40–41
  overmatching, 47
  pros/cons of, 43–48
Maximum likelihood method (MLE), 327–328
Mean difference, validity/reliability measure, 398
Medical surveillance bias, 127, 153–155
  causes of, 153–154
  prevention of, 154–155
Minimum Euclidean distance measure method, use of, 43
Minimum variance standard population, 270
Misclassification bias, 141–153
  and confounding variables, 151
  differential misclassification, 145–151
  nondifferential misclassification, 141–145
  prevention of, 152–153
Mixed design, cohort studies, 29
Model. *See* statistical models
Morbidity surveys, cross-sectional studies, 39
Multilevel analyses, purpose of, 18–19
Multiple linear regression, 290–297
  regression coefficient, 291–294
  uses of, 290
Multiple logistic regression, 297–306
  for case-control study, 305–306
  for cohort study, 299–304
  frequency-matched study, 314–315
  and predicted probabilities, 303–305
  uses of, 297, 304–305

Multiple-regression methods
  Cox proportional hazards model, 306–310
  linear regression, 281–297
  multiple logistic regression, 297–306
  ordinary least squares (OLS) method, 327–328
  Poisson regression, 310–314
  uses of, 280–281, 303–304, 337–339
Multiplicative interaction, 212, 216, 221–222
  detection of, 216–217, 221–222, 231–233
Multivariate analysis
  for case-cohort studies, 316–317
  conditional logistic regression, 314, 315–316
  and matched case-control studies, 314–315
  and multiple regression methods, 280–282
  for nested case-control studies, 315–317
  and statistical adjustment, 258
  uses of, 257
  use of term, 264
Multivariate trend test, 462

N

Negative confounding, 200–203
Negative interaction and weak associations, 249–250
  See also Antagonistic interaction
Negative predictive value, 366
Nested case-control studies, 33–38
  density sampling, 115–116
  multivariate analysis, 315–317
  See also Case-cohort studies
Noncausal associations. *See* Confounding
Non-concurrent studies, cohort studies, 29
Nondifferential misclassification, 141–145
  with multiple categories, 145
  with two categories, 141–145
Nonlinear relationships
  dummy variables, use of, 319–325
  J-shape relationship, 318–319
  linear regression for, 317–325
  scatter diagrams for, 325–326
Null hypothesis, test of, 433

O

Observational epidemiology, nature of, 4
Observational studies, confounding in,
  178–179
Observation, quality control monitoring,
  351–352
Observations
  censored observations, 58–62
  multiple observers, 140, 380
Observer bias, 139–140
  cause of, 139–140
  prevention of, 140
Occurrence of disease
  incidence rates, 58–84
  odds, 87–88
  prevalence rates, 85–88
Odds, 87–88
  definition of, 29, 87
  numerical representations for, 88
  and odds ratio, 106–107
  prevalence odds, 87–88
  and probability calculation, 87
Odds ratio, 93–98, 106–117
  absolute odds, 106–107
  advantages of, 97–98
  as approximation of relative risk, 95–98
  built-in bias, 96
  case-control studies, 29, 30, 106–117
  and cross-product ratio, 93, 106–107
  and incidence, 94–95
  in matched case-control studies, 110,
    277–278, 314–316
  logistic regression estimates of,
    299–303
  Mantel-Haenszel adjusted odds ratio,
    273–278
  multiple exposures, 116–117
  probabilities and, 94
  relative risk estimation, 95–98, 110–114
  standard error estimation, 440–443
One time scale, 76–77
Open cohorts, 70, 72, 75
Ordinal categorical variables, 324–325
Ordinary least squares (OLS) method. See
  Least squares method
Ordinate scale, of figures, 425–428
Outcome, definition of, 55
Outcome frequency. See Occurrence of
  disease
Outcome identification bias

observer bias, 139–140
respondent bias, 140–141
See also Medical surveillance bias
Overadjustment, 331–333
  example of, 332–333
  meaning of, 189–190, 331–332
Overmatching, 47, 332

P

Paired case-control data, Mantel-Haenszel
  adjustment method, 277–278
Paired t-test, validity/reliability measure,
  398
Pairwise comparison, 389
Pearson's linear (product-moment) correlation coefficient, 283–285, 392–395
  limitations of, 392–395
  validity/reliability measure, 389,
    391–394
Percent agreement
  Chamberlain's percent positive
    agreement, 375
  limitations of, 373–374
  percent positive agreement, 375
  statistical inference procedures,
    452–454
  validity/reliability measure, 371–375
Period effects, 8–16
  example of, 9–10
  and incidence rates, 14
  meaning of, 8–9, 10
  and prevalence rates, 10
Period prevalence
  cumulative lifetime prevalence, 85
  meaning of, 85
Person-time units, incidence rates, 67–81
  aggregate data, 69–70
  basic assumptions in, 71–72
  density/rate relationship, 72–75
  example studies, 68
  incidence density, 69
  individual data, 70–71
  multiple time scales, 77–79
  one time scale, 76–77
  reasons for use, 68–69
  stratification of person-time and rates,
    75–81
  time-dependent covariates, 79–81
Pilot study, quality assurance, 350
Point estimate, 417–419, 432
Point prevalence, 85–87

connection with incidence and
duration, 86–87
meaning of, 85
Point prevalence complement ratio bias,
156–157
Point prevalence rate ratio, cross-
sectional studies, 105–106
Poisson regression, 310–314
equation for, 310–311
log-linear model, 311
rate ratio, 311
regression coefficients, 311–312
uses of, 310
Population
cohort study selection, 91–92
standard population, 269–270,
272–273
Population attributable risk. *See* Levin's
population attributable risk calculation
Positive confounding, 200–203
Positive predictive value, 366
Prediction, and multiple-regression
methods, 281, 303–304
Predictive values, positive and negative,
366
Pretest, quality assurance, 349–350
Prevalence, 56
definition of, 56
effects on kappa, 384–388
event in, 56–57
Prevalence odds, 87–88
Prevalence rates, 85–88
and age effects, 4–8
and incidence, 85–87
and period effects, 10
period prevalence, 85
point prevalence, 85–87
Prevention
evidence needed, 207–208
primary prevention, 207
secondary prevention, 207
Primary prevention
evidence needed, 207, 208
meaning of, 207
Probability
adjusted difference, standard error
estimation, 445–447
and odds, 94
See also Odds; Odds ratio; Cumulative
incidence; Cumulative survival
Probability odds ratio. *See* Odds ratio

Proportional hazards model. *See* Cox
proportional hazards model
Publication bias, 169–173
causes of, 171–173
language bias, 173
prevention of, 173
Publications, assumptions of validity of,
170–171

Q

Qualitative confounding, 202
Qualitative interaction, 239–240
Quality assurance, 344–350
components of investigation, 345–347
data collection instruments, 348–349
definition of, 343
manuals of operation, 347–348
pilot study, 350
pretest, 349–350
staff training, 349
steps in, 350
study protocol, 344
Quality control
Bland-Altman plot, 399–401
coefficient of variability, 398–399
components of investigation,
345–347
intraclass correlation coefficient,
396–397
kappa statistic, 375–388
linear regression, 395–396
mean difference, 398
meaning of, 343
observation monitoring, 351–352
paired *t*-test, 398
Pearson's product-moment correlation
coefficient, 389, 391–394
percent agreement, 371–375
percent positive agreement, 375
reliability studies, 358–363
scatter diagram, 389
sensitivity/specificity indices of
validity, 363–370
Spearman correlation coefficient,
394–395
validity studies, 352–358
Youden's *J* statistic, 370–371
Quality control/quality assurance manual, 347–348
for blood pressure measurement,
468–471

for blood/urine collection and processing, 471–478
Quantitative interaction, 237–238

R

Random associations, random variability
  and confounding, 184
  and heterogeneity, interaction, 244
Rate ratio
  Poisson regression, 311
  standard error estimation, 438–440
Rate, use of term, 4
Ratio of incidence densities. *See* Rate ratio
Ratio of probabilities. *See* Relative risk
Readability, of epidemiologic reports, 414–416
Recall bias, 127–128, 136–138
  cause of, 136, 137
  prevention of, 136–138
Reductionism, 22
Regression coefficient
  confidence interval, 328, 451
  Cox regression, 308
  interpreting units of, 296–297
  linear regression, 287–289
  logistic regression, 299–302
  multiple linear regression, 291–294
  Poisson regression, 311–312
  standard error estimation, 450–452
Regression to the mean, effects of, 401
Relative differences
  multiplicative interaction, 212, 216–217, 221–222
  situations for use, 91, 92
Relative risk, 92–98
  approximation with odds ratio, 95–98
  odds ratio for estimation, 110–114
  standard error estimation, 436–438
Reliability
  definition of, 135
  meaning of, 343
  variability, sources of, 358–360
Reliability studies, 358–363
  for data collection activities, 360
  for laboratory determinations, 360–361
  limitations of, 361
  and sources of variability, 358–360
Reporting. *See* Epidemiologic reports
Representativeness of associations, and interaction, 251

Residual confounding, 42, 47, 199–200, 328–331
  causes of, 329–331
  exploring causal pathways, 186–187
  and heterogeneity of effects, 222
  and stratification, 263, 279–280
Respondent bias, 140–141
  cause of, 140
  prevention of, 140–141
Results section, epidemiologic reports, 408
Reverse causality, meaning of, 160
Risk factors
  exploring with interaction, 249–251
  reductionist approach, 22
Risk ratio, 92–93
  See also Relative risk
Risk-set sampling, use of, 34–35, 315
Rose questionnaire, 348

S

Scatter diagrams
  for nonlinear relationships, 325–326
  as validity/reliability measure, 389
Secondary prevention
  evidence needed, 207, 208
  meaning of, 207
Secular trends, lack of in studies, 67
Selection bias, 128–135
  case-based case-control studies, 32
  cause of, 128–132
  compensating bias, 133
  equalization of, 132–133
  in evaluation of screening, 162
  examples of, 129–131
  incidence-prevalence bias, 155–159
  meaning of, 126–127
  medical surveillance bias, 127, 153–155
  prevention of, 132–135
Sensitivity analysis, 339
Sensitivity and specificity
  definition of, 135
  index of validity, 363–370
  limitations of, 367–370
  statistical inference procedures, 452–454
Slope, regression coefficient, 287–289
Spearman correlation coefficient, validity/reliability measure, 394–395
Specificity

definition of, 135
    index of validity, 363–370
Staff training, quality assurance, 349
Standard error estimation, 432–433
    adjusted probabilities, 445–447
    attributable risk, 443–445
    cumulative survival estimate, 433–434
    incidence rates, 435–436
    kappa statistic, 454–456
    Mantel-Haenszel odds ratio, 448–450
    odds ratio, 440–443
    rate ratio, 438–440
    regression coefficient, 288, 450–452
    relative risk, 436–438
    standardized mortality ratio (SMR),
        447–448
    Youden's *J* statistic, 454
Standardized incidence ratio (SIR),
    calculation of, 272–273
Standardized mortality ratio (SMR)
    calculation of, 272–273
    standard error estimation, 447–448
Standardized pools, validity study,
    352–353
Standardized prevalence ratio (SPR), 272
Standard population
    and direct adjustment, 269–270
    and indirect adjustment, 272–273
    minimum variance standard
        population, 270
Statistical models
    concept, 333–337
    selection of model, 337–339
    types of, 264
Statistical significance
    assessing confounding, 203–205
    assessing correlation coefficient, 395
    common errors related to, 416–419
    and interaction, 243
    of regression coefficients, 326–328
Stratification-based adjustment
    basic assumptions in, 263–265
    direct adjustment, 265–271
    examples of, 258–263
    indirect adjustment, 271–273
    limitations of, 278–280
    Mantel-Haenszel method, 273–278
    and residual confounding, 263,
        279–280
Stratification, utility of, 198, 257

Study protocol, quality assurance, 344
Subcohorts, 316
Surveillance bias. *See* Medical surveillance
    bias
Survival analysis
    hazard rate in, 84
    See also Cumulative incidence
Survival bias, 156
Survival function
    Kaplan-Meier approach, 63
    See also Cumulative survival
Synergistic interaction, meaning of, 211

T

Tables, 420–423
    avoiding redundancy, 421–422
    between-group statistics compared, 421
    comparability with other reports, 421
    data presentation, 422–423
    labels/headings, 420
    shifting denominators, 422
    units, 421
Temporal bias, 159–161
    causes of, 159–160
    examples of, 160–161
    prevention of, 161
Threshold phenomenon, 318–319
Time-dependent covariates, 79–81
Time scales
    fixed and time-dependent covariates,
        79–81
    Lexis diagram, 78
    one time scale, 76–77
    two or more time scales, 77–79
Trends
    dose-response pattern, 459–462
    multivariate trend test, 462
Two-by-two table, 92

V

Validity
    construct validity, 330
    definition of, 135, 343
    sensitivity/specificity indices of
        validity, 363–370
    valid studies, elements of, 135
Validity studies, 352–358
    gold standard procedures, 352, 353,
        354, 355, 357
    importance of, 355–357

limitations of, 357–358
for positive responses only, 354
previous studies as, 355
of self-reports, 355
standardized pools for lab
    measurement, 352–353
Variability
    coefficient of, 398–399
    sources of, 358–360
Variables
    categorical dichotomous outcome
        variables, 55
    confounding variables, 40

continuous variables, 55
Vital statistics and incidence rates, 75, 82

W

Wald statistic, 328, 452
Weighted kappa, 380–384

Y

Yearly average rates, 82
Youden's *J* statistic
    standard error estimation, 454
    validity/reliability measure, 370–371

About the Authors

MOYSES SZKLO, MD, DRPH, is Professor of Epidemiology at the Johns Hopkins School of Hygiene and Public Health and is Director of its Chronic Disease Epidemiology Program. His current research focuses on risk factors for subclinical and clinical atherosclerosis. He is also Editor in Chief of the *American Journal of Epidemiology*.

F. JAVIER NIETO, MD, PHD, is Associate Professor of Epidemiology at the Johns Hopkins School of Hygiene and Public Health. His current research focuses on emerging risk factors for ischemic heart disease. He is also an Editor for the *American Journal of Epidemiology*.